Oral Health in America

Removing the Stain of Disparity

For access to digital chapters, visit the APHA Press bookstore (www.apha.org).

Oral Health in America

Removing the Stain of Disparity

Edited by
Henrie M. Treadwell, PhD
Caswell A. Evans, DDS, MPH

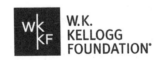

W.K.
KELLOGG
FOUNDATION®

Community Voices
HEALTHCARE FOR THE UNDERSERVED
Morehouse School of Medicine

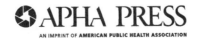

APHA PRESS
AN IMPRINT OF AMERICAN PUBLIC HEALTH ASSOCIATION

American Public Health Association
800 I Street, NW
Washington, DC 20001-3710
www.apha.org

Georges Benjamin, MD, Executive Director

Printed and bound in the United States of America
Book Production Editor: Maya Ribault
Typesetting: The Charlesworth Group
Cover Design: Alan Giarcanella
Printing and Binding: Sheridan Books

Library of Congress Cataloging-in-Publication Data

Names: Treadwell, Henrie M., editor. | Evans, Caswell A., Jr., editor. |
    American Public Health Association, issuing body.
Title: Oral health in America ; removing the stain of disparity / edited by
    Henrie M. Treadwell, and Caswell A. Evans.
Other titles: Oral health in America (Treadwell)
Description: Washington, DC : American Public Health Association, [2019] |
    Includes bibliographical references and index.
Identifiers: LCCN 2018050646 (print) | LCCN 2018052099 (ebook) | ISBN
    9780875533063 (ebook) | ISBN 9780875533056 (pbk.)
Subjects: | MESH: Oral Health | Health Status Disparities | Health Services
    Accessibility | United States
Classification: LCC RK61 (ebook) | LCC RK61 (print) | NLM WU 113 | DDC
    617.6--dc23
LC record available at https://lccn.loc.gov/2018050646

Contents

Preface

Oral health inequities persist among distinct population groups despite technical advances in the field of oral health. There is a need to embark on a journey toward health equity that includes access to innovations in quality and practice methodology, as well as culturally competent and racially diverse oral care for all. The observed inequities are the result of a myriad of factors including accessible care, limited workforce diversity and cadre stratification, limited and nonexistent coverage and affordability, disease prevention measures for populations and individuals, and, perhaps the most significant of all, social determinants of health. An extremely limited number of consolidated resources exist that address inequity in oral health.[1] This book presents these issues in clear focus and brings light to education, training, partnership, and policy solutions, with a focus on dental therapy, which is necessary to improve oral health and achieve oral health equity for all.

The W.K. Kellogg Foundation's Community Voices: Healthcare for the Underserved Initiative, initially funded in 1998 and now housed at the Morehouse School of Medicine, was the first coordinated national example of a comprehensive and integrated effort to support access to oral health care as a part of comprehensive health care. This initiative, implemented in 13 communities across the United States, resulted in the opening of services in underserved communities, many of which offered limited services for children and none for adults, but which have since expanded beyond original implementation due to community demand for health services.[2,3] The work initiated across the nation by Community Voices marked a deliberate and intentional focus on oral health in Kellogg Foundation programming that expanded over time. The evolution was actualized as support for an alternative, yet cost- and practice-effective, as well as validated, oral health care cadre—the dental health aide therapist—since it was evident there were workforce issues as measured by numbers and the racial and ethnic diversity of providers, which imposed an actual and cultural limit on access to care.

Paralleling this major effort at philanthropy, the federal government released *Oral Health in America: a Report of the Surgeon General,* which was published in 2000 under the leadership of Surgeon General David Satcher. The report pointed out that oral health and general health were integral and that any consideration of general health would be incomplete without inclusion of oral health. The report highlights that everyone has oral health factors, and these exist independently of whether or not access to and utilization of dental services can be achieved. The report also underlined that oral diseases and disorders in and of themselves affect health and well-being throughout a lifetime and that oral conditions are associated with other health problems. In addition, the report contained a highly troubling finding that drew a great deal of attention, summarized by the following quote: "There are profound and consequential oral health disparities within the US population."[4] A new Surgeon General's Report is forthcoming in 2020 from Surgeon General Jerome Adams.

In 2003, Surgeon General Richard H. Carmona released *A National Call to Action to Promote Oral Health.*[5] That document followed the outline of the Surgeon General's Report and proposed an action agenda to address the issues it raised with the objective to promote oral health. Increasing the oral health workforce's diversity, capacity, and flexibility was among its five key actions. The Surgeon General's Report and the Call to Action established themes and served as points of stimulation for subsequent reports. Among them, *Improving Access to Oral Health Care for Vulnerable and Underserved Populations* outlined the challenges and offered recommendations to improve access to care for underserved populations, all of which were defined by data that documented oral health inequities affecting those populations.[6]

Consonant with but independent from the federal reports, the W.K. Kellogg Foundation has worked continuously at the cutting edge to fully define pathways and solutions that tackle oral health inequities and consider the public's health and related health services. In June 2017, the *American Journal of Public Health* (*AJPH*) published an oral health supplement sponsored by the Morehouse School of Medicine with support from the Kellogg Foundation, which drew specific attention to oral health inequities with the intent of further informing communities, practitioners, and policy-makers regarding the continued existence and the impact of these inequities. The *AJPH* supplement, devoted to health justice, included articles advocating reconnecting the mouth to the body, as well as research on social factors, periodontitis in an older population, and lack of oral health care for adults in Harlem. This collection of articles situated oral health within the social justice mission of public health.[7,8,9]

The Kellogg Foundation launched a major initiative that has provided support for in-depth education and training of dental therapists.[10] Community Catalyst, a national nonprofit serves as the program office for the development of this cadre and attendant policies and began in Alaska but now is expanded across the nation.[11] A valuable online resource on dental therapy was developed in 2018 on the Kellogg Foundation Web site.[12] Articles in the *AJPH* supplement demonstrate the efficacy of dental therapists in providing quality care. The challenge is in reordering priorities in care delivery, which include addressing the needs of millions in this country who often cannot access care because no provider is available and the cost for the traditional dentist is prohibitive. Across the nation, states are beginning to integrate dental therapists into their workforce. This book, funded by the Kellogg Foundation, describes the successes in establishing dental therapy as a norm in every community, not only in isolated, rural communities, since data show that even those in major metropolitan cities are isolated from care.[6] Research studies are limited since many that need care are never seen in clinics due to their inability to pay or to the lack of available providers.

This book includes a number of chapters that previously appeared as articles in the *AJPH* supplement, as well as others that were subsequently solicited. Herein, the reader will find a rich collection of chapters exploring and depicting a wide range of issues related to oral health inequities, while addressing both the impact of as well as the solutions to inequities. The population groups represented in this volume vary in terms of ethnicity, geographical location, and demographic characteristics; they include children, older adults, incarcerated people, those with disabilities, as well as populations with specific health conditions. Some chapters delineate the issues with Medicaid and Medicare while delving into people's ability to access care with payment. Finally, research has validated the efficacy of dental therapists and dental therapy practices, as well as the relative cost savings that accrue when dental therapists are deployed to provide care and reduce human suffering.[13]

Among the challenges faced in all of the chapters is the general paucity of data regarding oral health. While there are national databases such as the National Health and Nutrition Examination Survey that include oral health data, many data collection endeavors do not include oral health data or data on those who simply do not or cannot access regular care. This challenge is particularly manifest in the attempts to outline the oral health condition of subpopulations cohorts within a larger database. There are also challenges around integration of databases: it is known that large numbers of some population groups are in the criminal justice system; however, their health data is not integrated into other sets used to set policy and programs. The chapters by Smith, Weatherspoon, and Makrides and Shulman highlight some of the populations and health issues not included in general health planning.

The book also focuses on emerging workforce models, paying particular attention to dental therapists and dental therapy practice, now legal in four states (Minnesota, Vermont, Maine, and Arizona) and practiced in three others (Alaska in the context of the Alaska Native Tribal Health Consortium, Washington at the Swinomish Indian Tribal Community clinic, and as a pilot in three tribal settings in Oregon). The chapters highlight changes and challenges in dental education regarding preparing an oral health workforce with appropriate diversity (racial/ethnic, with inclusive career laddering) and the capacity and flexibility to intervene effectively in addressing oral health inequities for underserved populations. There is no question that the current paradigm endorsed by professional organizations is inadequate and broken and advances first and foremost the profession, not the individuals in pain who are invisible to the systems that should be providing for their care.

The reader is advised that this book does not, nor could it, represent all of the issues related to oral health inequities. The purpose and intention of these chapters will be to stimulate ideas for subsequent research—for additional evaluation and methodology and for the creation of additional opportunities for data collection within existing initiatives to gather health data and others specifically focused on oral health. This book promotes the adoption of dental therapists into practices across the nation without these professionals being restricted to practice under the direct oversight of a dentist.

Oral health is a social justice issue and must incorporate the calls for inclusive structuring of policy practice leading to oral health for all. This call for equity is the central thesis of this book.[14] Science and chair-side technological innovations alone are not sufficient. This book provides an opportunity to identify and focus on the various factors. These must then be assembled into a portrait of need and a program of intervention that will serve all in this nation with quality and dignity. The chapters in this volume show that adopting the dental therapist model provides a pathway to equity. They demonstrate the wisdom of discarding traditional paradigms serving only a privileged few in favor of those paradigms that guarantee unfettered inclusion, as well as culturally competent and expedient, cost-effective quality care for all in this nation.

Special thanks to Jareese Stroud, Kiara Sims-Thrasher, and Starla Blanks from the Community Voices program, Satcher Health Leadership Institute, Morehouse School of Medicine. They have provided assistance and support over many months through the publication of the supplement and the development of this volume. We sincerely thank them.

Henrie M. Treadwell, PhD
Research Professor
Community Health and Preventive Medicine
Founding Director and Senior Advisor
Community Voices: Healthcare for the
Underserved
Morehouse School of Medicine

Caswell A. Evans, DDS, MPH
Associate Dean
Prevention and Public Health Sciences
College of Dentistry
University of Illinois at Chicago

REFERENCES

1. Northridge M. Oral health equity for minority populations in the United States. *Oxford Bibliographies in Public Health.* 2018

2. Le H, Hirota S, Liou J, Sitlin T, Le C, Quach T. Oral health disparities and inequities in Asian Americans and Pacific Islanders. *Am J Public Health.* 2017;107(suppl 1):S34–S35.

3. Harrell SN, Ro M, Hartsock LG. Improving Access to Oral Health Services Among Uninsured and Underserved Populations: FirstHealth Dental Care Centers. *Am J Public Health.* 2017;107(suppl 1):S48–S49.

4. US Department of Health and Human Services Oral Health Coordinating Committee. US Department of Health and Human Services Oral Health Strategic Framework, 2014–2017. *Public Health Reports*. 2016;131(2):242–257.

5. Office of the Surgeon General. National Call to Action to Promote Oral Health. Report no. 03-5303. Rockville, MD: National Institute of Dental and Craniofacial Research; 2003.

6. Institute of Medicine and National Research Council. Improving Access to Oral Health Care for Vulnerable and Underserved Populations. Washington, DC: The National Academies Press; 2011.

7. Treadwell HM, Formicola AJ. Improving the oral health of prisoners to improve overall health and well-being. *Am J Public Health*. 2008;98(suppl 1):S171–S172.

8. Braithwaite K. Health is a human right, right? *Am J Public Health*. 2008;98(suppl 1):S5–S7.

9. Satcher D, Higginbotham EJ. The public health approach to eliminating disparities in health. *Am J Public Health*. 2008;98(suppl 1):S8–S11.

10. W.K. Kellogg Foundation. https://www.wkkf.org/search/site?q=dental+therapist.

11. Community Catalyst. Dental therapists: expanding access to oral health care. Available at: https://www.communitycatalyst.org/resources/publications/document/DT-101-One-Pager_FINAL.pdf?1485901514. Accessed August 28, 2018.

12. W.K. Kellogg Foundation. Dental therapy: resource library. Available at: http://dentaltherapyresourceguide.wkkf.org. Accessed August 28, 2018.

13. Kim F. Economic viability of dental therapists. May 2013. Available at: https://www.communitycatalyst.org/doc-store/publications/economic-viability-dental-therapists.pdf. Accessed December 8, 2018.

14. Treadwell HM, Northridge ME. Oral health is the measure of a just society. *J Health Care Poor Underserved*. 2007;18(1):12–20.

I. RATIONALE

Dental Therapy: Communities Lead the Way for Improved Oral Health*

La June Montgomery Tabron

Growing up in a Yup'ik Native village in southwest Alaska 40 years ago, Valarie Davidson was terrified of the annual visit from the dentist. Children lined up and one by one were called in to have their teeth pulled; extraction was usually the only service available. Cavities weren't filled; no root canals or cleanings were performed for children who did not have regular dental care available in these communities.

In her own words, Davidson described her horrific experience in the 2012 Annual Report of the W.K. Kellogg Foundation (WKKF), a document that discussed the plight of vulnerable children and what communities could do to help them.

> As a child, I remember when the dentist came to our village once a year. As we waited in line to be seen, we could hear the screams behind the door as teeth were pulled from children ahead of us. The door would open and we'd see our crying brother, sister, cousin or friend holding a bloody gauze bandage to their mouth. We always asked how many teeth were pulled.
>
> Every year, one of the little ones would stand in line, terrified, and either wet themselves from fear or run out the clinic door. Our community health aide would wait five minutes to give the child time to calm down and then bring the child back. The 'runner' would move to the front of the line. For our children, going to see the dentist was truly traumatic. I have a cousin who still cannot be seen by a dentist unless she is under full anesthesia. Imagine how frightening it is for her to seek oral health care for her children.[1(p12)]

Today, with the support of the Kellogg Foundation and a growing movement led predominantly by communities, I'm pleased to report that there has been progress in expanding dental care and making it more accessible in some locations for more children to receive the care they need, when they need it.

In Alaska Native communities, a Dental Health Aide Therapy (DHAT) Program provides education and a college degree for dental therapists who are from the community, and are familiar with the residents and culture. The dental therapists provide education,

---

*This is a modified version of the article that appeared in the *American Journal of Public Health*. See: Montgomery Tabron LJ. Dental therapy: communities lead the way for improved oral health. *Am J Public Health*. 2017;107(suppl 1):S8–S9.

prevention, and treatment of patients and expand access to oral care. For more than 80 years, this model has been in place in more than 50 countries.

RACIAL/ETHNIC DISPARITIES

Yet, across the United States, data clearly show that low-income families and people of color continue to face barriers when it comes to improving oral health and their access to dental care. I find the racial/ethnic disparities so prominent that conscious and unconscious bias has to be considered a factor in the oral health patterns. Among children aged three to five years, 43.2% of American Indian/Alaska Natives have untreated tooth decay compared with 11.3% of White children. Tooth decay strikes 19.8% of Hispanic children in that age group, and 19.3% of African American children.[2] In fact, nationwide, 49 million Americans live in areas federally designated as shortage of dental providers (as of September 30, 2009, those 49 million Americans lived in one of 4,230 dental health professional shortage areas).[3]

Parents of children suffering from tooth decay, tribal residents and community leaders frequently overlook the signs that untreated dental problems are severely impacting overall health, lead to missed school or work days, and can cause life-threatening infections. And far too often, parents can't overcome the obstacle presented by the lack of access to dentists. As per the California Society of Pediatric Dentistry, "Untreated dental disease compromises the child's ability to eat well, sleep well, and function well at home and at school. The unaesthetic nature of untreated dental decay compromises the child's self-esteem and social development."[4] According to the Mayo Clinic, "Research suggests that heart disease, clogged arteries, and stroke may be linked to the inflammation and infections that oral bacteria can cause."[5]

To be sure, WKKF has been a leader in expanding access to dental care since 1930. The terrain has been difficult as entrenched laws, policies, and practices obstruct change, but we have seen progress. Moving forward it will take coalitions of civic, nonprofit, philanthropic, and public- and private-sector leaders to continue engaging with communities to address the practices, policies, and regulations that prevent dental therapists from caring for patients. Because dental therapists are members of the dental team, they allow dentists to care for more patients, focus on patients' most serious dental problems, and increase access to oral care.

EXPANSION ON THE DHAT PROGRAM

I believe the success of the community-driven DHAT program in Alaska can serve as a model that can be replicated in Native and non-Native communities in other states. The effectiveness of the DHAT has been thoroughly documented in studies. This model creates a pathway for community residents to become dental therapists, allowing people known in their communities to care for their children, a sharp contrast from the harrowing environment Davidson described. "Our children look up Davidson wrote in the Annual Report. "They are people that we know a of these close relationships, we are already changing the smiles of Ala dren."[1(p13)] Davidson is now Alaska's Commissioner of Health and Social Services, and her child-hood experiences led her to be a strategist for the DHAT program.

A 2010 study found that dental therapists provide safe, competent, appropriate care; are technically competent to perform the procedures within their scope of work; and are operating safely and appropriately.[6] Further more, a study by researchers at the University of Washington School of Dentistry will be publicly released in the summer of 2017. WKKF, a study cofunder, has received the results. The study focused on oral health outcomes of patients served by the Yukon-Kuskokwim Health Corporation (YKHC) between 2006 and 2015. YKHC cares for 25,000 Alaska Natives. Researchers found that for children, high exposure to dental therapists was associated with fewer extractions, less use of general anesthesia, and more preventive visits. Adults in communities with the highest DHAT visit days had fewer extractions and more preventive care visits.

The dental therapist model is gaining momentum, especially in Indian Country. The Swinomish Indian Tribal Community in Washington State has hired a dental therapist who is providing dental care in their clinic. And through the North-west Portland Area Indian Health Board, several tribes throughout the Northwest have launched a demon-stration program to send students to Alaska for DHAT training, and they return to their tribe to serve their communities. In addition, dental therapists now practice in Minnesota and will soon in Maine and Vermont. Other states, such as Kansas, Arizona, Massachusetts, Michigan, New Mexico, North Dakota, and Ohio, are exploring the use of dental thera-pists to improve and expand oral health care.

A VISION FOR ALL CHILDREN

For this vision to become real for all children, communities must acknowledge the role that race and ethnicity has played in oral health disparities, heal those wounds, and move forward to implement strategies that can allow dental therapists to provide much needed care to patients. It will take all segments of the community—people of all color, private and public sectors, non-profits, and others—to overcome the obstacles and enhance the quality of life for vulnerable children. Mr. Kellogg believed that it takes everyone in a community to address the health and well-being of children.

REFERENCES

1. Davidson V. At what point did you get involved? In: *Understanding Vulnerable Children: Who Knows What About Community?* W.K. Kellogg Foundation. Available at: https://www.wkkf. org/resource-directory/resource/annual-reports/2012-w-k-kellogg-foundation-annual-report. Accessed June 12, 2017.

Phipps KR, Ricks TL. Oral Health of American Indian and Alaska Native Children Aged 1–5 Years: Results of the 2014 IHS Oral Health Survey. Indian Health Service data brief. Rockville, MD: Indian Health Service. Available at: https://www.ihs.gov/doh/documents/IHS_Data_Brief_1-5_Year-Old.pdf. Accessed June 12, 2017.

3. Shortage Designation. HPSAs, MUAs & MUPs. Health Resources and Services Administration. US Department of Health and Human Services. Available at: https://data.hrsa.gov/tools/shortage-area. Accessed December 13, 2018.

4. The Consequences of Untreated Dental Disease in Children. The California Society of Pediatric Dentistry. Available at: https://www.cda.org/Portals/0/pdfs/untreated_disease.pdf. Accessed June 12, 2017.

5. Oral Health: A Window to Your Overall Health. Mayo Clinic. Available at: http://www.mayoclinic.org/healthy-lifestyle/adult-health/in-depth/dental/art-20047475. Accessed June 12, 2017.

6. Wetterhall S, Bader JD, Burrus BB, Lee JY, Shugars DA. Evaluation of the dental health aide therapist workforce model in Alaska. RTI International. Available at: http://www.rti.org/sites/default/files/resources/alaskadhatprogramevaluationfinal102510.pdf. Accessed June 12, 2017.

Oral Health and Medicine Integration: Overcoming Historical Artifact to Relieve Suffering*

Stephen A. Martin, MD, EdM, and Lisa Simon, DMD

"I haven't been able to kiss my wife in over a year."[1] Why? Kissing hurts her mouth too much. Why? Her teeth are fractured and painful. Why? Like many Americans, money is tight for this couple and American health care has failed them. Former US Surgeon General David Satcher, who published the landmark report *Oral Health in America* in 2000, recently observed, "Eighty percent of oral health problems affect about 20 percent of the population—the poor and minorities in this country."[2]

At massive weekend free clinics, dental care is the most in-demand service. Dental problems lead to underemployment, lower wages, and shame. Pain leads to both initial opioid misuse and substance use disorder relapse. A recent review concludes, "Poor oral health continues to serve as a primary physical, emotional, and psychological marker of social inequality."[3(p2173)]

This inequality stares at us. Look at celebrities, health care professionals, and lawmakers. Pearly white smiles are prerequisites for those with privilege. Most decision-makers will never have an untreated toothache or know the shame of being afraid to smile. Painful, cracked, broken, and missing teeth keep people down and out.[4]

Amid significant coverage gains, oral health is often ignored. Medicare, most adult Medicaid programs, and many private plans exclude dental care. Although children and some adults on Medicaid have limited dental benefits, fewer than one third of dentists accept public insurance; coverage alone is insufficient to provide access. Dental care joins other conditions that have been historically marginalized because of stigma: cancer, tuberculosis, HIV/AIDS, mental health, and substance use disorders.

Effective dental treatment exists at a far lower cost than many medical interventions. Yet, for too many, treatment remains unattainable without disposable income. We are stymied by the historical vagaries of excluding dentistry from the medical system and the fact that dental "insurance" is largely an indemnity plan, with coverage for prevention but not treatment.[5]

*This is a modified version of the article that appeared in the *American Journal of Public Health*. See: Martin SA, Simon L. Oral health and medicine integration: overcoming historical artifact to relieve suffering. *Am J Public Health*. 2017;107(suppl 1):S30–S31.

This "paradox of dental need" means vulnerable patients with the highest disease burdens are also least likely to receive necessary care. This leads to illogical and harmful outcomes, such as a patient with diabetes who receives a costly and life-saving kidney transplant but cannot repair dentition so poor that he eats only the softest, least nutritious foods.

An argument for dental care can be made on the grounds of improving systemic illness. Such care has even been found to be cost saving. Yet, that argument ignores the social, emotional, and physiological importance of oral health itself. Oral health equity should stem from not economic arguments but moral outrage with the system we have. Medical providers treat hundreds of healthy people with expensive medications for years to prevent one cardiovascular event, but we have not made it possible to help people actively suffering with dental decay and pain.

PUTTING THE MOUTH BACK IN THE BODY

We are encumbered with a sense of learned helplessness and historical artifact that keep dental care and health care apart. This separation obviously does not hold up to scrutiny. We take care of the brain and lung, mind and hormone, heart and eye in medicine. There is no rational reason we cannot take care of the mouth. Once we welcome the mouth back into the body, we can apply what works more generally for vulnerable populations who need timely, ongoing access to care (Table 2-1). Individual providers, health systems, and communities each play a role in prioritizing medically integrated oral health for all community members.

Central to this work is the patient's perspective: How can I get help for my teeth? A patient with pain from head trauma, appendicitis, or carcinoma can be cared for in a hospital or clinic. Patients seeking relief from dental pain in the health care system are often left with nothing but a palliative antibiotic and a directive to find a dentist. What is different when pain is in the mouth? The status quo tells us the mouth is different. Common sense tells us otherwise.

DOING THE WORK

Providers shoulder an increasing burden of unmet health needs because their geographic maldistribution is more inequitable than ever. The vast majority of dentists work in private practice in higher-income neighborhoods, where oral health need is relatively low. But changes to how dentists and medical providers practice can pave the way for a workforce more attuned to the need for oral health equity.

The number of dentists per capita is expected to increase in the coming decades, and these dentists are less likely to select traditional practice models. They may be more likely to work in medically integrated settings such as hospitals and emergency departments, where only one percent of dentists currently work. Dental schools have adopted successful programs to recruit students from rural and underserved areas, who are more likely to

CHAPTER 2

Table 2-1. Actions to Increase Oral Health Equity

Action	Providers	Health Systems	Communities
Improve coverage and payment systems for integrated oral health care.	Develop collaborative practice models that improve colocation and communication between providers.	Pioneer outcomes-based reimbursement that incentivizes oral health.	Increase coverage for dental treatment of adults under Medicaid, Medicare, and private insurance.
Enhance interactions between the medical and dental health systems.	Train providers to treat populations with complex multidisciplinary health needs.	Adopt interoperable electronic health records that include medical and dental information.	Adopt midlevel provider models that can provide dental care in novel settings.
Increase access to oral health for at-risk groups.	Train primary care locations to provide basic dental treatment such as fluoride varnish, sealants, and dental anesthesia.	Build referral systems that divert patients from emergency department utilization for preventable dental pain.	Continue expanding access to community water fluoridation.
Improve the experience of care for vulnerable patients.	Provide trauma-informed dental care, including appropriate anxiolytics.	Employ care navigators with knowledge of dental and medical systems to support patients.	Be advocates for vulnerable community members at risk for poor oral health.
Contextualize oral health within the social determinants of health.	Enhance diversity and cultural humility in medical and dental education and workforce.	Strengthen relationships of primary, dental, and specialist care with social services.	Destigmatize poor oral health and address challenges accessing care.

ose communities; expanding programs like the National Health Service ..ps can further strengthen dentists' ability to practice in these settings. The dentist of decades past, a solo private practice that accepts only private insurances, is on the wane.

Nor should dentists do the work alone. The creation of a dental therapist role, comparable to a nurse practitioner, would safely and significantly expand access to care; these clinicians would substantially increase meaningful dental access. Like organized medicine, the American Dental Association and state dental societies have been highly resistant to this practice innovation, and therapists currently only practice in Alaska and Minnesota. Increasingly bipartisan support has led Vermont and Maine to pass dental therapy legislation, with several other legislatures considering it. Community support and a growing evidence base must overcome obstruction by organized dentistry.

Medical practice must meet the needs it already faces but cannot fix. Dental problems lead to two percent of emergency visits and, in some areas, more than 10% of primary care visits. Basic procedures such as dental anesthesia and differential diagnosis of dental pain must be standard components of medical and nursing curricula, with elective opportunities to acquire additional dental skills, including tooth extraction. Many health professions schools have embraced interprofessional education, with dental and other health professions students working together in preparation for further collaboration in practice. Telehealth solutions have brought specialist expertise to patients in rural areas; teledentistry to connect medical and dental providers should be increasingly adopted.

Much of this work has been and is being pioneered by dedicated practitioners and community advocates, most often in community and federally qualified health centers.[6] Integrated care delivery models, with enhanced communication and task sharing between medical and dental providers, are being disseminated by groups such as the Marshfield Clinic and the Safety Net Medical Home Initiative, as well as by accountable care organizations.[7] The extension of dental services into long-term care facilities and schools has increased the reach of preventive care and treatment.

Medical and dental providers across the country have the privilege of seeing how transformative oral health is for their patients. But too many suffer for too long from an entirely preventable and treatable disease. As the dental workforce expands and evolves—including dentists, dental therapists, physicians, physician assistants, nurses, patient navigators, and more—our health system will finally have the opportunity to address the most prevalent disease in the country and put an end to the suffering it causes.

REFERENCES

1. Reichert J, Zaman F. Remote Area Medical [film]. 2013. Available at: http://remoteareamedicalmovie.com. Accessed December 12, 2016.

2. Scientific American. The case for oral health. 2016. Available at: https://www.scientificamerican.com/products/the-future-of-oral-health/the-case-for-oral-health/?wt.ac=SA_Custom_Colgate_RECRC. Accessed December 12, 2016.

3. Mertz EA. The dental–medical divide. *Health Aff (Millwood)*. 2016;35(12):2168–2175.

4. Treadwell HM, Northridge ME. Oral health is the measure of a just society. *J Health Care Poor Underserved*. 2007;18(1):12–20.

5. Simon L. Overcoming historical separation between oral and general health care: interprofessional collaboration for promoting health equity. *AMA J Ethics*. 2016;18(9):941–949.

6. Formicola AJ, Ro M, Marshall S, et al. Strengthening the oral health safety net: delivery models that improve access to oral health care for uninsured and underserved populations. *Am J Public Health*. 2008;98(9 suppl):S86–S88.

7. Glurich I, Acharya A, Shukla SK, Nycz GR, Brilliant MH. The oral-systemic personalized medicine model at Marshfield Clinic. *Oral Dis*. 2013;19(1):1–17.

II. DISPARITIES

Children's Oral Health Inequalities: Intersectionality of Race, Ethnicity, and Income

Karin Herzog, DDS, MSD, JoAnna Scott, PhD, and Donald L. Chi, DDS, PhD

Socioeconomically marginalized children, including racial and ethnic minorities and those from low-income families, are at increased risk for poor oral health.[1,2] The goal of health entitlement programs such as Medicaid is to address the needs of vulnerable families and children through no-cost health insurance. The federal Early and Periodic Screening, Diagnosis, and Treatment program mandates that state Medicaid programs include dental benefits for children. Subsequent research has demonstrated that no-cost dental insurance alone is insufficient in improving access to dental care and meeting the dental care needs of vulnerable enrollees.[3,4]

To improve access to dental care services, state Medicaid programs have implemented special dental initiatives to address barriers to care. Three examples are the Access to Baby and Child Dentistry (ABCD) program in Washington State, Into the Mouth of Babes in North Carolina, and I-Smile in Iowa. Similar initiatives have been introduced in other states.[5] Some states have reported higher dental utilization rates for children in Medicaid.[6] Less clear is the extent to which tooth decay rates have improved because of special Medicaid dental programs and other efforts such as increased dental reimbursement rates[7] and whether oral health inequalities persist for the most marginalized children.

Intersectionality is a framework originally developed to conceptualize inequalities experienced by Black women resulting from the intersection of race and sex.[8] While intersectionality has been used to uncover the roots of various social phenomena and health outcomes,[9–11] intersectionality has not been used as a framework to examine children's oral health inequalities. In the current study, our goal was to test the intersectionality hypothesis by evaluating tooth decay rates for marginalized children at the intersection of race, ethnicity, and income. Our study has important implications for future policies and interventions aimed at preventing dental disease, reducing inequality, and eventually achieving health equity.[12]

INTERSECTIONALITY AS A FRAMEWORK FOR RESEARCH ON CHILDREN'S DENTAL HEALTH

Analysis of the Data: Outcomes Measures, Model Covariates, and Statistical Analyses

We analyzed 2013–2014 National Health and Nutrition Examination Survey (NHANES) data for children aged 3 to 17 years.[13] This study was exempt from human participant approval by the University of Washington institutional review board.

Outcomes Measures

NHANES includes three tooth-level dental disease measures obtained through screenings: dental caries experience (defined as having a least one tooth with untreated dental decay or a dental restoration present), dental restoration (at least one tooth with a dental restoration present), and untreated dental decay (at least one tooth with untreated dental decay).

Model Covariates

There were two predictor variables. Race/ethnicity was a five-category variable: non-Hispanic White, non-Hispanic Black, Mexican American, other Hispanic, and other race. Income was calculated as a ratio of total family income divided by the federal poverty income, with larger ratios indicating higher household income: < 1.0, ≥ 1.0 to < 2.0, ≥ 2.0 to < 5.0, and ≥ 5.0. For subgroups analyses, we generated an additional indicator variable of whether the child had public health insurance (e.g., Medicaid, State Children's Health Insurance Program [SCHIP], military, other state health insurance).

Statistical Analyses

We used survey sampling weights to generate nationally representative prevalence estimates of the three dental disease measures. Next, we estimated dental disease rates by race, ethnicity, and income separately, restricting our analyses to White, Black, and Mexican American children because the remaining two race/ethnicity categories were nonspecific, making it difficult to interpret findings. Then, we examined race/ethnicity and income together, with the highest-income White children serving as the reference group. Finally, we conducted subgroup analyses restricted to publicly insured children to examine dental disease prevalence across race/ethnicity. We used Stata version 12.1 to complete all analyses (Stata Corp LP, College Station, TX).

RESULTS

Dental Disease Prevalence

About 45.8% of US children aged 3 to 17 years had dental caries experience (Table 3-1). About 36.7% of children had a dental restoration, and 16.9% had untreated tooth decay.

Racial/Ethnic Inequalities

Non-Hispanic White children had the lowest dental caries experience at 40.2% (Table 3-1). Non-Hispanic Black (48.4%) and Mexican American children (60.3%) had significantly higher caries experience rates than non-Hispanic White children. The dental restoration rate was significantly higher for Mexican American children compared with White children (49.8% and 32.5%, respectively), and untreated dental decay rates were significantly higher for non-Hispanic Black children (22.5%) and Mexican American children (21.4%) than for White children (14.8%).

Income-Related Inequalities

There were income gradients for all three outcomes, with children from the highest-income households presenting with the lowest rates of dental disease (Table 3-1). From highest to lowest income levels, dental caries experience ranged from 31.7% to 55.8%, dental restoration rates from 26.9% to 43.6%, and untreated dental decay rates from 11.2% to 23.4%. There were no statistically significant differences among the two highest-income subgroups, but rates were significantly lower in the highest- than in the lowest-income categories (Table 3-1). Similar income gradients were present within racial/ethnic groups in which the lowest-income children within each racial/ethnic group had the highest rates of dental caries experience, dental restorations, and untreated tooth decay (Table 3-2).

Intersection Between Race/Ethnicity and Income

Compared with the highest-income non-Hispanic White children, upper-middle–income non-Hispanic Black children had higher dental caries experience rates (32.6% and 47.9%, respectively; Table 3-2). Upper-middle–income and the lowest-income Black children also had significantly higher restoration rates. There were no significant differences between highest-income non-Hispanic White children and Mexican American children at all income levels for all three dental disease outcomes. Among non-Hispanic White children, dental caries experience and untreated decay rates were significantly higher for the lowest-income children.

Table 3-1. Prevalence of Dental Disease for All US Children Aged 3 to 17 Years and by Race, Ethnicity, and Income Level: National Health and Nutrition Examination Survey, 2013–2014

Chronic Health Condition	All Children, % (95% CI)	Race and Ethnicity					Income Level (Household Income to Poverty Ratio)						
		Non-Hispanic White (Ref), % (95% CI)	Non-Hispanic Black		Mexican American		≥ 5.0 (Ref), % (95% CI)	2.0 to < 5.0		≥ 1.0 to < 2.0		< 1.0	
			% (95% CI)	P	% (95% CI)	P		% (95% CI)	P	% (95% CI)	P	% (95% CI)	P
Dental caries experience[a]	45.80 (40.88, 50.81)	40.19 (33.56, 47.20)	48.42 (44.23, 52.64)	.029	60.32 (53.89, 66.41)	<.001	31.66 (23.80, 40.73)	40.78 (34.76, 47.10)	.076	52.16 (46.72, 57.55)	.001	55.79 (49.69, 61.72)	.001
Dental restoration[b]	36.71 (32.23, 41.43)	32.47 (25.82, 39.90)	35.71 (31.34, 40.34)	.481	49.82 (43.99, 55.65)	<.001	26.91 (19.40, 36.03)	32.18 (26.65, 38.27)	.201	42.46 (35.77, 49.43)	.004	43.64 (38.07, 49.38)	.009
Untreated dental decay[c]	16.88 (13.82, 20.45)	14.85 (11.05, 19.67)	22.52 (17.75, 28.13)	.006	21.44 (16.81, 26.94)	.038	11.22 (7.02, 17.48)	13.64 (9.15, 19.85)	.550	18.34 (16.32, 20.55)	.056	23.37 (19.02, 28.38)	.004

Source: Based on data from National Health and Nutrition Examination Survey, 2013–2014.[13]

Note: CI = confidence interval.

[a]At least one tooth with untreated dental decay or a dental restoration present.

[b]At least one tooth with a dental restoration present.

[c]At least one tooth with untreated dental decay.

Table 3-2. Prevalence of Dental Caries Experience, Dental Restoration, and Untreated Dental Decay at the Intersection of Race, Ethnicity, and Income for US Children Aged 3 to 17 Years: National Health and Nutrition Examination Survey, 2013–2014

Income	Non-Hispanic White		Non-Hispanic Black		Mexican American	
	% (95% CI)	P	% (95% CI)	P	% (95% CI)	P
Dental caries experience						
≥ 5.00	32.59 (23.22, 43.59)	Ref	21.02 (12.51, 33.12)	.044	26.62 (8.82, 57.63)	.634
≥ 2.00 to < 5.00	38.16 (29.91, 47.15)	.353	47.87 (35.86, 60.14)	.018	50.56 (37.72, 63.31)	.248
≥ 1.00 to < 2.00	49.64 (39.90, 59.40)	.036	42.11 (36.00, 48.47)	.482	64.43 (55.28, 72.62)	.181
< 1.00	49.07 (39.36, 58.87)	.036	54.29 (47.57, 60.86)	.060	65.49 (55.79, 74.05)	.132
Dental restoration						
≥ 5.00	27.80 (18.95, 38.82)	Ref	6.31 (1.52, 22.76)	.016	26.62 (8.82, 57.63)	.920
≥ 2.00 to < 5.00	30.07 (22.37, 39.08)	.627	35.53 (27.89, 43.99)	.016	37.32 (27.22, 48.65)	.533
≥ 1.00 to < 2.00	40.82 (29.38. 53.33)	.081	32.12 (24.96, 40.23)	.091	52.73 (44.37, 60.93)	.416
< 1.00	38.48 (26.45, 52.11)	.230	40.78 (34.06, 47.87)	.025	55.00 (46.12, 63.58)	.301
Untreated dental decay						
≥ 5.00	12.14 (7.07. 20.07)	Ref	14.71 (6.96, 28.43)	.656	8.50 (2.90, 22.41)	.508
≥ 2.00 to < 5.00	12.24 (6.87, 20.86)	.985	21.30 (9.71, 40.53)	.519	21.28 (10.73, 37.80)	.208
≥ 1.00 to < 2.00	18.65 (14.44, 23.75)	.183	15.65 (12.06, 20.08)	.442	23.72 (16.49, 32.87)	.267
< 1.00	22.90 (14.72, 33.82)	.042	26.71 (20.83, 33.54)	.976	21.93 (16.05, 29.21)	.558

Source: Based on data from National Health and Nutrition Examination Survey 2013–2014.[13]
Note: CI = confidence interval.

Subgroup Analyses

Among publicly insured children, Mexican American children had significantly higher dental caries experience and restoration rates compared with non-Hispanic White children (Table 3-3), with no significant differences between White and Black children across these measures. For untreated decay, the rates were significantly higher for Black children than for White children (25.3% and 18.3%, respectively).

Discussion of the Analyses

We analyzed nationally representative US oral health data to test the hypothesis that race, ethnicity, and income intersect to create oral health inequalities in children. Our analyses partially support the intersectionality hypothesis. There were two main findings.

Table 3-3. Prevalence of Dental Caries Experience, Dental Restoration, and Untreated Dental Decay at the Intersection of Race and Ethnicity for Publicly Insured US Children Aged 3 to 17 Years Based on National Health and Nutrition Examination Survey, 2013–2014

	Publicly Insured Children				
	Non-Hispanic White (Ref), % (95% CI)	Non-Hispanic Black		Mexican American	
		% (95% CI)	P	% (95% CI)	P
Dental caries experience	47.99 (39.43, 56.67)	54.20 (49.67, 58.67)	.250	64.84 (58.11, 71.03)	<.001
Dental restoration	39.36 (30.95, 48.45)	39.94 (34.23, 45.94)	.916	57.32 (50.94, 63.46)	<.001
Untreated dental caries	18.28 (14.15, 23.30)	25.33 (21.44, 29.65)	.016	19.26 (13.84, 26.16)	.698

Source: Based on data from National Health and Nutrition Examination Survey, 2013-2014.[13]
Note: CI = confidence interval.

First, we documented children's oral health inequalities based on the independent effects of race, ethnicity, and income. These findings are consistent with similar analyses conducted on NHANES III data from 1988 to 1994.[1] One explanation for persisting oral health inequalities is the lack of adequate attention to how social conditions affect health outcomes. The Fundamental Causes Theory posits that low socioeconomic status (SES) is the primary etiology of inequalities and that the mechanism by which SES affects outcomes such as health status is via differential access to resources, including money, knowledge, social networks, and social capital.[14] Suboptimal social conditions are likely to adversely affect oral health by constraining behaviors, a concept supported by related work on built environments and obesity outcomes.[15] For example, individuals living in low-income neighborhoods have fewer healthy food choices, and affordability barriers may further push these individuals to purchase less-healthy foods. These findings support intervention approaches that account for social conditions as well as broader social policies aimed at addressing poverty by ensuring equitable access to affordable housing, education, employment, clean water, healthy foods, and comprehensive health care, including mental health care services, prescription medications, and dental care.

Second, we found partial support for the intersectionality hypothesis in which Black and Mexican American children from the lowest-income households exhibited greater dental disease burden compared with the highest-income White children. This finding was magnified in the subgroup analyses focusing on publicly insured children. Collectively, these data support efforts to develop interventions that focus on racial and ethnic minorities and other high-risk subgroups within programs designed for low-income children. For instance, special dental Medicaid initiatives such as the ABCD program have improved overall dental utilization rates,[16] but the extent to which minority subgroups have benefitted is unclear. Subgroup analyses of our current NHANES data indicate similar findings across age subgroups (younger than 6 years, 6–11 years, and 12–17 years; data not shown). We would expect to observe dampened effects among young children because programs like ABCD focus on the youngest Medicaid enrollees. In addition, data from the I-Smile program in Iowa indicate that children with special health care needs within Medicaid may not benefit equally from such programs.[17] Continuing to rely on nontargeted approaches may limit improvements in health outcomes, widen inequalities, and move us farther away from health equity.[18] Future research should continue to test the intersectionality hypothesis by using data from state dental Medicaid programs to help guide the development targeted interventions that focus on meeting the needs of marginalized children within entitlement programs.

Because childhood tooth decay continues to be a highly prevalent disease, policies should continue to fully support publicly funded health entitlement programs, including Medicaid and SCHIP, which provide comprehensive dental benefits for children from low-income and working-poor households.[19,20] In addition, on the basis of the inherent limitations of dental care and the concomitant importance of optimizing other oral health–related behaviors, oral health researchers should continue to develop and test theory-based behavior change interventions aimed at improving fluoride exposure and diet for children. Programs like ABCD, Into the Mouth of Babes, and I-Smile do not contain explicit strategies to improve these oral health behaviors, which take place outside the dental office. This provides opportunities to develop and implement community- and home-based behavior change interventions within such special dental initiatives. Dentists also need training on effective chairside strategies that can be implemented within clinical settings to reinforce behavior change, which is an area in which additional research is needed.

LIMITATIONS OF THE STUDY

To our knowledge, this is the first study to test an intersectionality-based hypothesis to examine SES-related oral health inequalities in children. There are three main limitations. First, dental disease data from NHANES do not provide information on the extent to which treatment is necessary. For instance, untreated tooth decay may indicate need for definitive restorative treatment, such as fillings or crowns, or could be treated with commercially available caries-arresting medicaments such as silver diamine fluoride and monitored.[21]

Second, we included children identified as "other Hispanic" or "other race" in estimating dental disease prevalence rates, but did not include these children in the intersectionality analyses because the subgroups within these two categories are unclear. Although this approach is consistent with previous work,[1] it has the potential to overlook important high-risk subgroups including American Indian and Alaska Native children.[22]

National health surveys such as NHANES as well as state Medicaid programs should be mandated to collect race and ethnicity data to allow health monitoring and program planning. Special efforts will be needed to protect data collection standards on race, ethnicity, and primary language within Medicaid and SCHIP.[23]

Third, the income variable does not account for number of household members. However, this variable has been used in previous work, which allows direct comparisons with other studies.[24] Furthermore, we conducted subgroup analyses focusing on publicly insured children and the results were comparable.

CONCLUSIONS

We found that the lowest-income racial and ethnic minority children are disproportionately affected by dental caries and that minority children within health entitlement programs such as Medicaid may benefit from tailored approaches aimed at preventing dental disease, which is an important next step to address children's oral health inequalities and achieve health equity in the United States.

ACKNOWLEDGMENTS

The study was funded in part by the National Institute of Dental and Craniofacial Research Grant K08DE020856 and the William T. Grant Foundation Scholars Program.

REFERENCES

1. Vargas CM, Crall JJ, Schneider DA. Sociodemographic distribution of pediatric dental caries: NHANES III, 1988–1994. *J Am Dent Assoc.* 1998;129(9):1229–1238.

2. Dye BA, Li X, Thorton-Evans G. Oral health disparities as determined by selected Healthy People 2020 oral health objectives for the United States, 2009–2010. NCHS Data Brief No. 104. Hyattsville, MD: US Department of Health and Human Services; 2012:1–8.

3. Crall JJ. Improving oral health and oral health care delivery for children. *J Calif Dent Assoc.* 2011;39(2):90–100.

4. Chi DL, Raklios NA. The relationship between body system-based chronic conditions and dental utilization for Medicaid-enrolled children: a retrospective cohort study. *BMC Oral Health.* 2012;12(1):1–17.

5. US Department of Health and Human Services. Centers for Medicare and Medicaid. Keep kids smiling: promoting oral health through the Medicaid benefit for children & adolescents. 2013. Available at: https://www.medicaid.gov/Medicaid/Benefits/Downloads/Keep-Kids-Smiling.pdf. Accessed November 1, 2016.

6. Hakim RB, Babish JD, Davis AC. State of dental care among Medicaid-enrolled children in the United States. *Pediatrics.* 2012;130(1):5–14.

7. Beazoglou T, Douglass J, Myne-Joslin V, Baker P, Bailit H. Impact of fee increases on dental utilization rates for children living in Connecticut and enrolled in Medicaid. *J Am Dent Assoc.* 2015;146(1):52–60.

8. Crenshaw K. Demarginalizing the intersection of race and sex: a Black feminist critique of antidiscrimination doctrine. *Univ Chic Leg Forum.* 1989;1989(1):139–168.

9. Jackson JW, Williams DR, VanderWeele TJ. Disparities at the intersection of marginalized groups. *Soc Psychiatry Psychiatr Epidemiol.* 2016;51(10):1349–1359.

10. Veenstra G, Patterson AC. South Asian–White health inequalities in Canada: intersections with gender and immigrant status. *Ethn Health.* 2016;21(6):639–648.

11. Coley SL, Nichols TR, Rulison KL, Aronson RE, Brown-Jeffy SL, Morrison SD. Race, socio-economic status, and age: exploring intersections in preterm birth disparities among teen mothers. *Int J Popul Res.* 2015;2015:pii:617907.

12. Treadwell HM, Northridge ME. Oral health is the measure of a just society. *J Health Care Poor Underserved.* 2007;18(1):12–20.

13. US Department of Health and Human Services, Centers for Disease Control and Prevention. NHANES 2013–2014. Available at: https://wwwn.cdc.gov/nchs/nhanes/ContinuousNhanes/Default.aspx?BeginYear=2013. Accessed October 2, 2018.

14. Hill I, Benatar S, Howell E, et al. CHIP and Medicaid: evolving to meet the needs of children. *Acad Pediatr.* 2015;15(3 suppl):S19–S27.

15. Link BG, Phelan J. Social conditions as fundamental causes of health inequalities. In: Bird CE, Conrad P, Fremont AM, Timmermans S, eds. *Handbook of Medical Sociology.* 6th ed. Nashville, TN: Vanderbilt University Press; 2010:3–17.

16. Drewnowski A, Aggarwal A, Tang W, et al. Obesity, diet quality, physical activity, and the built environment: the need for behavioral pathways. *BMC Public Health.* 2016;16(1):1–12.

17. Lewis C, Teeple E, Robertson A, Williams A. Preventive dental care for young, Medicaid-insured children in Washington State. *Pediatrics.* 2009;124(1):e120–e127.

18. Chi DL, Momany ET, Mancl LA, Lindgren SD, Zinner SH, Steinman KJ. Dental homes for children with autism: a longitudinal analysis of Iowa Medicaid's I-Smile program. *Am J Prev Med.* 2016;50(5):609–615.

19. Wang YC, Bleich SN, Gortmaker SL. Increasing caloric contribution from sugar-sweetened beverages and 100% fruit juices among US children and adolescents, 1988–2004. *Pediatrics.* 2008;121(6):e1604–e1614.

20. Harrington ME. The Children's Health Insurance Program Reauthorization Act evaluation findings on children's health insurance coverage in an evolving health care landscape. *Acad Pediatr.* 2015;15(3 suppl):S1–S6.

21. White M, Adams J, Heywood P. How and why do interventions that increase health overall widen inequalities within populations? In: Babones S, ed. *Social Inequality and Public Health.* Bristol, UK: Policy Press; 2009:65–82.

22. Horst JA, Ellenikiotis H, Milgrom PL. UCSF protocol for caries arrest using silver diamine fluoride: rationale, indications and consent. *J Calif Dent Assoc.* 2016;44(1):16–28.

23. Phipps KR, Ricks TL, Manz MC, Blahut P. Prevalence and severity of dental caries among American Indian and Alaska Native preschool children. *J Public Health Dent.* 2012;72(3):208–215.

24. US Department of Health and Human Services. Improving the identification of health care disparities in Medicaid and CHIP: report to Congress. 2014. Available at: https://www.medicaid.gov/medicaid/quality-of-care/downloads/4302b-rtc-2014.pdf. Accessed November 10, 2016.

4

Perpetual Inequities in Access to Dental Care: Government or Professional Responsibility?

Oscar Arevalo, DDS, ScD, MBA, MS, and Scott L. Tomar, DMD, DrPH

Almost 40 years ago, Ralph Lobene described his frustration with the US dental care delivery system by stating, "The outdated philosophy that this service is a privilege to be enjoyed only by people affluent enough to afford it has long been tacitly accepted by the dental profession."[1] Oral health disparities adversely affect individuals who face greater barriers to health on the basis of socioeconomic status, racial or ethnic group, education, disability, mental health, geographic location, sexual orientation, and other characteristics historically associated with exclusion.[2,3] Disparities in oral health have been documented for the prevalence of dental caries, periodontal disease, tooth loss, cancer, and orofacial pain as well as to access to preventive and restorative services.[4-6] These inequities are partially the result of limited access to oral health care among individuals who have the greatest burden of disease, namely the poor, uninsured persons, racial and ethnic minorities, and Medicaid recipients.

From a macro perspective, two synergistic factors have led to these perpetual inequities in access to care: first, public policies that place low priority on oral health and attempt to control costs without a systematic assessment of their impact on access to care, and, second, a profession that is disengaged, does not represent the diversity of the patient population, and has failed to make the distribution of its services more equitable. This chapter attempts to provide a comprehensive overview of the contributing factors that have caused and perpetuated these disparities. We conclude by providing policy recommendations.

THE ROLE OF GOVERNMENT

Federal and state governments perform critical functions related to health care including financing and delivery, cost containment, and workforce issues.

Expenditures, Financing, and Delivery

Expenditures for dental care represent the importance that governments place on that particular service and serve as an indicator of the population's access to care. As the payors, the federal and state governments determine the funds to be allocated, eligibility,

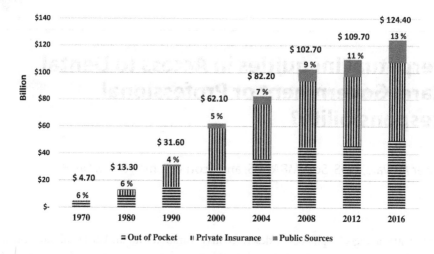

Source: Based on data from Centers for Medicare and Medicaid Services.[7]

Figure 4-1. Total Dental Services Expenditures and Percent by Payor, Selected Years, 1970–2016

benefits, and reimbursement levels. According to the Centers for Medicare and Medicaid Services, $124.4 billion was spent on dental services in 2016.[7] That figure is double the amount spent in 2000 and 25 times more than was spent in 1970 (Figure 4-1). Historically, most expenditures for dental care services have come from two sources: out of pocket and private insurance. As a percentage of total dental care expenditures, public expenditures represented 6% in 1970, 5% in 2000, and 13% in 2016. Through 2008, public expenditures represented less than 10% of total expenditures for dental care. Historically, total public funds for dental care have been small relative to other categories of services (Table 4-1).

Although the percentages of public expenditures for dentist and physician services have grown at similar rates since the 2000s, public expenditures for physician services represent a much larger percentage of total expenditures. The public share for hospital expenditures has decreased compared with the 2000s, perhaps as a result of more patient care being shifted from inpatient settings to outpatient facilities and nursing homes. In 2016, the federal and state governments paid for 64% of all expenditures for hospital-based care. Public expenditures for prescription drugs grew most sharply of all health care categories, increasing by 33% from 1970 to 2016. The limited allocation of public funds to dental care compared with other services suggests that access to oral health is a relatively low priority for legislators.

Medicaid, Children's Health Insurance Program, and Medicare

The Early and Periodic Screening, Diagnosis, and Treatment program was designed to ensure that Medicaid-enrolled children receive comprehensive health services, including comprehensive dental care, at no cost to the family. According to the Centers for Medicare

Table 4-1. National Health Expenditures, Public Expenditures as a Percentage of Total Expenditures 1970–2016

Category	1970%	1980%	1990%	2000%	2004%	2008%	2012%	2016%	Average
Dentists	5.4	5.8	3.9	5.5	7.3	8.7	11.3	13.4	7.7
Physicians				37.5	38.6	40.2	42.5	44.6	40.7
Hospitals	59.0	58.1	56.9	62.9	61.4	60.3	59.0	57.5	59.4
Prescription Drugs	9.0	13.7	16.3	21.6	25.7	34.1	39.1	42.9	25.3
Nursing Homes	51.0	58.2	53.5	59.3	63.9	64.2	65.6	63.9	60.0

Source: Based on data from Centers for Medicare and Medicaid Services.[7]

and Medicaid Services, in 2016, there were almost 46 million children enrolled in Medicaid and the state Children's Health Insurance Program (CHIP).[8] Studies have documented a steady increase in utilization of dental care services by children enrolled in these programs.[9,10] However, a major weakness of these analyses is that they reflect dental care utilization instead of treatment plan completion rates (i.e., a child may have visited a dentist for emergency, examination, or preventive services but her dental needs may have not been completely met).[8] Similarly, dental care utilization rates for children enrolled in Medicaid and CHIP remain lower than those of privately insured children. In 2013, 45.9% of children enrolled in Medicaid or CHIP reported a dental visit, compared with 57.1% of children with private dental insurance.[10] Children enrolled in Medicaid are more likely than children with private dental coverage to report unmet dental needs.[11]

While mandatory for children, dental benefits for Medicaid-enrolled adults are optional. States have substantial flexibility in determining the scope of dental services covered. As a result, Medicaid adult dental coverage varies widely among the states and may be limited to emergency services or to specific patient populations, such as pregnant women.[12] In contrast with the pediatric population, annual use of dental care among adults has declined gradually for both those living below and above federal poverty levels.[9]

According to the US Census Bureau, persons aged 65 years or older accounted for 15% of the US population in 2016 and are projected to account for 20% by 2029.[13] Medicare, the primary payer for health care for older adults in the United States, does not cover most dental care. In fact, these preclusions for dental benefits were part of the passage of the Social Security Act of 1965.[14] Policy attempts to add dental care to Medicare have, thus far, been unsuccessful. Therefore, for individuals receiving dental benefits through employer-sponsored insurance plans, retirement generally translates into a lack of dental care coverage.[15] In 2016, one half of all Medicare beneficiaries had incomes less than $26,200 per person and one quarter had incomes less than $15,250.[16] For those individuals, the financial burden becomes a significant barrier to accessing dental care. Although various bills seeking to expand dental benefits in the Medicare program have been introduced to the US House of Representatives and the US Senate during the past decade, those bills have not yet become law. The low priority of dental care within public funding mechanisms in the United States creates a particularly challenging situation for the working poor, low-income families, and older adults (i.e., paying out of pocket for dental care is prohibitive because of competing demands).

Cost Containment and Managed Care

Since the early 1980s, state governments have utilized various models of managed care to deliver and finance care for Medicaid enrollees, with the goals of controlling costs while simultaneously increasing access to care. A report by the Kaiser Family Foundation showed that the most commonly carved-out service is dental care, followed by inpatient and outpatient behavioral health care, nonemergency transportation, and pharmacy.[17] Despite its goals, managed dental care has failed as a strategy for improving patient care as a result of inadequate capitation payment rates leading to low fee-for-service reimbursement to providers, insufficient networks of providers to meet the dental needs of the enrolled population, or deficient state oversight of managed care programs. In instances in which states have not met their responsibility to provide children's dental services, advocates—including organized dentistry—have filed lawsuits for failure to meet federally mandated standards to ensure access to care. Of the 27 access-related lawsuits filed in 21 states, the states have lost or settled all but four.[18]

Responding to fiscal challenges, states reduced or eliminated Medicaid dental coverage for adults during the past decade, contributing to a 10% decline in oral health care utilization among low-income adults.[19,20] As a consequence, the use of hospitals' emergency departments for dental-related problems has increased nationally, doubling between 2000 and 2010.[21-23] In 2012, dental-related visits to the emergency department cost $1.6 billion to the US health care system, despite the inability of those facilities to effectively manage most dental conditions.[24] The absence of adult dental care coverage in Medicare and in most state Medicaid programs likely resulted in an inefficient and generally ineffective use of public dollars.

Workforce: Training and Availability of Providers

States are involved in the education and training of dental care professionals by appropriating funds to public educational institutions. In 2000, about one third of dental schools' funding—approximately $500 million—came from public sources[25] and the 36 states with public dental schools provided an average subsidy of $49,347 per dental student.[26] In the early 1990s, as state and local government support steadily declined, dental institutions focused their attention on alternative revenue sources—namely, increasing tuition and fees, clinical revenue, research funding, and gifts and endowments. An analysis of dental school revenues comparing 2004–2005 with 2011–2012 determined that public dental schools saw revenues from tuition and fees increase by 68.6% and state support decline by 17.2%, while for private schools, revenues from tuition and fees increased by 38.9% and university indirect subsidies declined by 77.9% over the same period.[27]

As dental schools became more dependent on tuition and fees, the increasing indebtedness of graduates became a major concern. According to the American Dental Education Association, the average educational debt for all indebted dental school graduates in the class of 2017 was $287,331. For dentists graduating from a public school, the average indebtedness was $239,895, with an average debt of $341,190 for graduates of private dental schools.[28] The rise in graduating student debt is a major concern because it hampers the recruitment of dentists to practice in underserved areas and limits their ability to participate in underfunded state Medicaid programs.[29–33]

With limited access to preventive or routine care, simple dental issues can progress to more severe conditions and expensive treatments, including use of hospital emergency departments. According to the Bureau of Health Professions, as of January 1, 2018, there were almost 63 million Americans who lived in 5,866 areas designated as Dental Health Professional Shortage Areas (DHPSAs).[34] An additional 10,802 providers were needed to remove DHPSA designations. Limited funding to incentivize providers contributed to the low number of graduates willing or able to practice in rural or urban underserved areas.[35]

THE ROLE OF THE PROFESSION

One important factor leading to disparities in access is the limited number of providers available to address the dental needs of the underserved. The lack of providers is the result of numerous factors including restrictive licensing practices, the business aspects of dentistry, a perceived lack of social responsibility, and a workforce that does not represent the racial or ethnic composition of the country.

Licensure and Regulation

It is claimed that dentistry in the United States operates on the concept of free markets and competition. This environment reportedly provides patients services of the greatest value, fostering innovation and adequate production while minimizing prices.[36] However, that claim fails to take into consideration the role of licensure. Licenses are granted by state boards of dentistry, which are dominated by dentists, enjoy a high degree of autonomy, and are rarely called upon to answer to the legislature.[37] State dental licensing boards require proof of educational attainment and successful completion of licensing examinations of dubious validity and poor reliability before a person can be considered for licensure. These requirements are defended on the grounds that they maintain the quality of care and ensure patients' safety. However, studies have demonstrated that occupational licensing has either no impact or even a negative impact on the quality of services provided to consumers by members of the regulated occupation, including dentistry.[37,38]

On the other side of the regulatory coin lies professional protectionism: when the number of licenses issued is restricted, the availability of providers can be controlled. Regulating the availability of licenses for practicing dentistry in a geographic area is one strategy for minimizing competition. Economic protectionism rather than protecting patient welfare frequently is the driver of the states' regulation of the practice of dentistry.[39] As long as the supply of dental services is limited by licensure, prices are kept higher and dentists enjoy higher incomes. Profits are maximized if the profession acts as a monopoly in determining who is allowed to practice. The demand for dental labor is derived from the demands for end-use final products (dental services), which suggests two further possibilities for raising dentists' income. First, it increases the price of labor substitutes, such as dental hygienists and midlevel dental providers whose prices can be made infinite by prohibiting them from rendering certain services, such as restorations, and, second, it increases the demand for dental services and, as a result, the dentist's income. For society, licensing control by dental boards translates into higher fees and difficulties in accessing dental care services. Although the viability of health care providers is an important issue for policymakers, it needs to be weighed against their responsibility to ensure access for all citizens.

The Business of Dentistry

From an economic perspective, dental offices are profit-making entities. Although dentists are highly trained professionals, in terms of economic structure and incentives, dentists operate as store owners. They take home at the end of the day a sum of money that is in part payment for their own services (in fact, they hire themselves) and in part pure profit, the reward for taking the risk of going into business. If dentists are categorized as businesspeople working in a market-based health care environment, ultimately their success is to be measured by the return on the investment. Therefore, compelling practitioners to provide care to individuals who cannot afford to pay or to serve patients who receive their dental benefits through underfunded Medicaid programs may be a daunting task. Unfortunately, business decisions that dentists make on a daily basis affect patients' access to care, primarily impacting the most vulnerable including the poor, uninsured persons, racial and ethnic minorities, and Medicaid recipients.[33]

Historically, provider participation in Medicaid dental programs is low in most states. The American Dental Association (ADA) estimated that in 2016 only 39% of dentists were enrolled in state Medicaid or CHIP.[40] However, that figure is likely an overestimate of current enrollment, and probably a tremendous overestimate of the number of dentists who actually participate in the programs. For example, the ADA reported that 30% of dentists in Florida participate in those public programs. However, Florida Department of Health's 2013–2014 workforce survey of dentists revealed that out of 11, practitioners only 1,544 (17.9%) were enrolled as Medicaid providers and only 10% oi dentists had seen more than 125 Medicaid-enrolled patients.[41] In the Florida Department of Health's 2015–2016 dental workforce survey, just 12.7% of the state's dentists expressed a willingness to accept Medicaid-enrolled children aged 0 to 20 years as new patients, compared with 68.2% willing to accept children in that age group overall.[42] Although financial and nonfinancial factors have been documented as the reasons for not participating, most studies report that low reimbursement is the main barrier.[31–33,43,44] States have implemented multiple strategies to increase participation in the Medicaid program but the common denominator is increasing reimbursement rates.[31,45–47]

Most dentists are small-business owners and, if they are to meet their financial obligations and keep their practices afloat, they must act like businesspeople. However, when higher value is attached to profit than to population benefit, professional credibility is eroded. In its principle of beneficence, the ADA's Code of Ethics and Professional Conduct states that the profession has the duty to promote the patient's welfare.[48] Nash's review and critique of these principles suggests that the community service code of conduct that falls under this principle should state that dental services are to be distributed not just based on merit or the ability to pay but also according to need.[49]

Social Responsibility and Altruism

The dental profession provides a considerable amount of uncompensated care.[50] However, there is a public perception that dentists are greedy and disconnected from their community and society at large.[51,52] Throughout its existence, organized dentistry has opposed many initiatives to increase access to dental services for the underserved. For example, the ADA opposed inclusion of dental benefits in Medicare in the 1960s, was unwilling to promote a dental mandate for children in CHIP in the 1990s, advocated "free-standing" dental insurance separate from medical insurance in the Affordable Care Act in the 2000s, and is currently opposed to the profession of dental therapy. Interestingly, in 2007, the ADA found in its annual survey that fewer than one half of nonparticipating providers would accept patients with Medicaid even if fees were raised to cover overhead costs.[53] More recently, more than two thirds of dentists responding to a survey in Florida reported they would not consider participating in Medicaid.[33] The same survey found that dentists would avoid participation in the Medicaid program owing to their perception of social stigma from other dentists.[54]

Despite its relevance, few publications have analyzed dentists' attitudes toward altruism and social responsibility.[55,56] One of those studies suggested that dentists experience conflict between their roles as business operators and their social responsibility as health care professionals.[56] However, it is possible that dental professionals' generally poor response to prevailing disparities may be partially the result of personal traits (e.g., lack of empathy or

determinants of health). In fact, the dental literature has documented
:tices and negative beliefs toward Medicaid-insured patients.[55,57-59]

The Role o⌐ ⌐Ɪe Academic Community

As the debate about oral health disparities in the nation progresses, advocates call for academicians to instill their graduates with strong values of social responsibility.[60] Academic institutions may find their goal to reshape values daunting if not impossible given the values and perceptions of individuals enrolling in dental schools, the lack of a unified voice among academicians, and the limited effectiveness of current approaches to shape socially sensitve practitioners.

Studies assessing the motivations for pursuing a dental career have consistently documented financial reward and income potential.[61-64] These incentives may be reinforced by some academicians whose opinions about access to care vary and are skeptical about the benefits of clinical experiences with underserved populations.[65-68] Multiple methodologies to yield a culturally sensitive professional compelled to care for the underserved have been used by academic institutions including social-learning experiences, community-based dental education, and ethics and professionalism courses. Although these efforts date back to the 1990s, the outcomes are somewhat disappointing; many graduating dental students do not consider access to care a problem and studies have found a decrease in idealistic attitudes toward caring for the underserved among dental students as they progress through dental school.[69-71]

As academicians, we are failing society in our role of addressing the disconnectedness between future dental professionals and underserved populations. Current efforts combining ethical and public health issues may lead future practititioners to reflect on their own interactions, beliefs, and preconceptions, which is an important component of a transformative learning process.[72] However, these self-assessments do not necessarily yield changes in beliefs, behaviors, and practices.[73] It may be time for admissions committees to use a more holistic approach during the selection process. Rather than placing the greatest weight on standardized tests and scores, admissions committees should assess personal traits that reflect the candidate's commitment to have a positive impact on communities through service, educational initiatives, cultural activities, and scholarly endeavors. These individuals will foster a culture of commitment to care for the underserved. The current criteria for selection seems to be self-defeating.

Ethnic Composition of the Workforce

A diverse workforce is important because it increases health care access, equity, and quality for minorities.[74] However, the dental workforce of the United States does not reflect equity in all racial and ethnic groups. As of 2016, Whites composed 62% of the US

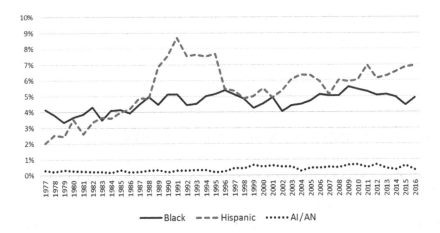

Source: Based on data from American Dental Education Association.[77]
Note: AI/AN = American Indian/Alaska Native.

Figure 4-2. Underrepresented Minority Graduates From Dental School, 1977–2016

population, yet they represented 74% of the dental professional workforce. Whereas Asian Americans were overrepresented, Hispanics, African Americans, and other groups were underrepresented. When combined, these groups represented 33% of the US population, yet these minorities composed only 11% of the dental workforce.[75] These disproportions are expected to become larger given current demographic trends. The US Census Bureau projects that between 2016 and 2060 the growth of underrepresented minorities (URMs; Hispanics, African Americans, and American Indians/Alaska Natives) will be 93%, 41%, and 37%, respectively, while there will be a decrease of 10% of Whites.[76]

Despite the demographic changes in the United States, 64% of dental school graduates in 2016 were White. Although URMs, particularly Hispanics and African Americans, experienced a large demographic growth during the last decade, they represented on average only 6% and 5%, respectively, of the classes graduating between 2006 and 2016. In 2016, URMs totaled 726 or 12% of the total number of graduates[77] (Figure 4-2). The low number of graduates is simply a reflection of the small size of the minority applicant pool to dental schools. Out of 12,508 dental school applicants during the 2015–2016 admission cycle, Hispanics, African Americans, and American Indians/Alaska Natives represented 9%, 6%, and 0.2% of total applicants, respectively, and 9%, 5%, and 0.1% of actual enrollees.[78] Increasing diversity in the health professions remains a challenge because of inequities in preprofessional education, an admission criterion heavily focused on standardized test scores, lack of role models in the profession, and inappropriate support and counseling from health sciences advisors.

It is important to stress that increasing the number of URMs alone will not solve access-to-care issues and address disparities for underserved populations. Racial affinity and altruism are cited as reasons that drive URM dentists to serve a particular patient population.[79-82] Although altruistic goals can help in the matching of caring health care professionals to underserved communities, this alone will not counter strong realities such as structural deficiencies, large rates of morbidity among the poor, and large uninsured and underinsured populations.

DISCUSSION AND POLICY RECOMMENDATIONS

Clearly there is no single or simple remedy for the nation's persistent and pervasive oral health disparities. However, improvements will only occur through concerted efforts and investments on the part of government and the dental profession. In theory, democratically elected government and self-regulated professional monopolies exist for only one reason: to promote the well-being of the public they serve. Historically, federal and state legislators have not established meaningful policy solutions. On the other hand, the dental profession has passed its responsibility away and onto the government by requiring unrealistic public expenditures. It is unlikely that we will see major infusions of funds to correct market deficiencies or provide comprehensive benefits for adults or senior citizens. However, if budgetary adjustments were possible, government and the profession should work together to allocate those resources to maximize their effectiveness while recognizing that compromise is essential.

Following are policy recommendations to help eliminate our nation's persistent and pervasive oral health access disparities. From a federal and state government perspective, additional resources should be allocated to enhancing or incorporating dental benefits in government-subsidized health insurance plans, increasing the availability of loan repayment programs, incorporating dental schools as part of the safety net, and strengthening community health center dental programs. Medicare and Medicaid programs should provide coverage for basic diagnostic, preventive, and restorative dental services for adults and senior citizens. Failure to do so will lead to continued squandering of public resources on inappropriate and avoidable use of hospital emergency departments. Older Americans suffer disproportionely from oral diseases and the problem is particularly serious for those living in long-term-care facilities.

Incentives such as educational loan repayment programs make it more feasible and attractive for health care providers to practice and remain in underserved areas.[83-85] Alternatively, graduates of publicly supported dental schools could be required to repay some of that taxpayer investment by practicing in DHPSAs or meaningfully participating in state Medicaid programs.

Although dental schools play a vital role in providing access for the Medicaid and the uninsured and underinsured patient populations, they are not entitled to public subsidies like federally qualified health centers are for treating disadvantaged individuals. The cost of treating patients has a tremendous impact on the cost of dental education, and schools find it difficult to sustain their missions of education and research when resources are funneled to subsidize the care of patients. Public funding for these services would significantly reduce the need for tuition and fee increases. A few states including New York, Missouri, and North Carolina provide their dental schools with additional Medicaid resources. Relief from educational debt would allow dental graduates to participate in the dental Medicaid program or practice in underserved areas.

Federally qualified health centers and community health center dental clinics are important components of the dental safety net. Because they serve the most vulnerable patients and communities, appropriate staffing is crucial. Unfortunately, those health centers struggle with issues of recruitment and retention. In a 2010 survey, 39% of executive directors reported having at least one dentist vacancy and, of those vacancies, 52% were of greater than six months duration.[86] In 2017, these facilities provided oral examinations and preventive services to 5.2 million individuals, restorative treatment to 1.8 million individuals, and emergency and surgical care to approximately 1.2 million individuals.[87] However, even collectively, the dental safety net is unable to meet the oral health needs of the millions of Americans who are underserved.[88,89] Therefore, any meaningful increase in access will require the participation of private practitioners.

The dental profession has the knowledge, expertise, and capacity to address the oral health needs of those Americans who routinely seek care. However, addressing oral health disparities in the United States will require re-engineering the dental care delivery system to maximize output (i.e., services provided). For example, dental hygiene professionals could be much more effective and efficient in preventing and managing disease if allowed to function at the top of their scope of care, without the burden of dentist supervision levels that increase costs without enhancing patient safety or outcomes.

Similarly, emerging midlevel providers such as dental therapists have great potential in allowing private practitioners, community health centers, and isolated areas to deliver services in a more cost-effective manner. The scientific literature and current experiences in Alaska and Minnesota—early US adopters of that model—suggest dental therapists can provide technically competent care and enhance access in a state with very low Medicaid reimbursement rates.[90,91] The ADA has advocated the introduction of the community dental health coordinator, a community health worker who provides health promotion, outreach, and prevention services. The rationale behind that midlevel provider is to make the dental safety net more efficient. However, as noted earlier, the dental safety net does not have the capacity to address the needs of the millions of Americans who are underserved. In addition, the limited clinical scope of this individual does not allow her or him to serve as a substitute for a dentist in the provision of certain services. Economic efficiency dictates that, while controlling for the quality of output, services should be provided by the least costly provider. If both legislators and the dental profession were willing to re-engineer the delivery system and focus on health outcomes rather than simply regulating the supply of services, we could have a more equitable system.

CONCLUSIONS

In our introduction, we opened with a controversial statement related to inequities in access to dental care. Sadly, 40 years later, this statement still holds true. We acknowledge that some of the issues and suggestions presented here are contentious. Rather than pointing fingers, our objective has been to challenge the status quo and illustrate major synergistic and persistent factors that, unless addressed, will impede progress in the elimination of disparities in access to care. Both legislators and organized dentistry must agree that access to oral health is a matter of social justice and a priority for this country. Once government and the dental profession share that common goal, both sectors must be willing to share the responsibility, relinquish some control, and make the choices that are inevitable to eliminate oral health disparities.

REFERENCES

1. Lobene R. *The Forsyth Experiment: An Alternative System for Dental Care.* Cambridge, MA: Harvard University Press; 1979.

2. Lee JY, Divaris K. The ethical imperative of addressing oral health disparities: a unifying framework. *J Dent Res.* 2014;93(3):224–230.

3. Vargas CM, Arevalo O. How dental care can preserve and improve oral health. *Dent Clin North Am.* 2009;53(3):399–420.

4. Dye BA, Li X, Thorton-Evans G. Oral health disparities as determined by selected Healthy People 2020 oral health objectives for the United States, 2009–2010. NCHS Data Brief. 2012;104:1–8.

5. Thomson WM. Social inequality in oral health. *Community Dent Oral Epidemiol.* 2012;40(suppl 2):28–32.

6. Chattopadhyay A. Oral health disparities in the United States. *Dent Clin North Am.* 2008;52(2):297–318.

7. Centers for Medicare and Medicaid Services. National Health Expenditure Data. Available at: https://www.cms.gov/Research-Statistics-Data-and-Systems/Statistics-Trends-and-Reports/NationalHealthExpendData/NationalHealthAccountsHistorical.html. Accessed July 12, 2018.

8. Centers for Medicare and Medicaid Services. Children enrolled in Medicaid and CHIP. Available at: https://www.medicaid.gov/chip/reports-and-evaluations/index.html. Accessed June 16, 2018.

9. Nasseh K, Vujicic M. Dental care utilization rate continues to increase among children, holds steady among working-age adults and the elderly. Health Policy Institute Research Brief. American Dental Association. October 2015. Available at: http://www.ada.org/~/media/ADA/Science%20and%20Research/HPI/Files/HPIBrief_1015_1.ashx. Accessed June 19, 2018.

10. Medicaid and CHIP Payment and Access Commission. Medicaid access in brief: children's dental services. June 2016. Available at: https://www.macpac.gov/wp-content/uploads/2016/06/Childrens-access-to-dental-services.pdf. Accessed June 16, 2018.

11. Kenney GM, McFeeters JR, Yee JY. Preventive dental care and unmet dental needs among low-income children. *Am J Public Health.* 2005;95(8):1360–1366.

12. Yarbrough C, Vujicic M, Nasseh K. More than 8 million adults could gain dental benefits through Medicaid expansion. Health Policy Institute Research Brief. American Dental Association. February 2014. Available at: https://www.ada.org/~/media/ADA/Science%20and%20Research/HPI/Files/HPIBrief_0214_1.pdf?la=en. Accessed May 19, 2018.

13. Colby SL, Ortman JM. The baby boom cohort in the United States: 2012 to 2060. Current Population Reports, P25-1141. US Census Bureau. 2014. Available at: https://www.census.gov/prod/2014pubs/p25-1141.pdf. Accessed May 7, 2018.

14. Social Security Administration. Social Security Amendments of 1965 Volume 1. Available at: https://www.ssa.gov/history/pdf/Downey%20PDFs/Social%20Security%20Amendments%20of%201965%20Vol%204.pdf. Accessed August 13, 2018.

15. Manski RJ, Moeller J, Schimmel J, et al. Dental care coverage and retirement. *J Public Health Dent.* 2010;70(1):1–12.

16. Kaiser Family Foundation. Income and assets of Medicare beneficiaries, 2016–2035. Available at: https://www.kff.org/medicare/issue-brief/income-and-assets-of-medicare-beneficiaries-2016-2035. Accessed May 7, 2018.

17. Kaiser Commission on Medicaid and the Uninsured. A profile of Medicaid managed care programs in 2010: findings from a 50-state survey. 2011. Available at: https://kaiserfamily-foundation.files.wordpress.com/2013/01/8220.pdf. Accessed May 12, 2018.

18. Perkins J. National Health Law Program: docket of Medicaid cases to improve dental access. Available at: http://www.healthlaw.org/issues/child-and-adolescent-health/epsdt/docket-of-medicaid-cases-to-improve-dental-access-august-2007#.WpCSrFrwZhE. Accessed April 23, 2018.

19. National Conference of State Legislatures. Health cost containment and efficiencies: NCSL briefs for state legislators. 2014. Available at: http://www.ncsl.org/documents/health/IntroandBriefsCC-16.pdf. Accessed May 27, 2018.

20. American Dental Association. Dental care utilization declined among low-income adults, increased among low-income children in most states from 2000 to 2010. Available at: http://www.ada.org/~/media/ADA/Science%20and%20Research/HPI/Files/HPIBrief_0213_3.ashx. Accessed February 20, 2018.

21. Wall T, Nasseh K. Dental-related emergency department visits on the increase in the United States. Chicago, IL: American Dental Association, Health Policy Institute; 2013.

22. Okunseri C, Okunseri E, Thorpe JM, Xiang Q, Szabo A. Patient characteristics and trends in nontraumatic dental condition visits to emergency departments in the United States. *Clin Cosmet Investig Dent.* 2012;4:1–7.

23. Davis EE, Deinard AS, Maiga EW. Doctor, my tooth hurts: the costs of incomplete dental care in the emergency room. *J Public Health Dent.* 2010;70(3):205–210.

24. Wall T, Vujicic M. Emergency department use for dental conditions continues to increase. Health Policy Institute Research Brief. American Dental Association. April 2015. Available at: http://www.ada.org/~/media/ADA/Science%20and%20Research/HPI/Files/HPIBrief_0415_2. ashx. Accessed June 12, 2018.

25. Byck GR, Kaste LM, Cooksey JA, Chou CF. Dental student enrollment and graduation: a report by state, census division, and region. *J Dent Educ.* 2006;70(10):1023–1037.

26. Bailit HL, Beazoglou TJ. State financing of dental education: impact on supply of dentists. *J Dent Educ.* 2003;67(12):1278–1285.

27 Bailit HL, Beazoglou T. Trends in financing dental education, 2004–05 to 2011–12. *J Dent Educ.* 2017;81(8):eS1–eS12.

28. American Dental Education Association. Educational debt. Available at: http://www.adea. org/GoDental/Money_Matters/Educational_Debt.aspx#sthash.gModF2Nm.dpbs. Accessed July 5, 2018.

29. Osborne PB, Haubenreich JE. Underserved region recruitment and return to practice: a thirty-year analysis. *J Dent Educ.* 2003;67(5):505–508.

30. Saman DM, Arevalo O, Johnson AO. The dental workforce in Kentucky: current status and future needs. *J Public Health Dent.* 2010;70(3):188–196.

31. Al Agili DE, Pass MA, Bronstein JM, Lockwood SA. Medicaid participation by private dentists in Alabama. *Pediatr Dent.* 2007;29(4):293–302.

32. Shulman JD, Ezemobi EO, Sutherland JN, Barsley R. Louisiana dentists' attitudes toward the dental Medicaid program. *Pediatr Dent.* 2001;23(5):395–400.

33. Logan HL, Guo Y, Dodd VJ, Seleski CE, Catalanotto F. Demographic and practice characteristics of Medicaid-participating dentists. *J Public Health Dent.* 2014;74(2):139–146.

34. Bureau of Health Workforce. Designated health professional shortage areas. Available at: https://datawarehouse.hrsa.gov/tools/hdwreports/Reports.aspx. Accessed July 13, 2018.

35. Henry Kaiser Family Foundation. Dental care health professional shortage areas (HPSAs). Available at: https://www.kff.org/other/state-indicator/dental-care-health-professional-shortage-areas-hpsas/?currentTimeframe=0&sortModel=%7B%22colId%22:%22Loca-tion%22,%22sort%22:%22asc%22%7D. Accessed June 12, 2018.

36. Guay A, Wall T. Considering large group practices as a vehicle for consolidation in dentistry. Health Policy Institute Research Brief. American Dental Association. April 2016. Available at: http://www.ada.org/~/media/ADA/Science%20and%20Research/HPI/Files/HPIBrief_0416_1. pdf. Accessed July 7, 2018.

37. Shepard L. Licensing restrictions and the cost of dental care. *J Law Econ.* 1978;2(1):187–201.

38. Kleiner MM. Licensing occupations: ensuring quality or restricting competition? Kalamazoo, MI: W. E. Upjohn Institute; 2006.

39. Friedland B, Valachovic RW. The regulation of dental licensing: the Dark Ages. *Am J Law Med*. 1991;17(3):249–270.

40. American Dental Association. Dentist participation in Medicaid or CHIP. Available at: https://www.ada.org/~/media/ADA/Science%20and%20Research/HPI/Files/HPIGraphic_0318_1.pdf?la=en. Accessed August 5, 2018.

41. Florida Department of Health. Report on the 2011–2012 Florida Workforce Survey of Dentists. April 2014. Available at: http://www.floridahealth.gov/programs-and-services/community-health/dental-health/reports/florida-workforce-survey-of-dentists-2011-2012.pdf. Accessed July 15, 2018.

42. Florida Department of Health. 2015–2016 workforce survey of dentists. January 2017. Available at: http://www.floridahealth.gov/programs-and-services/community-health/dental-health/reports/_documents/florida-workforce-survey-dentists-2015-2016.pdf. Accessed July 15, 2018.

43. Nebeker CD, Briskie DM, Maturo RA, Piskorowski WA, Sohn W, Boynton JR. Michigan dentists' attitudes toward Medicaid and an alternative public dental insurance system for children. *Pediatr Dent*. 2014;36(1):34–38.

44. Borchgrevink A, Snyder A, Gehshan S. The effects of Medicaid reimbursement rates on access to dental care. National Academy for State Health Policy. 2008. Available at: https://nashp.org/wp-content/uploads/sites/default/files/CHCF_dental_rates.pdf. Accessed July 11, 2018.

45. Beazoglou T, Douglass J, Myne-Joslin V, Baker P, Bailit H. Impact of fee increases on dental utilization rates for children living in Connecticut and enrolled in Medicaid. *J Am Dent Assoc*. 2015;146(1):52–60.

46. Nasseh K, Vujicic M, Yarbrough C. A ten-year, state-by-state, analysis of Medicaid fee-for-service reimbursement rates for dental care services. Health Policy Institute. American Dental Association. October 2014. Available at: https://www.ada.org/~/media/ADA/Science%20and%20Research/HPI/Files/HPIBrief_1014_3.pdf?la=en. Accessed July 11, 2018.

47. Nietert PJ, Bradford WD, Kaste LM. The impact of an innovative reform to the South Carolina dental Medicaid system. *Health Serv Res*. 2005;40(4):1078–1091.

48. American Dental Association. Principles of Ethics and Code of Professional Conduct. 2018. Available at: https://www.ada.org/~/media/ADA/Publications/Files/ADA_Code_of_Ethics_2018.pdf?la=en. Accessed May 15, 2018.

49. Nash DA. Ethics in dentistry: review and critique of Principles of Ethics and Code of Professional Conduct. *J Am Dent Assoc*. 1984;109(4):597–603.

50. Chattopadhyay A, Slade GD, Caplan DJ. Professional charges not reimbursed to dentists in the US: evidence from Medical Expenditure Panel Survey, 1996. *Community Dent Health*. 2009;26(4):227–233.

51. Christensen GJ. The credibility of dentists. *J Am Dent Assoc.* 2001;132(8):1163–1165.

52. Rule JT, Welie JV. The dilemma of access to care: symptom of a systemic condition. *Dent Clin North Am.* 2009;53(3):421–433.

53. American Dental Association. 2007 Survey of Current Issues in Dentistry: selected results. Chicago, IL: American Dental Association; 2008.

54. Logan HL, Catalanotto F, Guo Y, Marks J, Dharamsi S. Barriers to Medicaid participation among Florida dentists. *J Health Care Poor Underserved.* 2015;26(1):154–167.

55. McKernan SC, Reynolds JC, Momany ET, et al. The relationship between altruistic attitudes and dentists' Medicaid participation. *J Am Dent Assoc.* 2015;146(1):34–41.

56. Dharamsi S, Pratt DD, MacEntee MI. How dentists account for social responsibility: economic imperatives and professional obligations. *J Dent Educ.* 2007;71(12):1583–1592.

57. Lam M, Riedy CA, Milgrom P. Improving access for Medicaid-insured children: focus on front office personnel. *J Am Dent Assoc.* 1999;130(3):365–373.

58. Mofidi M, Rozier RG, King RS. Problems with access to dental care for Medicaid-insured children: what caregivers think. *Am J Public Health.* 2002;92(1):53–58.

59. Kelly SE, Binkley CJ, Neace WP, Gale BS. Barriers to care-seeking for children's oral health among low-income caregivers. *Am J Public Health.* 2005;95(8):1345–1351.

60. Davis EL, Stewart DC, Guelmann M, et al. Serving the public good: challenges of dental education in the twenty-first century. *J Dent Educ.* 2007;71(8):1009–1019.

61. Scarbecz M, Ross JA. Gender differences in first-year dental students' motivation to attend dental school. *J Dent Educ.* 2002;66(8):952–961.

62. Scarbecz M, Ross JA. The relationship between gender and postgraduate aspirations among first- and fourth-year students at public dental schools: a longitudinal analysis. *J Dent Educ.* 2007;71(6):797–809.

63. Crossley ML, Mubarik A. A comparative investigation of dental and medical student's motivation towards career choice. *Br Dent J.* 2002;193(8):471–473.

64. Hawley NJ, Ditmyer MM, Sandoval VA. Predental students' attitudes toward and perceptions of the dental profession. *J Dent Educ.* 2008;72(12):1458–1464.

65. Eaton KA, de Vries J, Widström E, et al. "Schools without walls?" Developments and challenges in dental outreach teaching: report of a recent symposium. *Eur J Dent Educ.* 2006;10(4):186–191.

66. Gray MJ, Ondaatje EH, Fricker R, et al. Combining service and learning in higher education. Santa Monica, CA: RAND Education; 1999.

67. Hood JG. Service-learning in dental education: meeting needs and challenges. *J Dent Educ.* 2009;73(4):454–463.

68. Graham BS. Educating dental students about oral health care access disparities. *J Dent Educ.* 2006;70(11):1208–1211.

69. Chmar JE, Weaver RG, Valachovic RW. Annual ADEA survey of dental school seniors: 2005 graduating class. *J Dent Educ.* 2006;70(3):315–339.

70. Holtzman JS, Seirawan H. Impact of community-based oral health experiences on dental students' attitudes towards caring for the underserved. *J Dent Educ.* 2009;73(3):303–310.

71. Sherman JJ, Cramer A. Measurement of changes in empathy during dental school. *J Dent Educ.* 2005;69(3):338–345.

72. Stone JR. Healthcare inequality, cross-cultural training, and bioethics: principles and applications. *Camb Q Healthc Ethics.* 2008;17(2):216–226.

73. Cranton P. *Understanding and Promoting Transformative Learning: A Guide for Educators of Adults.* San Francisco, CA: Jossey-Bass Publishers; 1994.

74. Bristow LR, Butler AS, Smedley BD, eds. *In the Nation's Compelling Interest: Ensuring Diversity in the Health-Care Workforce.* Washington, DC: National Academies Press; 2004.

75. Health Policy Institute, American Dental Association. Racial and ethnic diversity among dentists in the US. 2016. Available at: https://www.ada.org/~/media/ADA/Science%20 and%20Research/HPI/Files/HPIgraphic_1117_6.pdf?la=en. Accessed August 4, 2018.

76. Vespa J, Armstrong DM, Medina L. Demographic turning points for the United States: population projections for 2020 to 2060. Current Population Reports, P25-1144. US Census Bureau. 2018. Available at: https://www.census.gov/content/dam/Census/library/publications/2018/ demo/P25_1144.pdf. Accessed August 4, 2018.

77. American Dental Education Association. Minority graduates of US dental schools, 1977–2016. Available at: http://www.adea.org/data/students. Accessed August 4, 2018.

78. Wanchek T, Cook BJ, Valachovic RW. US dental school applicants and enrollees, 2016 entering class. *J Dent Educ.* 2017;81(11):1373–1382.

79. Sullivan LW. Missing persons: minorities in the health professions, a report of the Sullivan Commission on Diversity in the Healthcare Workforce. 2004. Available at http://health-equity.lib.umd.edu/40/1/Sullivan_Final_Report_000.pdf. Accessed June 15, 2018.

80. Solomon ES, Williams CR, Sinkford JC. Practice location characteristics of Black dentists in Texas. *J Dent Educ.* 2001;65:571–574.

81. Brown LJ, Wagner KS, Johns B. Racial/ethnic variations of practicing dentists. *J Am Dent Assoc.* 2000;131(12):1750–1754.

82. Okunseri C, Bajorunaite R, Abena A, Self K, Iacopino AM, Flores G. Racial/ethnic disparities in the acceptance of Medicaid patients in dental practices. *J Public Health Dent.* 2008; 68(3):149–153.

83. Goodfellow A, Ulloa JG, Dowling PT, et al. Predictors of primary care physician practice location in underserved urban or rural areas in the United States: a systematic literature review. *Acad Med.* 2016;91(9):1313–1321.

84. Opoku ST, Apenteng BA, Lin G, Chen LW, Palm D, Rauner T. A comparison of the J-1 visa waiver and loan repayment programs in the recruitment and retention of physicians in rural Nebraska. *J Rural Health.* 2015;31(3):300–309.

85. Daniels ZM, Vanleit BJ, Skipper BJ, Sanders ML, Rhyne RL. Factors in recruiting and retaining health professionals for rural practice. *J Rural Health.* 2007;23(1):62–71.

86. National Network for Oral Health Access. Survey of health center oral health providers. Available at: http://www.nnoha.org/nnoha-content/uploads/2013/07/Survey-of-Health-Center-Oral-Health-Providers.pdf. Accessed August 7, 2018.

87. US Department of Health and Human Services, Health Resources and Services Administration. Selected diagnoses and services rendered, national summary for 2017. Available at: https://bphc.hrsa.gov/uds/datacenter.aspx?q=t6a&year=2017&state=. Accessed August 13, 2018.

88. Bailit HL, Beazoglou T, Demby N, McFarland J, Robinson P, Weaver R. Dental safety net: current capacity and potential for expansion. *J Am Dent Assoc.* 2006;137(6):807–815.

89. Institute of Medicine, National Research Council. *Improving Access to Oral Health Care for Vulnerable and Underserved Populations.* Washington, DC: The National Academies; 2011.

90. Bader JD, Lee JY, Shugars DA, Burrus BB, Wetterhall S. Clinical technical performance of dental therapists in Alaska. *J Am Dent Assoc.* 2011;142(3):322–326.

91. Minnesotta Department of Health. Dental therapy in Minnesota—issue brief. 2018. Available at: http://www.health.state.mn.us/divs/orhpc/workforce/oral/2018dtbrief.pdf. Accessed August 5, 2018.

5

Promoting an Understanding of Dental Health Disparities in a Midwestern Latino Population Through a Community-Based Research Collaboration

Daniel J. Kruger, PhD, Adreanne Waller, MPH, Charo Ledón, and Mikel Llanes, MD

Dental health is significantly associated with an individual's overall quality of life, including her/his ability to speak, eat, and work as well as significant health issues, including diabetes,[1,2] hypertension,[2] coronary artery disease,[2] atherosclerosis,[2] preterm delivery,[3] depression,[4] and anxiety.[4] Long-term oral health is affected greatly by utilization of dental care.[5] Minority children in general suffer higher rates of long-term dental care deficits as a result of a lack of access.[6]

Latinos in the United States face barriers to utilization of dental services with disparities related to income, education, gender, and lack of health insurance.[7] Education and having dental insurance were the most important factors in determining use of dental care among Mexican Americans, Cuban Americans, and Puerto Ricans in the early 1980s, whereas acculturation was a lesser factor.[8] Those with lower acculturation had a greater number of decayed and missing teeth; however, this effect was accounted for by age, gender, education, and income status.[9] Most migrant farmworkers in a southern Illinois community reported access-to-care barriers and episodic or lack of dental services and about half reported signs of periodontal disease.[10] Dental decay is more prevalent in Mexican Americans and non-Hispanic Blacks than in other races or ethnicities in the United States.[11,12] Children of parents/guardians who are Hispanic with less than a high-school education were found to have the highest rates of several early childhood caries, placing them at a greater risk of tooth loss later in life.[13] Specialized practices for Hispanics and Spanish-language information have been cited as potentially beneficial tools in reducing the amount of time between dental visits.[14]

This chapter documents how a community-based participatory health survey can promote a better understanding of the origins of local disparities in dental health. Planning, implementing, and evaluating policies and interventions as well as promoting community health require high-quality and highly relevant local data. However, there are few sources of health data at the community level, leaving many communities to rely on state and regional estimates to facilitate local efforts. We examined predictors of permanent tooth loss among residents of a Midwestern US Latino community. Data were collected via a community-based participatory research (CBPR) process to generate the first, to our knowledge, systematic health assessment of Latinos in the local population. Dental health was identified by community members as a priority concern.

COMMUNITY-BASED PARTICIPATORY RESEARCH

CBPR is an approach to local data collection that can promote the understanding of community health issues and increase the relevance, usefulness, and applicability of the data for intervention research and improve the research and program development capacity of all partners.[15,16] CBPR involves a partnership in which community representatives are actively engaged in research with representatives from academic institutions. Ideally, CBPR involves all partners equitably in the research process and recognizes the unique strengths that each brings.[17] Participation by local stakeholders makes the research and results more relevant to the community and provides academics with insights known by local stakeholders that may not be apparent to external individuals.

CBPR often begins with a needs assessment process to characterize a community's health from multiple perspectives and to identify and address community health concerns. Frequently, there is a focus on a research topic identified as important to the community. The research process typically includes the goal of providing knowledge that will facilitate social and policy change to improve health outcomes and eliminate health disparities.[17]

Washtenaw County, Michigan, has a small but rapidly growing Latino community, comprising about 5% of the local population. However, Latinos were underrepresented in existing county-level health assessments. The Washtenaw County Public Health Department's Health Improvement Plan survey was conducted solely in English through telephone landline and cell phone interviews. Unlike in other Midwestern areas such as Detroit, Michigan, and Chicago, Illinois, there are no specific neighborhoods in Washtenaw County that are associated with a high concentration of Latino residents. Although the Latino proportion of residents does vary across neighborhoods, Latinos are geographically distributed across the entire county; have ancestries ranging across North, Central, and South America; and range socioeconomically from unskilled laborers to tenured university professors.

Collaborators at the Washtenaw County Public Health Department, the University of Michigan, and Casa Latina, a community-based organization engaged with the local Latino community, designed and implemented *Encuesta Buenos Vecinos* (the Good Neighbors Survey) through a CBPR process to better understand the health of the Washtenaw County Latino population. Consistent with the CBPR principle of collaboration on all major phases of the research process,[17] the entire project was guided by the Community Leadership Team, which identified dental health as a priority issue. The survey incorporated several items on dental health access, utilization, barriers, and outcomes. These data were utilized to identify factors predicting permanent tooth loss, an important indicator of health status.

METHODS

Community partners were involved in all phases of *Encuesta Buenos Vecinos*, including the creation and review of the survey instrument. The director of *Casa Latina* (now director of *Encuesta Buenos Vecinos*) was a coinvestigator and representative on the three-member Project Leadership Team, along with the health department and academic coinvestigators. The project was also guided by the Community Leadership Team, a diverse group of members of the local Latino community, including a physician, a business owner, a community college student, a mother and homemaker, and health department staff, as well as representatives of organizations serving the local Latino community. Several members of the Community Leadership Team served as survey interviewers. A broader group of consultants provided feedback at critical stages of the project, such as identifying priority topics, reviewing the complete survey instrument draft, and informing data collection procedures.

The survey was conducted in Spanish or English, online or face to face, by trained members of the local Latino community in door-to-door or community-based group sessions. Inclusion criteria included being aged 18 years or older, identifying as Hispanic or Latino/a, and living in Washtenaw County. A total of 487 Latinos participated in the survey from September 2013 to January 2014.

Investigators began by considering the demographic composition of census tracts in Washtenaw County with the greatest proportion of Latino residents. During data collection, investigators steered data collection toward underrepresented groups and geographic areas. The research team monitored survey respondents on an ongoing basis to ensure that the sample closely reflected age, gender, and educational composition of the focus population. The resulting sample is considered by Washtenaw County Public Health to provide the best and most representative depiction of Latinos in Washtenaw County.

The survey was designed to provide a robust baseline measure of health status and social determinants of health among Latinos while increasing the capacity of *Encuesta Buenos Vecinos* partners to engage in health-promoting research and intervention. The survey included a broad range of topics, including health-related knowledge, attitudes, beliefs, health behaviors, access to health care, sources of health information, family planning, child health, social support and conflict, social and neighborhood conditions, immigration issues, and economic opportunities. The survey contained questions (slightly adapted or reprinted) from the US Centers for Disease Control and Prevention Behavioral Risk Factor Surveillance System (BRFSS)[18] and other sources.[19,20]

Dental health questions on the survey were the following[18]:

- How many of your permanent teeth have been removed because of tooth decay or gum disease? (Not including wisdom teeth or teeth lost in an injury. Include teeth lost to infection.)
- How long has it been since you visited a dentist or a dental clinic for any reason?
- In the past 12 months, did you need to see a dentist but could not because of the cost?

BRFSS general health items were the following[18]:

- Is your health. . .
  - Excellent
  - Very good
  - Fair
  - Poor
- During the past 30 days, how many days did you feel . . . your physical health was not good? (physical health includes physical illness and injury); your mental health was not good? (mental health includes stress, depression, and problems with emotions); poor physical or mental health kept you from doing your usual activities, such as self-care, work, or recreation?

Health coverage and access items were the following[18]:

- Do you have any kind of health care coverage, including health insurance, prepaid plans such as HMOs, or government plans such as Medicare or Washtenaw Health Plan?
- Have you ever been refused health care?

The survey contained four items from The Everyday Discrimination Scale[19]:

- "In your day-to-day life how often have any of the following things happened to you? . . . You are treated with less respect than other people; People act as if you are not as good as they are; You are called names or insulted; You are threatened or harassed."

English fluency was assessed by three items[20]:

- "How well do you speak English?"
- "How well do you read English?"
- "How well do you write in English? (Not at All, Poorly, Fairly Well, Very Well, Excellently)"

Demographics included age in years, gender, highest level of education attained, and years lived in the United States.

We compared rates of permanent tooth loss among *Encuesta Buenos Vecinos* participants with those of 1692 non-Hispanic Whites included in the 2010 Washtenaw County Health Improvement Plan survey. A forward stepwise linear regression predicted the number of permanent teeth removed as a continuous measure on the basis of demographics, dental health items, coverage and access items, everyday discrimination, and English fluency. We also investigated the extent to which permanent tooth loss was an indicator of general health status by examining associations with BRFSS general health items, controlling for demographics.

RESULTS

For a summary of participant demographics and descriptives, see Table 5-1. Nearly half (47%) of respondents (n = 387 with complete data) had at least one permanent tooth removed, a rate higher than permanent tooth loss for non-Hispanic Whites in

Table 5-1. Participant Demographics and Descriptives (n = 387): *Encuesta Buenos Vecinos*, Washtenaw County, Michigan; September 2013 to January 2014

Descriptive	% or Mean (SD)	Range
Gender	. . .	. . .
Women	57	. . .
Men	43	. . .
Age in years	36 (14)	18–88
Years of education	12 (4)	0–20
English fluency	4 (2)	1–6
Years in United States	16 (11)	1–69
Everyday discrimination	3 (4)	0–20
No health care coverage	22	. . .
Cost was a barrier to dental care	39	. . .
Ever been refused health care	6	. . .
Time since dental visit	. . .	. . .
Less than a week	3	. . .
Less than a month	13	. . .
Less than a year	48	. . .
One to 5 years	18	. . .
More than 5 years	8	. . .
Never visited a dentist	10	. . .
Permanent tooth removed	2 (4)	0–32

Washtenaw County (32%; $\chi^2_{(1)}$ = 105.02; P < .001; Table 5-2). At the bivariate level, older age, lower levels of education, greater time since most recent dental visit, cost as a barrier to dental care, being refused health care, and lower levels of English fluency predicted greater permanent tooth loss (Table 5-3). The forward stepwise linear regression identified older age, longer time since respondents' most recent dental visit, and financial cost as a barrier to dental health care as unique predictors of permanent tooth loss (Table 5-4). These predictors explained 18% of the variance in permanent tooth loss. Once these factors were accounted for, participants' gender, English fluency, experiences of everyday discrimination, having health care coverage, and years lived in the United States did not account for additional variance in permanent tooth loss. In bivariate relationships, greater permanent tooth loss predicted worse self-reported health ($r_{(386)}$ = .219; P < .001), and more days in the past 30 when physical health was not good ($r_{(368)}$ = .206; P < .001). When age in years, gender, and education in years were controlled, the number of permanent teeth removed predicted the number of days in the past 30 when physical health was not good ($r_{(352)}$ = .164; P = .002).

DISCUSSION OF THE RESULTS

Latinos in Washtenaw County reported greater permanent tooth loss than non-Hispanic Whites. As expected, the extent of permanent tooth loss was associated with known social determinants of health, such as educational level and English fluency. However, in addition to older age, the unique predictors of greater permanent tooth loss were indicators of access to dental care. The greater the time elapsed since a participant's most recent dental visit and needing dental care but being unable to receive it because of the financial cost, the worse was a participant's dental health. Also, as

Table 5-2. Permanent Tooth Loss Among *Encuesta Buenos Vecinos* Study Participants and Non-Hispanic Whites in Washtenaw County, Michigan; September 2013 to January 2014

	EBV Participants, % (n = 387)	Non-Hispanic Whites, % (n = 1692)
Permanent tooth loss	. . .	. . .
None	53	78
1-5	41	14
≥ 6 but not all	6	6
All	1	1

Source: Data for non-Hispanic Whites in Washtenaw County are based on the 2010 Washtenaw County Health Improvement Plan survey.[21]
Note: EBV = *Encuesta Buenos Vecinos* (Good Neighbors Survey).

Table 5-3. Bivariate Correlations Among Variables (n = 387): *Encuesta Buenos Vecinos*, Washtenaw County, Michigan; September 2013 to January 2014

	2	3	4	5	6	7	8	9	10
1. Tooth loss	.384‡	−.067	−.172‡	.038	.123*	.136†	.143†	−0.025	−.209‡
2. Age	1	−.064	−.130*	.352†	−.104*	.024	.098	−.138†	−.278‡
3. Gender		1	−.011	.033	.103*	.024	−.010	−.048	.076
4. Education			1	.157†	−.173‡	−.110*	−.036	−.005	.616‡
5. Years in United States				1	−.188‡	−.102*	.061	.078	.349‡
6. Time since dental visit					1	.173‡	.066	.039	−.220‡
7. Cost as a barrier						1	.124*	.179†	−.220†
8. Refused health care							1	.040	−.030
9. Perceived discrimination								1	−.054
10. English fluency									1

*P < .05; †P < .01; ‡P < .001.

expected, the extent of permanent tooth loss was associated with general physical health status.

This project makes several contributions to the understanding of health disparities. Most notably, it identifies mechanisms associated with Latino dental health, thus providing insights into the underlying causes of disparities in dental health outcomes documented in the current and previous research and surveillance efforts. Remarkably, the findings suggest that tightly focused efforts to increase Latino/a access to, and utilization of, dental care would be effective in improving Latino health outcomes. Direct indicators of dental care access accounted for the associations between permanent tooth loss and social determinants of health. This provides a reassuring message, as increasing the availability of dental services may be easier to accomplish than altering the structural parameters of populations, such as reducing educational and income inequality or eliminating other social determinants of health such as discrimination. The Washtenaw County Health Department has since opened a dental clinic that is highly utilized by Latino residents.

Ameliorative efforts should be directed toward both child and adult dental care, as early implementation of regular dental care is the most effective method of ensuring long-term oral health care. Enhancements in dental care access would include insurance coverage for consistent dental visits, literature on oral health care in Spanish throughout one's lifespan, and an increase in Hispanic-friendly dental offices as means of ensuring information is effectively disseminated and complemented with culturally appropriate services. Increasing dental care accessibility will decrease oral diseases and well as improve overall health in this vulnerable population.

Table 5-4. Predictors of Number of Permanent Teeth Removed (n = 387): *Encuesta Buenos Vecinos,* Washtenaw County, Michigan; September 2013 to January 2014

	Unstandardized Coefficients		Standardized Coefficients		
	b	SE	B	t	P
(Constant)	−5.19	0.90	...	−5.80	.001
Age in years	0.12	0.01	.397	8.54	.001
Time since dental visit	0.49	0.16	.146	3.11	.002
Cost as a barrier	0.84	0.39	.101	2.15	.032

Most research on US Latino health is conducted in large coastal cities or border regions with large and more socially established Latino populations. These communities often have more extensive infrastructure available and accessible to local Latinos—for example, Spanish-speaking health professionals. The current study was conducted in a community where Latinos are a small yet growing proportion of an increasingly diverse population. Local Latinos are diverse in socioeconomic characteristics, regions of origin, and geographical distribution. Thus, the current sample may be more representative of Latinos in the wide geography of middle America than in areas with highly concentrated and/or historically longstanding Latino populations.

Third, this project demonstrates the effectiveness of CBPR in understanding health issues in populations that are difficult to access with traditional research methods. The extensive involvement of Latino community members facilitated the success of the project by providing guidance in every phase of the project. This input ensured that the project addressed the issues of greatest concern to the study population, that the content and wording of items generated understanding consistent with the intended design, that recruitment efforts generated a sample that was representative of the local population, and that the products of the research process were consistent with community goals. In addition, the results of the project were made available to the community of study through public presentations and forums, as well as summaries in freely available electronic documents.

CONCLUSIONS

Results demonstrate the magnitude of dental health issues in the Washtenaw County Latino population and identify access to dental care as the primary predictor of dental health outcomes. Latinos are the largest and fastest-growing ethnic minority group in the United States. Policymakers and health planners should work to ensure access to dental for US Latinos to address a central aspect of health and well-being.

ACKNOWLEDGMENTS

The *Encuesta Buenos Vecinos* study was supported by grant funds from the US Department of Housing and Urban Development: Sustainable Communities Project, The University of Michigan's Michigan Institute for Clinical & Health Research: Community University Research Partnership (grant 2UL1TR000433-06), Michigan Department of Community Health: Health Equity Capacity Building Project, and Washtenaw County Public Health. The University of Michigan's Institutional Review Board for Health Sciences and Behavioral Sciences reviewed and approved the research before data collection.

REFERENCES

1. Patel MH, Kumar JV, Moss ME. Diabetes and tooth loss: an analysis of data from the National Health and Nutrition Examination Survey, 2003–2004. *J Am Dent Assoc.* 2013;144(5):478–485.

2. Castillo R, Fields A, Qureshi G, Salciccioli L, Kassotis J, Lazar JM. Relationship between aortic atherosclerosis and dental loss in an inner-city population. *Angiology.* 2009;60(3): 346–350.

3. Hwang SS, Smith VC, McCormick MC, Barfield WD. The association between maternal oral health experiences and risk of preterm birth in 10 states, Pregnancy Risk Assessment Monitoring System, 2004–2006. *Matern Child Health J.* 2012;16(8):1688–1695.

4. Okoro CA, Strine TW, Eke PI, Dhingra SS, Balluz LS. The association between depression and anxiety and use of oral health services and tooth loss. *Community Dent Oral Epidemiol.* 2011;40(2):134–144.

5. Huang DL, Park M. Socioeconomic and racial/ethnic oral health disparities among US older adults: oral health quality of life and dentition. *J Public Health Dent.* 2014;75(2):85–92.

6. Ackerman MB, Perlman MP, Waldman HB. Increasing use of dental services by children, but many are unable to secure needed care. *J Clin Pediatr Dent.* 2014;39(1):9–11.

7. Eke PI, Jaramillo F, Thornton-Evans GO, Borgnakke WS. Dental visits among adult Hispanics— BRFSS 1999 and 2006. *J Public Health Dent.* 2011;71(3):252–256.

8. Stewart DC, Ortega AN, Dausey D, Rosenheck R. Oral health and use of dental services among Hispanics. *J Public Health Dent.* 2002;62(2):84–91.

9. Ismail AI, Szpunar SM. Oral health status of Mexican-Americans with low and high acculturation status: findings from southwestern HHANES, 1982–84. *J Public Health Dent.* 1990; 50(1):24–31.

10. Lukes SM, Miller FY. Oral health issues among migrant farmworkers. *J Dent Hyg.* 2002; 76(2):134–40.

11. Northridge ME, Ue FV, Borrell LN, et al. Tooth loss and dental caries in community-dwelling older adults in northern Manhattan. *Gerodontology.* 2012;29(2):e464–e473.

12. Liu Y, Li Z, Walker MP. Social disparities in dentition status among American adults. *Int Dent J*. 2014;64(1):52–57.

13. Weatherwax JA, Bray KK, Williams KB, Gadbury-Amyot CC. Exploration of the relationship between parent/guardian sociodemographics, intention, and knowledge and the oral health status of children/wards enrolled in a Central Florida Head Start Program. *Int J Dent Hyg*. 2015;13(1):49–55.

14. Lugo I, Arteaga S, Sanchez V. Oral health status, perceptions, and access to dental care in the Hispanic population. *Gen Dent*. 2014;62(4):24–30.

15. Israel BA, Schulz AJ, Parker EA, Becker AB. Review of community-based research: assessing partnership approaches to improve public health. *Annu Rev Public Health*. 1998;19:173–202.

16. Schulz AJ, Parker EA, Israel BA, Becker AB, Maciak BJ, Hollis R. Conducting a participatory community-based survey: collecting and interpreting data for a community health intervention on Detroit's east side. *J Public Health Manag Pract*. 1998;4:10–24.

17. Israel BA, Eng E, Schulz AJ, Parker EA. *Methods in Community-Based Participatory Research for Health*. San Francisco, CA: Jossey-Bass; 2005.

18. National Center for Chronic Disease Prevention and Health Promotion. *2011 Behavioral Risk Factor Surveillance System (BRFSS)*. Atlanta, GA: US Department of Health and Human Services, Centers for Disease Control and Prevention; 2012.

19. Williams DR, Yu Y, Jackson JS, Anderson NB. Racial differences in physical and mental health: socioeconomic status, stress, and discrimination. *J Health Psychol*. 1997;2(3):335–351.

20. Alegria M, Takeuchi D. National Latino and Asian American Study (NLAAS), 2002–2003 (ICPSR 191). September 18, 2013. Available at: https://www.icpsr.umich.edu/icpsrweb/ICPSR/studies/00191. Accessed December 12, 2018.

21. Hembroff LA. *The Washtenaw County Behavioral Risk Factor Survey, 2010: Methodological Report*. East Lansing, MI: Office for Survey Research of the Institute for Public Policy and Social Research (IPPSR) at Michigan State University; 2011.

6

The Oral Health Needs of the Incarcerated Population: Steps Toward Equal Access*

Nicholas S. Makrides, DMD, MA, MPH, and Jay D. Shulman, DMD, MA, MSPH

REPORT OF THE SURGEON GENERAL ON ORAL HEALTH IN AMERICA

On May 25, 2000, Assistant Secretary of Health and Surgeon General David Satcher issued the first report ever written on the oral health of Americans, *Oral Health in America: A Report of the Surgeon General.* Within the dental community, this was a significant milestone as it brought to light the difficulties that millions of Americans suffer because of poor oral health.[1] The report described the burden of disease experienced by Americans as a "silent epidemic." Moreover, it affirmed the importance of oral health with respect to general health and well-being.[1]

The Surgeon General's report demonstrated the inextricability of oral health from general health, in particular the association between oral infections and conditions including diabetes and cardiovascular disease. Moreover, the report noted that the burdens of oral disease weigh most heavily on disadvantaged populations and underrepresented minority groups.[1] Although the report served as a springboard for many initiatives targeting noninstitutionalized populations, it did not address the oral health needs of institutionalized individuals.

HEALTHY PEOPLE 2020 AND ORAL HEALTH IN AMERICA

Healthy People 2020, initiated in 2010, identified the nation's 10-year health goals and objectives:

- Attain high-quality, longer lives free of preventable disease, disability, injury, and premature death.
- Achieve health equity, eliminate disparities, and improve the health of all groups.

*This is a modified version of the article that appeared in the *American Journal of Public Health*. See: Makrides NS, Shulman JD. The oral health needs of the incarcerated population: steps toward equal access. *Am J Public Health*. 2017;107(suppl 1):S46–S47.

- Create social and physical environments that promote good health for all.
- Promote quality of life, healthy development, and healthy behaviors across all life stages.[2]

These objectives, although addressing disparities according to race, ethnicity, and education, did not address the incarcerated because, unlike the case with the general population, there are no national data sets on which to base goals and evaluation metrics.

As with the Surgeon General's report, *Healthy People* relies heavily on national surveys such as the National Health and Nutrition Examination Survey (NHANES), the National Health Interview Survey, and Behavioral Risk Factor Surveillance System. Although data from these sources have been useful in quantifying the oral health burden in community-dwelling populations, again, they provide no data on institutionalized populations such as the incarcerated.

INCARCERATED POPULATIONS, ILLNESS, AND ORAL HEALTH CARE

According to the Bureau of Justice Statistics, approximately 7 million Americans are supervised by correctional jurisdictions, of whom almost 4.55 million are on parole or probation. At the end of 2016, an adjusted total of 2,162,400 individuals—approximately the population of Houston, Texas—were incarcerated. This equates to roughly 1% of the adult population of the United States. State, federal, and private prisons housed 1,505,400 inmates, whereas county and local jails housed 740,700.[3]

Inmates come from all walks of life. As with the general population, there has been a demographic shift to an older population. Many come from disadvantaged backgrounds and enter prison with histories of substance abuse and mental illness. High rates of chronic disease and unmet dental needs are common.[4] Little is known about the health status of inmates, as there are few nationally representative data sets available. This population is, for all intents and purposes, invisible, which is particularly problematic given that inmates are the only individuals in the United States with a constitutionally established right to health care. They are not necessarily guaranteed to receive good care; rather, they have only the right to receive care that is free from deliberate indifference to serious medical needs, a low bar indeed (see *Estelle v Gamble*[5]). Simply put, care need only be minimally adequate.

To the extent that there are available health care data on incarcerated populations, they are derived from periodic surveys reported by the Bureau of Justice Statistics. One of these surveys revealed that 38.5%, 42.8%, and 38.7% of inmates in federal prisons, state prisons, and local jails, respectively, suffered from chronic medical conditions.[4] The burden of infectious disease, chronic disease, and mental illness weighs heavily on the incarcerated as a result of poverty and drug abuse.[6]

Similarly, one of the few studies in which prisoners' oral health was compared with that of an age- and race-matched population (from NHANES) showed that North Carolina prisoners had a substantially higher dental disease prevalence than their study counterparts.[7] This is not surprising given that a disproportionate number of inmates come from disadvantaged communities where access to dental care is limited.[8]

RECOMMENDATIONS FOR PROVIDING IMPROVED ORAL HEALTH CARE TO INCARCERATED POPULATIONS

Removing correctional dentistry and the oral health needs of inmates from obscurity requires that the public health community recognize the importance of oral health to overall health. Although it is generally known that the oral health of prisoners is poorer than that of noninstitutionalized populations, there are no reliable data sets that administrators, academics, and managers can use to describe and monitor inmates' oral health. We offer the following recommendations to increase awareness of inmates' oral health and to enhance available national data on which to base oral heath objectives:

- Include prisoners in nationally collected data sets such as NHANES.
- Increase the information technology infrastructure in correctional facilities to include electronic health records.
- Establish standardized oral health program outcome measures for correctional facilities.
- Include oral health in clinical guidance and health care policies for primary care providers.
- Improve working relationships with dental directors at the state and correctional department levels.
- Develop a correctional oral health infrastructure by providing clinical opportunities as part of dental hygiene and graduate dental training programs.

CONCLUSIONS

Because of the paucity of national data, the health care needs of the incarcerated are often unnoticed given their status in society. Finding advocates to champion inmate health care, much less oral health care, is difficult because this invisible demographic must compete with the interests of the unincarcerated population. Our recommendations are just a beginning step in revealing the oral health needs of this overlooked and vulnerable population.

We are not naive about the challenges ahead. The most difficult part of improving the health care and oral health of inmates will be convincing legislators and the American public that inmate health care is important. Although others have eloquently defended legal, ethical, social, and public health reasons why prisoners must and should be provided health care, the words of Fyodor Dostoyevsky resonate with us[9,10]: "The degree of civilization in a society can be judged by entering its prisons."[11]

ACKNOWLEDGMENTS

The comments and recommendations made by the authors are their own. They do not necessarily represent the views and opinions of the Federal Bureau of Prisons, the US Department of Health and Human Services, the US Public Health Service, the Baylor College of Dentistry, or Texas A&M University.

REFERENCES

1. US Department of Health and Human Services. Oral health in America: a report of the Surgeon General. Rockville, MD: National Institute of Dental and Craniofacial Research, National Institutes of Health; 2000.

2. US Department of Health and Human Services. About Healthy People. Available at: https://www.healthypeople.gov/2020/About-Healthy-People. Accessed November 5, 2018.

3. Kaeble D, Cowhig M. Correctional populations in the United States, 2016. Bureau of Justice Statistics. April 2018. Available at: https://www.bjs.gov/content/pub/pdf/cpus16.pdf. Accessed November 2, 2018.

4. Wilper AP, Woolhandler S, Boyd JW, et al. The health and health care of US prisoners: results of a nationwide survey. *Am J Public Health*. 2009;99(4):666–672.

5. *Estelle v Gamble*, 429 US 97 (1976).

6. Greifinger R. *Public Health Behind Bars: From Prisons to Communities*. New York, NY: Springer Science and Business Media; 2007.

7. Clare JH. Dental status, unmet needs and utilization of dental services in a cohort of adult felons at admission and after three years' incarceration. *J Correct Health Care*. 2002;9(1):65–76.

8. Shulman JD, Makrides NS, Lockhart A. The organization of a correctional dental program. *Correct Health Care Rep*. 2015;16(4):49–61.

9. Paris JE. Why prisoners deserve health care. *Virtual Mentor*. 2008;10(2):113–115.

10. Treadwell HM, Northridge ME. Oral health is the measure of a just society. *J Health Care Poor Underserved*. 2007;18(1):12–20.

11. Wikiquote. Fyodor Dostoyevsky. Available at: https://en.wikiquote.org/wiki/Fyodor_Dostoyevsky. Accessed January 4, 2017.

7

The Largest Minority Population With Unmet Oral Health Needs: Individuals With Disabilities

H. Barry Waldman, DDS, PhD, MPH, and
Steven P. Perlman, DDS, MScD, DHL (Hon)

The report on disability produced by the World Health Organization and the World Bank in 2011 detailed that more than a billion people had some form of disability, of whom nearly 200 million experience considerable difficulties in functioning.[1] In the years ahead, disability will be an even greater concern because its prevalence is on the rise. For example, in the United States, about 1 in 59 children has been identified with autism spectrum disorder, according to estimates from Centers for Disease Control and Prevention's (CDC's) Autism and Developmental Disabilities Monitoring Network.[2] In addition, increases will occur as populations age and as a result of the higher risk of disability in older people, as well as the global increase in chronic health conditions such as diabetes, cardiovascular disease, cancer, and mental health disorders.

CURRENT DISABILITY RATES IN THE UNITED STATES

In the United States, 56 million residents exhibit varying levels of disabilities including the following:

- Of the civilian noninstitutionalized population, **40.7 million or 12.8%** have a severe disability.
- In West Virginia, of the civilian noninstitutionalized population in 2016, **20.1%** had a disability—among the highest rates in the nation. Utah, at 9.9%, had the lowest rate.
- A total of **7.5 million** of the total civilian noninstitutionalized population aged 18 to 64 years is employed with a disability.
- The median earnings in the past 12 months (in 2016 inflation-adjusted dollars) of the civilian noninstitutionalized population aged 16 years and older with earnings and a disability was **$22,047**.[3]

Table 7-1. Civilian Noninstitutionalized Population in 1,000s Rounded With Disabilities: United States, 2016

Population	No. (%)
Total	39,273 (12.5)
Male	18,948 (12.4)
Female	20,324 (12.7)
Race and Hispanic origin	
White alone	29,932 (13.0)
Black alone	5,448 (14.0)
American Indian/Alaska Native	421 (16.9)
Asian alone	1,139 (6.9)
Native Hawaiian/other Pacific Islander	57 (10.4)
Other race alone	1,216 (8.1)
Two or more races	1,059 (11.0)
White alone, not Hispanic	4,799 (8.8)
Age, years	
<5	155 (0.8)
5–17	2,887 (5.4)
18–34	4,350 (6.0)
35–64	15,837 (12.9)
65–74	6,629 (25.4)
≥75	9,413 (50.0)
Disability type	
Hearing difficulty	11,089 (3.5)
Vision difficulty	7,232 (2.3)
Cognitive difficulty	14,807 (5.0)
Ambulatory difficulty	20,609 (7.0)
Self-care difficulty	7,878 (2.7)
Independent living difficulty	13,941 (5.6)

Source: Adapted from US Census Bureau.[4]

In 2016, the proportion of the US population with disabilities increased dramatically by age from 5.4% for children aged 5 to 17 years to 50.0% for seniors aged 75 years or older (Table 7-1). There are marked differences by race and ethnicity in the proportion of US residents with disabilities, ranging from 6.9% for Asians to 14.0% for Blacks and 16.6% for American Indians and Alaska Natives (Table 7-1).

REALITIES OF DISABILITY: HEALTH, ILLNESS, AND HEALTH CARE OPTIONS

People with disabilities generally have poorer health, lower education achievement, fewer economic opportunities, and higher rates of poverty than people without disabilities. This is largely because of the lack of services available to them that most of us take for granted, and the many obstacles they face in their everyday lives. Disability is part of the human condition. Almost everyone will be temporarily or permanently impaired at some point in their life, and those who survive to old age will experience increased difficulties in functioning. Most extended families have a member with a disability and many nondisabled people take responsibility for supporting and caring for their relatives and friends with disabilities.

Responses to disabilities have changed since the 1970s, prompted largely by the self-organization of people with disabilities and by the growing tendency to see disability as a human rights issue. Historically, people with disabilities have largely been provided for through solutions that segregate them, such as residential institutions and special schools. Policy has now shifted toward community and educational inclusion, and medically focused solutions have given way to more interactive approaches that recognize that people can be disabled by environmental factors as well as by their bodies.

People with disabilities develop the same health problems that affect the general population. Some may be more susceptible to developing chronic conditions because of the influence of behavioral risk factors such as increased physical inactivity. They also may experience earlier onset of these conditions. These difficulties are exacerbated in less-advantaged communities.

The disability experience resulting from the interaction of health conditions, personal situations, and environmental factors varies greatly. Persons with disabilities are diverse and heterogeneous, well beyond the stereotypical views of disability that emphasize wheelchair users and a few other "classic" groups such as blind and/or deaf people. Disability encompasses the child born with a congenital condition such as cerebral palsy, the young soldier who loses his leg to a land mine, the middle-aged woman with severe arthritis, or the older person with dementia, among many others. Health conditions can be visible or invisible, temporary or long term, static, episodic, degenerating, painful, or inconsequential.

The health behaviors practiced by some adults with disabilities can differ in degree from those of the general population. People with disabilities are more likely to be overweight or obese and to smoke. In particular, persons with intellectual disabilities also are prone to hypokinetic conditions (lack of movement), which could develop into diabetes, cancer, and stroke. In addition, persons with intellectual and developmental disabilities tend to be affected by an extended series of comorbid conditions, such as seizure disorders, dysphagia (difficulty in swallowing), aspiration pneumonia, osteoporosis, sensory processing disorders, and polypharmacy (overuse of medication and multiprescribers who do not communicate with each other).

People with disabilities are at greater risk of violence than those without disabilities. The prevalence of sexual abuse against people with disabilities has been shown to be higher, especially for institutionalized men and women with intellectual disabilities, intimate partners, and adolescents. People with disabilities are at higher risk of nonfatal unintentional injury from road traffic crashes, burns, falls, and accidents related to assistive devices; as a result, they have a higher risk of premature death. Mortality rates for people with disabilities vary depending on the health condition. In some instances, mortality rates for people with disabilities have decreased in developed countries.[2]

Individuals with disabilities report seeking more inpatient and outpatient care than people without disabilities. Women seek care more often than men, as do female individuals with disabilities. The proportion of individuals seeking care in high-income countries increases with age; the results vary for low-income countries. Respondents with disabilities in low-income countries show higher rates of not receiving care than respondents in high-income countries. Needs and unmet needs exist across the spectrum of health services—promotion, prevention, and treatment. The oral health of many people with disabilities is poor, and access to dental care is limited.[2]

DENTAL CARE SERVICE FOR THOSE WITH DISABILITIES

Barriers to Care Faced by Special Needs Populations

The ability to pay for care remains the primary obstacle to obtaining oral health care for this population. Many individuals with special needs are without private health insurance and are reliant on government programs such as Medicare and Medicaid to pay for their medical and dental services. For those with private insurance, policies may not cover dental care or the cost of treatment sometimes required by patients with special needs. Other barriers include the following:

- Language: communication difficulties between the individuals with disabilities and the providers of oral health services;
- Sensory impairments: for example, vision, hearing, and learning problems;
- Psychological issues: for example, low oral health literacy, dental anxiety, and past negative experiences;
- Limited transportation;
- Accessibility: for example, dental offices that are not wheelchair-accessible;
- Cultural barriers: differing attitudes regarding the cause of disabilities and the treatment of individuals with disabilities;
- Educational behavior: for example, health providers with limited training in competency and/or treating patients with special needs.[5]

Although many dental practitioners do provide care for the legions of patients with disabilities, planning is essential to prepare the broad base of practitioners for the provision of needed services. For example, it was not until 2004 that the US Commission on Dental Accreditation (CODA) adopted a new standard (with implementation in 2006) stating that "Graduates from U.S. dental schools *must* [italics added] be competent in assessing the treatment needs of patients with special needs."[6] The standard does not require clinical experience during dental school training. Unfortunately, it was only through subterfuge (carried out by one of the authors of this chapter [HBW]) that the Commission adopted a new standard for 2006, that educational programs in dental and dental hygiene schools in the United States were required to include some aspects of the preparation for the care of individuals with disabilities.[7] The literature reports that academic dental institutions have a history of underpreparing students to deal with the increasing population of individuals with special needs.

The reality is that the issues of inadequate preparation of dental school students to provide care for patients with disabilities and the frequent reluctance of practitioners to supply the services for patients with special needs is not just a US problem. The situation exists throughout many parts of the world. For example, students from Greece, Belgium, Ireland, Germany, Brazil, Saudi Arabia, Jordan, Germany, Nigeria, Indonesia, China, and the Caribbean and Latin America repeat the drumbeat of limited or, at best, varying levels of dental school preparation and the inadequate access to dental treatment for individuals with disabilities.[8]

In addition, there are barriers in preparing current practitioners to provide care to individuals with special needs (i.e., the dentists who graduated from dental schools before implementation of the CODA modified programmatic standard). The reality is that few, if any, continuing education programs provide sessions dedicated to the care of individuals with disabilities.

Dental practitioners must carry out preparatory procedures similar to those of a physician (e.g., history taking, medication listings related to the particular disability), and cooperation of the patient over an extended period is necessary (the use of general anesthetics carries with it added concerns).

Another issue is that it may not be an easy task to find a dentist who is trained, willing, and able to treat children and adults with disabilities. Many studies have demonstrated the reality that the more significant the disabilities, the more difficult it is to find a dental professional who is willing to provide the needed care. In addition, as noted previously, limitations in insurance coverage, the restrictions of the Medicaid system (e.g., the elective inclusion of dental service coverage for youngsters as they reach their adult years), and the general lack of funding for state programs provide additional barriers for care.

UNMET DENTAL NEEDS

The US Department of Health and Human Services National Survey of Children with Special Health Care Needs stated the following in 2007:

> Overall, 16 percent of [children with special heath care needs] were reported to need at least one health care service that they did not receive in the past year, and 6 percent needed more than one service that they did not receive. *The service most commonly reported as needed but not received was preventive dental care* [italics added]. [9]

Although there are increasing general national reports on the oral health needs of individuals with disabilities, few detail their findings in terms of racial and/or ethnic demographics. Nevertheless, overall reports for particular demographic groups do infer the expected variations of unmet dental needs for individuals with special needs. For example, in national studies, the proportion of demographic groups with untreated dental caries varies greatly by race and ethnic origin:

- In all age groups, the Asian-only population has the lowest rate of untreated dental caries, compared with the highest rates for the Black-only and Mexican-origin Hispanic populations.
- In all age groups younger than 65 years living below the poverty level, the Black-only population has the highest rate of untreated caries.
- In all age groups living above the poverty level, the Black-only and Hispanic populations have the highest rates of untreated dental caries (Table 7-2).

Table 7-2. Percentage of Persons With Untreated Dental Caries by Selected Characteristics: United States, 2011–2014

	Age 5–19 y	Age 20–44 y	Age 45–64 y	Age ≥65 y
Total	18.6%	31.6%	27.2%	21.8%
Race and Hispanic origin				
White-only	16.7%	27.1%	23.4%	18.6%
Black-only	23.4%	46.1%	45.4%	40.7%
Asian-only	15.4%	20.5%	17.4%	27.6%
Hispanic	21.7%	37.8%	35.9%	34.4%
Mexican origin	23.8%	40.0%	40.8%	46.3%
Percentage of poverty level				
White-only				
<100%	24.5%	47.4%	52.2%	47.6%
≥100%	14.8%	23.0%	20.9%	17.9%
Black-only				
<100%	27.5%	56.0%	71.7%	52.9%
≥100%	19.3%	41.3%	37.9%	38.6%
Asian-only				
<100%	24.2%[a]	24.6%	26.2%[a]	
≥100%	13.6%	19.9%	15.4%	26.7%
Hispanic				
<100%	23.6%	43.4%	45.6%	39.0%
≥100%	19.7%	33.3%	33.6%	33.1%
Mexican origin				
<100%	23.1%	44.4%	49.9%	58.7%
≥100%	23.7%	35.8%	38.5%	42.3%

Source: Adapted from National Center for Health Statistics.[10]

Note: y = years.

[a]Estimate considered unreliable.

Now add the realities of the barriers to care that are faced by the populations with special needs. Is it any wonder that the "Largest population in the US without adequate dental care"[11] is individuals with disabilities? These numbers will only increase in the future.

PROJECTED FUTURE DISABILITY RATES

The projected estimated proportion and number of individuals with severe disabilities are not available for 2030. A projection of 45.8 million residents with severe disabilities was developed by using Census Bureau general total national population and state projections for the year 2030:

- In 2015: The proportion of individuals with disabilities ranged from 9.9% in Utah and 10.3% in Colorado, to 19.4% in West Virginia and 21.4% in Puerto Rico. The estimated number of individuals with severe disabilities ranged from 71,000 in Wyoming and 76,000 in the District of Columbia, to 3,126,000 in Texas and 4,097,000 in California.[12]
- In 2030: On the basis of both the total number of state residents and proportion with disabilities for 2015, the estimated number of residents with severe disabilities ranged from 65,000 in North Dakota and Wyoming to 3,865,000 in Texas and 4,382,000 in California.[12]

CONCLUSIONS

The dental profession is undergoing dramatic changes as it responds to (1) the evolving delivery system for a diversifying population and (2) reports of the stagnation of economics of dental practices.[13] At these times, surely individual practitioners and the general profession cannot overlook the oral health necessities of the tens of millions of children and adults with disabilities.

REFERENCES

1. Centers for Disease Control and Prevention. Autism spectrum disorder. Available at: https://www.cdc.gov/ncbddd/autism/data.html. Accessed July 27, 2018.

2. World Health Organization, World Bank. World Report on Disability. WHO Library Cataloguing-in-Publication Data. 2011. Available at: http://www.who.int/disabilities/world_report/2011/en. Accessed July 20, 2018.

3. US Census Bureau. American Community Survey. Community facts. Available at: https://factfinder.census.gov/faces/nav/jsf/pages/index.xhtml. Accessed July 25, 2018.

4. US Census Bureau. American Community Survey. Available from: https://factfinder.census. gov/faces/tableservices/jsf/pages/productview.xhtml?pid=ACS_16_5YR_S1810&prodType= table. Accessed July 25, 2018.

5. Moore TA. Dental care for patients with special needs. Decisions in Dentistry. 2016. Available at: http://decisionsindentistry.com/article/dental-care-patients-special-needs/print. Accessed July 25, 2018.

6. Commission on Dental Accreditation. Accreditation for dental education. Chicago, IL: American Dental Association; 2014.

7. Waldman HB. I'm a liar and proud of it! Or, my introduction to reality. *Exceptional Parent Magazine*. 2012;42(12):20–21.

8. Waldman HB, Wong A, Raposa K, Perlman SP. Preparing current Massachusetts dentists to provide care of individuals with disabilities. *J Massachusetts Dent Soc*. 2017;55(2):24–26.

9. The National Survey of Children With Special Health Care Needs. Chart book 2005–2006. Rockville, MD: US Department of Health and Human Services, Maternal and Child Health Bureau; 2007.

10. *Health, United States, 2016 With Chart Book on Long-term Trends in Health*. Hyattsville, MD: National Center for Health Statistics; 2017.

11. Waldman HB, Perlman SP, Wong A. Largest minority population in US without adequate dental care. *Spec Care Dentist*. 2017;37(4):159–163.

12. Waldman HB, Perlman SP, Wong A. Children with disabilities are among the largest minority population without adequate oral health care. *Exceptional Parent Magazine*. 2017;488(8):36–39.

13. Vujicic M. Solving dentistry's "business" problem. *J Am Dent Assoc*. 2015;146(8):641–643.

8

Oral Health and Aging*

Carol Raphael, MPA, MEd

Oral diseases and conditions that are associated with aging concomitantly result in an increased need for preventive, restorative, and periodontal dental care. This is particularly true of seniors aged 65 years and older who are economically disadvantaged, who are members of racial/ethnic minority groups, and who are institutionalized, disabled, or homebound.

Nearly 19% of seniors no longer have any natural teeth. Loss of teeth increases with age and varies by race/ethnicity.[1] According to 2011–2012 data reported by the National Center for Health Statistics, adults aged 75 years and older (26%) were twice as likely to be edentulous as those aged 65 to 74 years (13%). Non-Hispanic Blacks (29%) were significantly more likely to be edentulous compared with Hispanics (15%) and non-Hispanic Whites (17%). A Massachusetts survey revealed that 34% of seniors in nursing homes have urgent and major dental health needs.[2]

Tooth loss has multiple impacts on health and well-being. Seniors who have lost all or most of their teeth often end up avoiding fresh fruits and vegetables—basic elements of a healthy diet. Relying on soft foods that are easily chewable results in a decline in nutrition and health. In addition to causing pain and difficulty in speaking, toothlessness often leads to embarrassment and a loss of self-esteem contributing to loneliness and social isolation.

More than half (53%) of seniors have moderate or severe periodontal disease. There is increasing evidence of the association of periodontal disease with chronic conditions including diabetes, heart disease, and stroke. Oral health conditions among seniors with chronic conditions are often exacerbated by use of medications. About 400 commonly used medications can cause dry mouth, which heightens the risk of oral disease.[3]

DENTAL INSURANCE COVERAGE

About one half of seniors do not go to the dentist.[4] More than one in five Medicare beneficiaries have not visited a dentist in five years.[5] Cost is the major reason why seniors do not seek or utilize dental care. Approximately 70% of older Americans lack dental

*This is a modified version of the article that appeared in the *American Journal of Public Health*. See: Raphael C. Oral health and aging. *Am J Public Health*. 2017;107(suppl 1):S44–S45.

insurance. The remainder are covered through employer sponsored plans, Medicaid, or self-purchased supplemental insurance.

For its 55 million beneficiaries, traditional Medicare does not cover routine dental care. Medicare Part A (hospital insurance) covers very limited "medically necessary" benefits related to certain dental services provided during a hospital stay.

Medicare Advantage plans that do offer dental coverage provide minimal benefits. According to the Medicare Rights Center, most beneficiaries do not realize that dental services are not covered and express concern about how to access and afford needed dental services. Under Medicaid, states have the option of providing adult dental coverage. As a consequence, four states do not offer a dental benefit and 15 states offer emergency-only coverage.[6] Access is further hampered because 80% of dentists do not accept Medicaid because of low reimbursement rates.

Upon retirement, seniors often lose their dental insurance. Only two percent of retirees retain dental coverage.[7] With supplemental dental insurance, the coverage cap on claims generally ranges from $1,000 to $1,500 per year and has not increased in 30 years.

SYSTEM BARRIERS TO CARE

Many seniors incur high out-of-pocket dental expenses. For example, the average cost of an implant is $4,000 or more if bone graft and anesthesia are needed. For the large segment of seniors who live on fixed incomes, this is unaffordable. Seniors below 150% of the federal poverty level are three times as likely to report unmet dental needs compared with those with incomes over 300% of the federal poverty level.

Complicating this situation are overall and regional shortages of dental practitioners willing to treat seniors. More than 60% of states have substantial provider shortages and racial/ethnic diversity of providers is lacking. Only six percent of dentists are racial/ethnic minorities.[7]

ADDRESSING THE NEEDS

To address the oral health needs of seniors, a multiyear, multipronged approach is needed. This includes tackling two cultural norms: First, we must challenge the concept that oral health care is optional rather than an integral part of health care. Second, we cannot yield to the ageist view that accepts less than optimal oral health or asserts that seniors should be resigned to losing their teeth and living with oral disease.

A successful approach encompasses the following components:

1. A vigorous education campaign that will get this issue on the public's radar screen. The campaign must demonstrate why society should care about this issue and how it would benefit if these issues were addressed.

2. A broad and potent coalition that builds broad support particularly among credible groups with no financial stake in the outcome. It should include national stakeholders, collaborators, and champions in executive and legislative branches.

3. A set of financially and politically feasible options that includes essential benefits and supports quality care and value-based outcomes with the additional goal of reducing costs. A recent study by Avalere (2016) for the Pacific Dental Services Foundation estimated the cost and savings of a new Medicare Part B benefit covering the initial and ongoing treatment of periodontal disease for beneficiaries with diabetes, coronary artery disease, or stroke. It concluded that this new benefit would generate a net savings for Medicare of $63.5 billion from 2016 to 2025.

4. At the same time, it may be advisable to work with private-sector insurers and providers establishing risk-based coordinating entities such as accountable care organizations. These organizations would have more flexibility in benefit design and in applying the results of retrospective claims research demonstrating the link among oral health, periodontal disease treatment, and medical costs in practice environments.

5. New models of delivery are needed to treat the increasing population of older adults who are retaining more of their teeth and have multiple chronic conditions that require multiple medications. In addition, new delivery models are needed to address the needs of the homebound and long-term-care populations in nursing homes and assisted living sites. Mobile technology, tele-dentistry adoption of oral health teams, and integration with geriatric and primary care offer opportunities for significant improvements in care delivery models.

CONCLUSIONS

The population of older adults is growing and is increasingly diverse. Dental practice and dental systems can and should be transformed to ensure the oral health of all seniors. Focusing on the oral health of seniors benefits not only those who are seniors today but also seniors in the future.

REFERENCES

1. Dye BA, Thorton-Evans G, Li X, Iafolla TJ. Dental caries and tooth loss in adults in the United States, 2011–2012. NCHS data brief 197. National Center for Health Statistics. 2015. Available at: https://www.cdc.gov/nchs/data/databriefs/db197.pdf. Accessed March 9, 2017.

2. A path to expanded dental access in Massachusetts. Philadelphia, PA: Pew Charitable Trusts; 2015.

3. Oral health for older Americans. Centers for Disease Control and Prevention. 2006. Available at: https://www.cdc.gov/oralhealth/publications/factsheets/adult_oral_health/adult_older.htm. Accessed January 3, 2017.

4. Manski R. Access to oral care and the impact of retirement. Lecture presented at: Expanding Oral Healthcare for America's Seniors: A Sante Fe GroupSalon; September 29, 2016; Arlington VA.

5. Oral health and Medicare beneficiaries. *Coverage, Out-of-Pocket Spending and Unmet Need.* Washington, DC: Kaiser Family Foundation; 2012.

6. *Medicaid Adult Dental Benefits: An Overview.* Hamilton, NJ: Center for Health Care Strategies; 2015.

7. State of decay. *Are Older Americans Coming of Age Without Oral Healthcare?* Chicago, IL: Oral Health America; 2013.

9

Dental-Related Use of Hospital Emergency Departments by Hispanics and Non-Hispanics in Florida*

Claudia A. Serna, DDS, PhD, MPH, Oscar Arevalo, DDS, ScD, MBA, MS, and Scott L. Tomar, DMD, DrPH

Health disparities are profound in the United States for many groups defined by race, ethnicity, socioeconomic status, gender, age, and geographic location. Hispanics constitute the nation's largest and fastest growing racial/ethnic minority group, making up 17% of the US population (53 million in 2012).[1] More than one half of the Hispanic population in the United States resides in just 3 states: California, Texas, and Florida. In 2015, there were 4.8 million Hispanics in Florida, accounting for 24.4% of the state's population.[2]

Disparities in dental care and dental disease burden exist among racial and ethnic groups. Among ethnic groups, Hispanics face measurable disadvantage when it comes to oral health. In 2008, 31% of Hispanic adults reported fair or poor oral health.[3] Periodontal disease occurs 10 times more frequently in Hispanics than in Whites.[4,5] The percentage of Hispanic adults who had at least 1 dental visit in the past year was 49.9% compared with 66.8% of non-Hispanic White adults. In addition, Mexican Americans have the lowest utilization rate and poorest oral health status of all Hispanic subgroups.[6]

For Hispanics, some of the barriers for not seeking needed dental care include high cost, fear of the dentist, long waiting time, transportation difficulties, language barriers, and lack of available facilities.[6] As a result, the hospital emergency department (ED) may become a place where many receive dental care. For example, in 2014, there were 21,204 visits to an ED by Hispanics and 142,702 visits by non-Hispanics in Florida for a dental condition.[7] Most hospitals do not have the facilities or trained staff to provide comprehensive dental care. As a consequence, many patients receive only palliative care such as antibiotics or pain medication, but the underlying dental problem is not addressed. In too many cases, the patient returns to the ED with the same problem—or worse.[8–12] There is little research focused on ED utilization for dental conditions by ethnic groups in Florida.

---

*This is a modified version of the article that appeared in the *American Journal of Public Health*. See: Serna CA, Arevalo O, Tomar SL. Dental-related use of hospital emergency departments by Hispanics and Non-Hispanics in Florida. *Am J Public Health*. 2017;107(suppl 1):S88–S93.

Oral health is essential to the general health and well-being of individuals and the population. Yet significant oral health disparities persist in the US population attributable to complex cultural and social processes that affect both oral health status and access to effective dental health care.[13] Major risk factors for poor oral health in the United States include unhealthy diet, tobacco use, frequent alcohol use, poor access to dental services, and lack of dental insurance.[14] Of all ethnic groups in the United States, non-Hispanic Blacks, Hispanics, American Indians, and Alaska Natives generally have the poorest oral health.[15] As Hispanics have become the largest minority group in the United States, this has resulted in an increased demand for oral health care.[4] According to the Hispanic Community Health Study/Study of Latinos, the mean number of decayed or filled tooth surfaces, missing teeth, and measures of periodontitis varied among different Hispanic or Latino subgroups.[16-18] Many Hispanics lack either access to routine dental care or financial resources, and for that reason they may rely on the ED as a source of dental care. Currently, the use of the hospital ED for dental conditions is a large and growing phenomenon in the United States.[19] However, EDs are neither the most appropriate setting for dental care nor are they generally equipped to provide definitive treatment of dental conditions.[20] The number of dental-related ED visits in Florida has grown annually, from 104,646 in 2005 up to 163,906 in 2014.[7]

Each year, many Americans seek dental care at EDs. Florida is one of the most ethnically diverse states and, in particular, Hispanics face many barriers when it comes to access to dental care. The purpose of this study was to examine differences between Hispanics and non-Hispanics in dental-related use of hospital EDs to determine ways to reorient care for better individual and community outcomes.

METHODS

We drew data for this study from ambulatory ED discharge records compiled by Florida's Agency for Health Care Administration. The data included all ED visits in Florida in which ED registration occurred for the years 2013 through 2015. The data for the study included patient demographic characteristics; the *International Classification of Diseases, Ninth Revision, Clinical Modification (ICD-9-CM)* and *International Classification of Diseases, Tenth Revision, Clinical Modification (ICD-10-CM)*[21,22] codes for the dental condition; principal payer; patient visit by weekday; and hour of arrival at the ED.

We merged data for 3 calendar years (2013, 2014, and 2015) to ensure adequate sample size for the main purpose of the analysis, differences in dental-related use of hospital EDs between Hispanics and non-Hispanics in Florida. Presently, Florida is the nation's third most populated state. To identify areas with higher number and rate of dental-related ED visits,[7] we used the patient's county of residency at the time of the claim to divide the state into 8 geographic regions (Northwest, Northeast, North Central, Central West, Central East, Central, Southwest, and Southeast). Also, we defined the visits for dental-related reasons for this study by the patient's reported reason for seeking care (admitting diagnosis) or the ED physician's primary diagnosis by using *ICD-9-CM* and *ICD-10-CM* codes. The *ICD-9-CM* was used for 2013, 2014, and the first 3 quarters of 2015, after which the Florida Agency for Health Care Administration switched to *ICD-10-CM*. For purposes of this analysis, we operationally defined a dental-related ED visit as one in which the primary or admitting diagnosis was coded as *ICD-9-CM* or *ICD-10-CM* codes 520–526.9, 528–528.9, 784.92, V52.3, V53.4, V58.5, V72.2, K00–K14.9, Z46.3, or Z46.4. Some of these codes have been used in a recent analysis of the state and national ED data.[7,23]

We calculated rates by ethnicity and region by age group (0–18 years, 19–64 years, and >65 years) and gender. We calculated the dental ED rates per 10,000 population as the total number of dental-related ED visits that occurred by merging 3 calendar years (2013, 2014, and 2015), divided by the population estimates available from Florida Charts[2] by region for the 3 years, multiplied by 10,000. We used the χ^2 test to investigate statistical differences among regions and among Hispanics and non-Hispanics for the age ranges. We considered a *P* value of .05 or less to be statistically significant.

Finally, we calculated the percentage distribution of dental-related ED visits for Hispanics and non-Hispanics by primary payer (Medicare, Medicaid, commercial, self-pay, and other), day of the week, and hour of arrival (12AM to 11PM). We defined non-business hours as from 5PM to 8AM on Monday to Friday and on weekends. We used a Pearson χ^2 analysis to investigate whether the distribution of hour of arrival at the ED differed significantly between Hispanics and non-Hispanics.

RESULTS

After we merged calendar years 2013, 2014, and 2015, Hispanics represented 24% of the state population and non-Hispanics accounted for 76%. Based on these 3 years, the total number of ED visits for dental complaints was 489,262 with 64,100 or 13% of ED visits made by Hispanics and 425,162 or 87% made by non-Hispanics. Overall, the rate for ED dental-related visits was 45.5 per 10,000 population for Hispanics and 95.2 per 10,000 population for non-Hispanics. (Note that all rates are reported per 10,000 population, but for purposes of simplicity the denominator is not reported in the following paragraphs.)

The geographic regions with the highest ED rates for dental-related visits were Central Florida for Hispanics with 73.8 and Northwest Florida for non-Hispanics with 136.1 (Table 9-1). Southeast Florida was the region with the lowest ED rate for dental-related visits for both Hispanics (30.0) and non-Hispanics (63.8). That region comprised the following counties: Martin, Palm Beach, Broward, Miami-Dade, and Monroe.

Regarding age, rates for dental-related ED visits for adults aged 19 to 64 years were higher compared with the other age groups at 52.9 for Hispanics and 139.3 for non-Hispanics. By region, the highest rates for Hispanics were in the Southwest with 48.7 for those aged 0 to 18 years, Central with 95.4 for those aged 19 to 64 years, and Central East with 25.4 for those aged 65 years or older. For non-Hispanics, the highest ED dental-related visit rates were in the

Table 9-1. Number and Rate per 10,000 Hispanic vs. Non-Hispanic Persons of Dental-Related Visits to Hospital Emergency Departments by Region: Florida, 2013–2015

Florida Region	Total ED Visits for Dental Complaints		Total Population		ED Visits for Dental Complaints per 10,000 Residents	
	Hispanic	Non-Hispanic	Hispanic	Non-Hispanic	Hispanic	Non-Hispanic
NW	702	39,742	178,282	2,919,892	39.4	136.1
NE	1,799	49,091	381,575	4,3383,34	47.1	113.2
NC	886	33,614	202,314	2,565,123	43.8	131.0
CW	9,931	72,690	1,868,095	9,547,044	53.2	76.1
CE	3,591	42,468	569,155	4,012,969	63.1	105.8
C	18,392	80,251	2,491,896	7,973,972	73.8	100.6
SW	4,443	23,935	788,431	2,873,462	56.4	83.3
SE	22,823	66,446	7,607,111	10,410,040	30.0	63.8
Unknown	1,533	16,925	...	...	...	....
Total	64,100	425,162	14,086,859	44,640,836	45.5	95.2

Note: C = Central (Marion, Sumter, Lake, Seminole, Orange, Osceola, Polk, Hardee, Highlands); CE = Central East (Volusia, Brevard, Indian River, Okeechobee, St Lucie); CW = Central West (Citrus, Hernando, Pasco, Pinellas, Hillsborough, Manatee, Sarasota, DeSoto); ED = emergency department; NC = North Central (Gadsden, Leon, Wakulla, Jefferson, Madison, Taylor, Hamilton, Suwannee, Lafayette, Dixie, Columbia, Union, Bradford, Gilchrist, Alachua, Levy); NE = Northeast (Baker, Nassau, Duval, Clay, St Johns, Putnam, Flagler); NW = Northwest (Escambia, Santa Rosa, Okaloosa, Walton, Holmes, Washington, Bay, Jackson, Calhoun, Liberty, Gulf, Franklin); SE = Southeast (Martin, Palm Beach, Broward, Miami-Dade, Monroe); SW = Southwest (Charlotte, Glades, Lee, Hendry, Collier).

Northwest with 69.5 for those aged 0 to 18 years and 192.3 for those aged 19 to 64 years, followed by North Central with 17.8 for those aged 65 years or older. There were statistically significant differences between Hispanics and non-Hispanics across all regions and age groups ($P < .001$) except among those aged 0 to 18 years in Central West region ($P = .23$; Table 9-2).

Overall, female patients had higher rates than male patients both among Hispanics (48.0 vs. 43.2) and non-Hispanics (104.2 vs. 86.0). The highest rate for Hispanic male patients was in Central Florida at 67.6 and for non-Hispanic male patients was in the Northwest Region at 113.4. For female patients, the region with the highest rate for Hispanics was Central Florida (80.4) and the Northwest for non-Hispanics (159.5).

Regarding the percentage distribution of dental-related ED visits by primary payer, Medicaid was the largest payer for dental-related ED visits for both Hispanics (45.2%) and non-Hispanics (38.1%), followed by self-pay for Hispanics at 30.2% and for non-Hispanics at 35.9%. Commercial insurance was the third-largest primary payer at 12.8% for Hispanics versus 12.9% for non-Hispanics. Other primary payer was the fourth-largest payer at 6.9% for Hispanics and 7.1% for non-Hispanics. Medicare was the smallest payer for ED dental-related visits at 4.7% for Hispanics versus 5.0% for non-Hispanics.

Table 9-2. Number and Rate per 10 000 Hispanic vs. Non-Hispanic Persons of Dental-Related Visits to Hospital Emergency Departments, by Age: Florida, 2013–2015

Florida Region	Aged 0-18 Years		Aged 19-64 Years		Aged ≥ 65 Years	
	Hispanic, Frequency (Rate)	Non-Hispanic, Frequency (Rate)	Hispanic, Frequency (Rate)	Non-Hispanic, Frequency (Rate)	Hispanic, Frequency (Rate)	Non-Hispanic, Frequency (Rate)
NW	187 (30.8*)	4,539 (69.5)	507 (46.5*)	34 359 (192.3)	8 (9.3*)	844 (17.5)
NE	404 (31.2*)	5,569 (54.6)	1,358 (60.1*)	42,400 (160.6)	37 (14.0*)	1,122 (16.6)
NC	234 (39.3*)	3,298 (60.0)	635 (67.9*)	29,641 (181.1)	17 (16.4*)	675 (17.8)
CW	2,523 (42.3)	7,688 (42.5)	7,158 (65.0*)	62,720 (113.8)	250 (16.5*)	2,282 (10.2)
CE	712 (37.5*)	3,916 (52.3)	2,744 (84.0*)	37,201 (161.6)	135 (25.4*)	1,351 (14.0)
C	3,663 (46.2*)	8281 (49.6)	14,295 (95.4*)	69,862 (148.8)	434 (21.4*)	2,108 (13.0)
SW	1,296 (48.7*)	2,535 (55.3)	3,027 (64.2*)	20,427 (135.3)	120 (23.3*)	973 (10.7)
SE	6,566 (37.1*)	10,498 (46.9)	14,951 (31.0*)	53,033 (87.4)	1,306 (12.7*)	2,915 (13.8)
Unknown	250 (...)	1,319 (...)	1,201 (...)	14,513 (...)	82 (...)	1,093 (...)
Total	15,835 (40.8)	47,643 (52.1)	45,876 (52.9)	364,156 (139.3)	2,389 (15.5)	13,363 (14.3)

Note: C = Central (Marion, Sumter, Lake, Seminole, Orange, Osceola, Polk, Hardee, Highlands); CE = Central East (Volusia, Brevard, Indian River, Okeechobee, St Lucie); CW = Central West (Citrus, Hernando, Pasco, Pinellas, Hillsborough, Manatee, Sarasota, DeSoto); NC = North Central (Gadsden, Leon, Wakulla, Jefferson, Madison, Taylor, Hamilton, Suwannee, Lafayette, Dixie, Columbia, Union, Bradford, Gilchrist, Alachua, Levy); NE = Northeast (Baker, Nassau, Duval, Clay, St Johns, Putnam, Flagler); NW = Northwest (Escambia, Santa Rosa, Okaloosa, Walton, Holmes, Washington, Bay, Jackson, Calhoun, Liberty, Gulf, Franklin); SE = Southeast (Martin, Palm Beach, Broward, Miami-Dade, Monroe); SW = Southwest (Charlotte, Glades, Lee, Hendry, Collier). There were statistically sig- nificant differences between Hispanics and non-Hispanics, across all regions and age groups.

*P < .001 except among those aged 0–18 years in the CW region (P = .23).

In terms of the frequency of dental-related ED visits by day, the distribution was similar for the 2 groups. The majority of visits occurred on Sunday for both Hispanics at 15.8% and non-Hispanics at 15.4%. However, for Hispanics, the second-most frequent day was Saturday whereas for non-Hispanics it was Monday, both at 15.1%. During the remaining days of the week the visits ranged from 13.1% to 14.8% for Hispanics versus 13.4% to 14.5% for non-Hispanics.

Concerning arrival times, most individuals in both groups arrived between 9AM and 6PM—specifically, 53.5% of Hispanics and 56.8% of non-Hispanics. After this time, the frequency of visits to the ED dropped through the late night and early morning and started to increase at 6AM. For Hispanics, the hour with the largest percentage of visits was 7PM whereas for non-Hispanics it was 11AM. A Pearson χ^2 analysis showed that the distribution of hour of arrival at the ED differed significantly between Hispanics and non-Hispanics ($P < .001$).

DISCUSSION

The findings in this study are consistent with earlier reports indicating high use of EDs for dental problems in the United States[19,23,24] and in Florida.[7] This study found that Hispanics' rate of use of EDs for dental complaints was lower than the rate for non-Hispanics. In addition, the Southeast region, which has the largest Hispanic population in Florida, had the lowest rate of ED visits for dental complaints among the state's regions. These results are similar to those of other studies. For example, in California, Mexican-born immigrants were less likely to have used the ED in the past year compared with the US-born Mexican Americans.[25] In other studies, Hispanics presented a significantly lower odds of ED use for oral conditions[19,24] and Hispanic adults were less likely than non-Hispanic White adults to have visited the ED.[26] Possible explanations could be cultural norms and attitudes about oral hygiene and dental care-seeking behavior.[24] Contrary to popular perception, the least-acculturated Hispanic individuals were the least likely to use the ED. As Hispanics become more acculturated to the United States, they might also become more accustomed to US knowledge and beliefs surrounding the use of the ED as a convenient alternative to access care.[27]

The rate of ED visits for dental complaints was not uniform across the state. The analysis shows that ED dental visits rates for Hispanics in the Central, Central East, and Southwest regions were higher that elsewhere. For non-Hispanics, the higher rates were in the Northwest, Northeast, and North Central regions.

We found that hospital ED visits for dental conditions occurred more often on Saturdays and Sundays for Hispanics and Sundays and Mondays for non-Hispanics. The findings are consistent with other studies regarding Hispanics as they have found that Hispanics visited the ED for dental care more often on Saturdays and Sundays as well as during night hours.[28] The analysis by hour revealed that both groups tended to visit the

ED mostly at regular hours of operation for dental offices (i.e., 8AM to 5PM). This finding is consistent with previous studies and reports that documented that the ED is the regular source of care for individuals who are uninsured, underinsured, or face difficulties accessing dental care.[8-10] Although our analysis showed that the arrival time to the ED differed significantly between Hispanics and non-Hispanics, one caveat is that even small differences can be highly statistically significant when one is analyzing a large sample. Whether the difference is really meaningful is a judgment call; based on the plot, the curves actually look fairly similar.

There were statistically significant differences between Hispanics and non-Hispanics across all regions and age groups, except for those aged 0 to 18 years in the Central West region. This finding is particularly interesting as this age group is entitled to dental benefits under Medicaid. We hypothesize their higher utilization may be explained by low number of participating providers in the Medicaid program. Adults aged 19 to 64 years were more likely than other groups to use the ED for dental care. This finding is consistent with a previous study in which adults aged 18 to 64 years had significantly higher rates of making ED visits, whereas children aged younger than 18 years and adults aged 65 years and older did not show significant differences in their visit rates.[24,29] An analysis of a national survey indicated that adults aged 18 to 64 years enrolled in Medicaid were generally in poorer health than people with private insurance coverage and the uninsured.[26] In addition, women were more likely than men to use the ED. This finding is consistent with previous studies in Florida and nationwide.[7,26]

We also found that Medicaid was the most common primary payer for dental-related ED visits. Other studies have reported that individuals visiting the ED for dental as compared with medical problems were significantly more likely to indicate Medicaid or self-pay as the payer rather than private insurance.[24,30] It is possible that these patients were not able to access dental care because of geographic maldistribution of dentists, inadequate number of dentists accepting Medicaid enrollees, and the limited dental coverage for adults within the state.[9,31] Improved Medicaid reimbursement, together with other measures such as expansion of dental provider hours, and increasing racial and ethnic minority workforce to match local demographics could possibly decrease ED visits for dental care and improve the health of patients.

LIMITATIONS

The results presented here must be interpreted in light of their limitations. First, the study used state data from defined geo-graphic areas, which cannot be considered nationally representative. Therefore, the study results may not be generalizable to other areas of the United States. Second, the analysis was limited to the patient's reported reason for the visit (admitting diagnosis) and the clinician's principal diagnosis code. People may visit the ED because they perceived they have an oral health problem and later the condition may be diagnosed as being not dental-related. In addition, medical providers in the ED typically address symptoms of pain and infection, often without a good understanding of the causes and appropriate treatment of the oral health problems underlying these symptoms. The lack of oral health knowledge by clinicians and factors such as reimbursement may influence coding consistency across physician and facilities across Florida.

Third, the information on race/ethnicity was collected via the patient's self-report. Fourth, the study did not take into account variables such as patients' level of education, occupation, employment status, or marital status. These factors may have had an important impact on the number of ED visits for dental complaints. Fifth, each ED visit was a unique record, and records for a person with multiple ED visits cannot be linked in the data set used in this study. Without knowing whether a specific ED visit was an initial visit or a repeat visit by a patient, the extent of repeated visits to the ED could not be quantified in this study.

Sixth, previous publications have documented that illegal status can deter individuals from seeking care because of fear they will not receive care or that they will be deported.[32-34] In 2014, Florida ranked as the state with the third-largest unauthorized immigrant population—approximately 850,000.[35] Although we may hypothesize that this may explain the lower utilization of EDs by Hispanics, legal status was not a variable of interest in this study. Despite these limitations, this study provides the first-known examination of differences in dental-related use of hospital EDs between Hispanics and non-Hispanics in Florida.

PUBLIC HEALTH IMPLICATIONS

Emergency departments have become a regular source of care for individuals with dental problems, particularly for individuals who are on Medicaid or who are self-payers. A major driver of dental-related ED visits is a failure to ensure that disadvantaged people have access to routine preventive and restorative care from dentists and other providers. Many persons in the United States experience barriers to health care. Among these barriers are lack of insurance, high cost, lack of understanding about how to navigate the health care system, limited knowledge on nutrition and the importance of preventive care, transportation difficulties, and lack of available facilities providing dental services. Among US persons, Hispanics have lower rates of insurance coverage, face communication difficulties if their primary language is not English, and consequently may have a greater unmet need for dental care. From a public health perspective, documenting and understanding ethnic minorities'—especially Hispanics'—use of EDs is important for policy and program development as well as for setting priorities and goals to improve access to dental care.

Effective interventions need to be developed in the context of a social—ecological model to better understand factors such as health, economics, and education, among others. Understanding and intervening with the individual, communities, and policy could help to modify behaviors and improve access to dental care. At the individual level, messages need to be targeted for specific ethnic minorities. For example, Hispanics may have specific beliefs and attitudes, language and literacy barriers, culturally specific foods, and particular community outreach problems. These characteristics need to be taken into consideration when one is developing health educational programs. At the community level, interventions should focus on efforts to better implement coordination between oral care and general medical care. The need to create strategies to improve access to care among ethnic minorities in the state may include training ED physicians in the management of dental conditions in EDs; the creation of ED diversion programs, including a better referral system to target one-time users so they do not become multiple users of the ED for dental care; the provisions of urgent care clinics for dental care; and the implementation of culturally competent case managers to assist in appointment scheduling and follow-up.

Moreover, at the policy level, interventions must include expanding policies that value prevention and provide care for low-income and uninsured persons. The establishment of a comprehensive Medicaid benefit in Florida may result in a reduction of dental-related ED visits. Enhanced educational repayment programs may help to recruit dental professionals to Federally Qualified Health Centers, which are designed to meet the demand of the uninsured and those with Medicaid coverage. Future work should focus on understanding the complex interactions among the sociodemographic, health status, and health care access factors among ethnic minorities that appear to be associated with visits to the ED.

ACKNOWLEDGMENTS

The authors are solely responsible for the analysis and interpretation of the emergency department discharge data. The Florida Agency for the Health Care Administration specially disclaims responsibility for analysis, interpretations, or conclusions that may be created as a result of the limited data set.

REFERENCES

1. US Department of Commerce. Profile America. Facts for features: Hispanic heritage month 2013: Sept. 15–Oct. 15. 2013. Available at: http://www.census.gov/newsroom/facts-for-features/2013/cb13-ff19.html. Accessed July 18, 2016.

2. Florida Charts. Florida population estimates. 2015. Available at: http://www.floridacharts.com/flquery/population/populationrpt.aspx. Accessed August 23, 2016.

3. Bloom B, Simile CM, Adams PF, Cohen RA. Oral health status and access to oral health care for US adults aged 18–64: National Health Interview Survey, 2008. *Vital Health Stat 10.* 2012; 47(253):1–22.

4. Mejia GC, Kaufman JS, Corbie-Smith G, Rozier RG, Caplan DJ, Suchindran CM. A conceptual framework for Hispanic oral health care. *J Public Health Dent*. 2008;68(1):1-6.

5. Ramos-Gomez F, Cruz GD, Watson MR, Canto MT, Boneta AE. Latino oral health: a research agenda toward eliminating oral health disparities. *J Am Dent Assoc*. 2005;136(9): 1231-1240.

6. Castañeda X, Ruiz Ruelas M, Ramos-Gomez F, Ojeda G. Oral health and Latinos in the US (fact sheet). Berkeley, CA: Health Initiative of America, School of Public Health, University of California Berkeley; 2010.

7. Tomar SL, Carden DL, Dodd VJ, Catalanotto FA, Herndon JB. Trends in dental-related use of hospital emergency departments in Florida. *J Public Health Dent*. 2016;76(3):249-257.

8. Pennycook A, Makower R, Brewer A, Moulton C, Crawford R. The management of dental problems presenting to an accident and emergency department. *JR Soc Med*. 1993;86(12): 702-703.

9. Pajewski NM, Okunseri C. Patterns of dental service utilization following nontraumatic dental condition visits to the emergency department in Wisconsin Medicaid. *J Public Health Dent*. 2014;74(1):34-41.

10. Davis EE, Deinard AS, Maiga EW. Doctor, my tooth hurts: the costs of incomplete dental care in the emergency room. *J Public Health Dent*. 2010;70(3):205-210.

11. Cohen LA, Bonito AJ, Eicheldinger C, et al. Comparison of patient visits to emergency departments, physician offices, and dental offices for dental problems and injuries. *J Public Health Dent*. 2011;71(1):13-22.

12. Cohen LA, Harris SL, Bonito AJ, et al. Low-income and minority patient satisfaction with visits to emergency departments and physician offices for dental problems. *J Am Coll Dent*. 2009;76(3):23-31.

13. Patrick DL, Lee RS, Nucci M, Grembowski D, Jolles CZ, Milgrom P. Reducing oral health disparities: a focus on social and cultural determinants. *BMC Oral Health*. 2006;6(suppl 1):S4.

14. US Department of Health and Human Services. *Oral Health in America: A Report of the Surgeon General—Executive Summary*. Rockville, MD: National Institutes of Health, National Institute of Dental and Craniofacial Research; 2000.

15. Centers for Disease Control and Prevention. Disparities in oral health. Available at: http://www.cdc.gov/oralhealth/oral_health_disparities. Accessed June 9, 2016.

16. US Department of Health and Human Services. *Hispanic Community Health Study/Study of Latinos Data Book: A Report to the Communities*. Bethesda, MD: National Institutes of Health, National Heart, Lung, and Blood Institute; 2013. NIH publication 13-7951.

17. Beck JD, Youngblood M, Atkinson JC, et al. The prevalence of caries and tooth loss among participants in the Hispanic Community Health Study/Study of Latinos. *J Am Dent Assoc*. 2014;145(6):531-540.

18. Jiménez MC, Sanders AE, Mauriello SM, Kaste LM, Beck JD. Prevalence of periodontitis according to Hispanic or Latino background among study participants of the Hispanic Community Health Study/Study of Latinos. *J Am Dent Assoc.* 2014;145(8):805–816.

19. DeLia D, Lloyd K, Feldman CA, Cantor JC. Patterns of emergency department use for dental and oral health care: implications for dental and medical care co-ordination. *J Public Health Dent.* 2016;76(1):1–8.

20. Okunseri C, Okunseri E, Thorpe JM, Xiang Q, Szabo A. Medications prescribed in emergency departments for nontraumatic dental condition visits in the United States. *Med Care.* 2012;50(6):508–512.

21. *International Classification of Disease, Ninth Revision, Clinical Modification.* Hyattsville, MD: National Center for Health Statistics; 1980. Available at: https://www.cdc.gov/nchs/icd/icd9cm.htm. Accessed October 15, 2016.

22. *International Classification of Disease, Tenth Revision, Clinical Modification.* Hyattsville, MD: National Center for Health Statistics; 2000. Available at: https://www.cdc.gov/nchs/icd/icd10cm.htm. Accessed October 21, 2016.

23. Wall T, Nasseh K. Dental-related emergency department visits on the increase in the United States. Chicago, IL: American Dental Association, Health Policy Institute; 2013.

24. Okunseri C, Okunseri E, Thorpe JM, Xiang Q, Szabo A. Patient characteristics and trends in nontraumatic dental condition visits to emergency departments in the United States. *Clin Cosmet Investig Dent.* 2012;4:1–7.

25. Ortega AN, Fang H, Perez VH, et al. Health care access, use of services, and experiences among undocumented Mexicans and other Latinos. *Arch Intern Med.* 2007;167(21):2354–2360.

26. Gindi RM, Black LI, Cohen RA. Reasons for emergency room use among US adults aged 18-64: National Health Interview Survey, 2013 and 2014. *Natl Health Stat Report.* 2016;(90): 1–16.

27. Allen L, Cummings J. Emergency department use among Hispanic adults: the role of acculturation. *Med Care.* 2016;54(5):449–456.

28. Okunseri C, Okunseri E, Fischer MC, Sadeghi SN, Xiang Q, Szabo A. Nontraumatic dental condition-related visits to emergency departments on weekdays, weekends and night hours: findings from the National Hospital Ambulatory Medical Care survey. *Clin Cosmet Investig Dent.* 2013;5:69–76.

29. Tang N, Stein J, Hsia RY, Maselli JH, Gonzales R. Trends and characteristics of US emergency department visits, 1997–2007. *JAMA.* 2010;304(6):664–670.

30. Cohen LA, Manski RJ. Visits to non-dentist health care providers for dental problems. *Fam Med.* 2006;38(8):556–564.

31. Wall T, Vujicic M. Emergency department use for dental conditions continues to increase. Health Policy Institute Research Brief. Chicago, IL: American Dental Association; 2015.

32. Berk ML, Schur CL, Chavez LR, Frankel M. Health care use among undocumented Latino immigrants. *Health Aff (Millwood)*. 2000;19(4):51–64.

33. Campbell RM, Klei AG, Hodges BD, FismanD, Kitto S. A comparison of health access between permanent residents, undocumented immigrants and refugee claimants in Toronto, Canada. *J Immigr Minor Health*. 2014;16(1):165–176.

34. Hacker K, Anies M, Folb BL, Zallman L. Barriers to health care for undocumented immigrants: a literature review. *Risk Manag Healthc Policy*. 2015;8:175–183.

35. Passel JS, Cohn D. Overall number of US unauthorized immigrants holds steady since 2009. Washington, DC: Pew Research Center; 2016.

10

The Oral Health Status of Black Men in the United States: A Need for Upstream Research and Multilevel Intervention

Patrick D. Smith, DMD, MPH

HEALTH, ILLNESS, AND MORTALITY AMONG BLACK MEN

Black men in the United States are vulnerable to poor health outcomes. Life expectancy at birth of Black men consistently lags behind that of White men. Although the gap has lessened in recent years, White men can still expect to live nearly 4.5 years longer than Black men.[1] Disparities in life expectancy between communities are greater depending on geographic distinctions of low socioeconomic status and racial factors.[2,3] Black men also have the highest death rates among men of other racial groups from cerebrovascular disease, cancer, and heart disease.[1] In addition, they experience higher incidences of HIV infection[4] and are 50% more likely than White men to have been diagnosed with diabetes by a physician. As a result, Black men are more likely to suffer from visual impairment, end-stage renal disease, and death as a result of diabetic complications.[5]

As it relates to oral health, the only conclusive evidence of significant morbidity and mortality from oral disease is the low 5-year survival of Black men from oral cancer.[6] Although data show that White men have higher incidences of oral cavity and oral pharyngeal cancers, in 2014, the 5-year survival of Black men was 47.2% compared with 66.0% for White men.[7] This trend is consistent for both early and late-stage cancers and is in spite of White men having higher incidences of oral and pharynx cancers than Black men since 2007.[7] Lower incidences of oral cancer among Blacks may correlate with the lower prevalence of tobacco use among Blacks.[8] Yet, literature suggests that causes for the disparity in mortality are knowledge gaps of oral cancer-related lesions and symptoms and difficulty accessing care, leading to late-stage diagnosis.[9,10]

RISK FACTORS FOR ORAL DISEASE AMONG BLACK MEN

Despite a lack of evidence of oral disease incidence, prevalence, and outcomes, a case can be made that the collective oral health status of Black men is likely poor based on their experiences with racial health disparities, oral health–related chronic diseases, challenges accessing dental care, and a lack of social protective factors.

For example, Black adults experience more periodontal disease, untreated tooth decay, and tooth loss than White adults.[11,12] Uncontrolled diabetic patients are at increased risk for dental infections,[13] while other associations of poor oral health and disease morbidity exist for cardiovascular disease, cancer, chronic kidney disease, and HIV infection.[14-18] In addition, according to the Medical Expenditure Panel Survey,[19] in 2015, 75.4% of all non-Hispanic Blacks included in the study had some form of dental insurance. However, only 30.4% had a dental visit compared with 48.7% of non-Hispanic Whites, and Blacks had the fewest total dental visits of all racial and ethnic groups.

ACCESS AND FINANCIAL BARRIERS TO DENTAL CARE

At the center of Black men's vulnerability to oral disease is access to care.[20,21] Regardless of age, income level, and type of insurance, financial barriers to dental care are significant for the US population in general.[1,22,23] Nearly 60% of adults cite cost as a reason for not visiting the dentist,[24] and individuals with higher incomes report lower rates of untreated dental caries.[1] For Black men, financial barriers may be more pronounced. As of June 2018, the unemployment rate of Black men in the United States aged 20 years and older was 6.2%—twice the rate for White men.[25] Among men who are employed, the median usual weekly earnings of Black men is consistently lower than that of White and Asian men, and slightly higher than that of Hispanic men.[26] Also, in 2016, the median household income among Blacks was $39,490 compared with $81,431 for Asian households, $65,041 for White households, and $47,675 for Hispanic households.[27] In addition, the poverty rate for Blacks that year was 22% compared with 8.8% for non-Hispanic Whites, 10.1% for Asians, and 19.4% for Hispanics.[27] Comparisons of wealth between the two groups reveal that in 2016 the median and mean net worth of White families in the United States was $171,000 and $933,700, respectively, compared with $17,600 and $138,200, respectively, for Black families.[28] The impact of such economic disparity is that Blacks, on average, may have less financial resiliency to manage unforeseen circumstances such as job loss, living expense hikes, and sudden medical or dental ailments that may require additional income or savings to overcome. Gaps in employment, earnings, and wealth suggest that comparatively more Black men have difficulty accessing dental care and more dental disease for financial reasons alone.

LACK OF GOVERNMENT FINANCIAL SUPPORT FOR DENTAL CARE

Among other issues related to dental care utilization trends among Blacks is a lack of public assistance for low-income adults to receive dental care. Medicare does not offer dental benefits for routine oral health prevention and maintenance, and Medicaid benefits for adults are limited.[29,30] Despite the Patient Protection and Affordability Care Act not including dental coverage as an essential health benefit for adults, many adults were able to obtain dental care through Medicaid expansion programs.[31,32] However, several states have not opted to expand Medicaid eligibility, leaving many low-income, working-class Americans to fall into coverage gaps based on affordability. The impact of such outcomes disproportionately affects Black populations.[33] Even among states that do provide Medicaid dental benefits, lack of dental providers in low-income and rural areas is an additional barrier to care.[34]

Finally, Black dentists play an important role in improving access to care among the Black US population, particularly among underserved and medically compromised patients.[35] However, Black dentists make up only 3.3% of all dentists while Blacks make up roughly 13.5% of the US population.[35] A large majority of Black dental providers in the United States also practice in states that have not opted to expand Medicaid, further minimizing potential to improve access to care among Blacks in those states.

EDUCATION AND ORAL HEALTH

The significance of education is also substantial for Black men. It is known that adults aged 35 to 44 years with less than a high-school education are three times more likely to experience untreated tooth decay and periodontal disease than adults with some college education.[11] In 2015, the status dropout rate for Black males was 6.4% compared with a national rate of 5.0%.[36] In addition, the 4-year graduation rate of Blacks in the United States is 76%, compared with 88%, 79%, and 91% for Whites, Hispanics, and Asians, respectively.[37] Furthermore, although smoking prevalence is lower among Blacks than among Whites,[8] smoking rates increase as levels of education attainment decrease,[1] placing those individuals at higher risk for oral cancers and periodontal disease.[38]

ASSESSMENT OF ORAL HEALTH AMONG BLACK MEN

Despite what can be inferred regarding the oral health status of Black men, the true oral health status of Black men in the United States is difficult to assess. The National Health and Nutritional Examination Survey (NHANES), National Health Interview Survey (NHIS), Behavioral Risk Factor Surveillance System (BRFSS), and National Oral Health

Surveillance System (NOHSS) provide data surveillance to describe oral health status for populations according to social and demographic variables of age, gender, race, ethnicity, income, education, and insurance type, among other things.[39–42]

SOURCES OF ASSESSMENT DATA

NHANES provides the most extensive list of oral health measures. Questions regarding access to care, quality of life, periodontal condition, pain experience, hygiene habits, and access to information about cigarettes, diabetes, and oral cancer are assessed among other things. Time since an individual's last dental visit or whether or not an individual has had a dental visit in the past year is a common measure for oral health status among NHANES, BRFSS, NHIS, and NOHSS surveillance programs. BRFSS asks participants about oral disease experience with the question "How many of your permanent teeth have been removed because of tooth decay or gum disease?"[41] NHIS asks questions regarding tooth loss in addition to types of cancer.[40] NOHSS is a combination of data from BRFSS, the Surveillance Epidemiology and End Results data, American State and Territorial Dental Directors, and State Oral 101 Health Surveys, but mostly maintains data for children's oral health.

The main indicator for oral health in NOHSS data for adults aged 18 years and older is "whether or not an individual has had a dental visit."[42] However, other data indicators for adults aged 65 years and older have recently been prioritized. Such indicators include questions about tooth loss, untreated dental caries for individuals in long-term care or skilled nursing facilities, and dental treatment among adults aged 65 years and older who attend congregate meal sites. Objectives from *Healthy People 2020* have also determined priorities for measuring oral health status of adults[43]; of those are indicators of untreated decay, tooth loss, periodontal disease, and oral and pharyngeal cancer. However, those objectives, with the exception of oral and pharyngeal cancer detection, do not prioritize disease measurement of individuals aged 18 to 35 years. None of the data provide clinical context for true assessment of oral disease incidence, prevalence, and severity among this population. Challenges for obtaining more population-based data to characterize oral health status among this population could be attributable to low sample sizes, low response rates, and health pessimism of self-reported data.[44–47]

LIMITATIONS OF ASSESSMENT DATA

Although some surveys ask questions of neighborhood context and health-seeking behavior,[39,40] there is a lack of social and structural context within national data surveillance to support upstream interventions.[48] Any acceptance of the social determinants of health as having significant influence on poor oral health must embrace efforts that delve into the social experiences of Black men in American society. A 2018 report in the

New York Times highlighted that Black boys raised in economic 1% have the same chances of growing up poor as White boys raiseᴅ ing $36,000 per year.[49] In addition, one in three Black males born being incarcerated in his lifetime.[50] Blacks make up 13.4% of the U 37.7% of all federal inmates in US prisons are Black.[51,52] Of all federaᴵ ₃, 93.0% are male.[53] The rationales for such outcomes are complex and data suggest that they are influenced by, but not directly correlated with, income, education, or neighborhood disadvantage alone.[54] High incarceration rates among Black men exclude a disproportionate number of them from participating in national data surveillance programs. There is also a lack of oral health data among incarcerated individuals despite high levels of oral health need.[55]

Finally, independent variables in national data sets of age, income, and education do not reflect a portrait of how race and gender intersect upstream for Black men. Being college educated, married, and having high levels of social support have been shown to increase oral health utilization among Black men.[21] In addition, living in disadvantaged neighborhoods, having more material hardship, and exposure to chronic stressors have been associated with negative self-assessments of oral health status among Black men.[56-60] Such findings mirror other studies that show how after adjusting for income, education, age, and insurance, socioeconomic position may be more predictive of health outcomes, regardless of race.[6,61]

CONCLUSIONS

Collectively, the social and life experiences of Black men have profound negative effects on their opportunities for maintaining good oral health. If the end result of data surveillance is to inform policy and programs for health protection and promotion of vulnerable groups within the US population, efforts to obtain more data for Black men are needed to support multilevel interventions. Such data should intentionally inform an upstream logic of identifying and reporting health outcomes, health-seeking experiences, life experience outcomes, social and environmental influences, and structural policies that have downstream effects.

ACKNOWLEDGMENTS

The authors would like to thank Todd Ester, DDS, MS, Assistant Dean for Diversity, Equity, and Inclusion, University of Michigan School of Dentistry, Bruce Dye, DDS, MPH, Director, National Institute of Dental and Craniofacial Research, and Caswell A. Evans, DDS, MPH, Associate Dean, Prevention and Public Health Sciences, College of Dentistry, University of Illinois at Chicago.

ERENCES

1. National Center for Health Statistics. Health, United States, 2016: with chartbook on long-term trends in health. 2017: 116–117. Available at: https://www.cdc.gov/nchs/data/hus/hus16.pdf. Accessed July 21, 2018.

2. Dwyer-Lindgren L, Bertozzi-Villa A, Stubbs R, et al. Inequalities in life expectancy among US counties, 1980 to 2014: temporal trends and key drivers. *JAMA Intern Med.* 2017;177(7):1003–1011.

3. Center on Society and Health, Virginia Commonwealth University. Mapping life expectancy. September 26, 2016. Available at: https://societyhealth.vcu.edu/work/the-projects/ mapping-life-expectancy.html. Accessed July 22, 2018.

4. Centers for Disease Control and Prevention. Estimated HIV incidence and prevalence in the United States, 2010–2015. HIV Surveillance Supplemental Report. 2018;23(1). Available at: http://www.cdc.gov/hiv/library/reports/hiv-surveillance.html. Accessed July 22, 2018.

5. US Department of Health and Human Services, Office of Minority Health. Diabetes and African Americans, 2016. Available at: https://minorityhealth.hhs.gov/omh/browse.aspx?lvl= 4&lvlid=18. Accessed July 22, 2018.

6. Surveillance and Epidemiology End Results Program, National Cancer Institute. Cancer stat facts: oral and pharynx cancer. Available at: https://seer.cancer.gov/statfacts/html/oralcav. html. Accessed July 22, 2018.

7. Noone AM, Howlader N, Krapcho M, et al., eds. SEER cancer statistics review, 1975–2015. National Cancer Institute. 2018. Available at: https://seer.cancer.gov/csr/1975_2015. Accessed July 25, 2018.

8. Centers for Disease Control and Prevention. African Americans and tobacco use. 2017. Available at: https://www.cdc.gov/tobacco/disparities/african-americans/index.htm. Accessed July 25, 2018.

9. Howell J, Sheppard J, Logan H. Barriers to oral cancer screening: a focus group of rural Black adults. *Psychooncology.* 2013;22(6):1306–1311.

10. Sheppard J, Logan J, Howell J. A survey of barriers to screening for oral cancer among rural Black Americans. *Psychooncology.* 2014;23(3):276–282.

11. Centers for Disease Control and Prevention. Disparities in oral health. 2018. Available at: https://www.cdc.gov/oralhealth/oral_health_disparities/index.htm. Accessed July 22, 2018.

12. Dye B, Thornton-Evans G, Li X, Iafolla T. Dental caries and tooth loss in adults in the United States, 2011–2012. NCHS Data Brief. 2015: 197. Available at: https://www.cdc.gov/nchs/data/ databriefs/db197.pdf. Accessed July 25, 2018.

13. Lamister I, Lalla E, Borgnakke W, Taylor G. The relationship between oral health and diabetes mellitus. *J Am Dent Assoc.* 2008;139:19S–24S.

14. Akar H, Akar G, Carrero J, Stenvinkel P, Lindholm B. Systemic consequences of poor oral health in chronic kidney disease patients. *Clin J Am Soc Nephrol.* 2011;6(1):218–226.

15. Patton L. Progress in understanding oral health and HIV/AIDS. *Oral Dis.* 2014;20(3):223–225.

16. Kholy K, Genco R, Van Dyke T. Oral infections and cardiovascular disease. *Trends Endocrinol Metab.* 2015;26(6):315–321.

17. Najafipour H, Malek Mohammadi T, Rahim F, Haghdoost AA, Shadkam M, Afshari M. Association of oral health and cardiovascular disease risk factors: "results from a community based study on 5900 adult subjects." *ISRN Cardiol.* 2013;2013:782126.

18. Fitzpatrick S, Katz J. The association between periodontal disease and cancer: a review of the literature. *J Dent.* 2010;38(2):83–95.

19. Agency for Healthcare Research and Quality. Medical Expenditure Panel Survey. Research findings #38: dental services: use, expenses, source of payment, coverage, and procedure type, 1996–2015. 2017. Available at: https://meps.ahrq.gov/data_files/publications/rf38/rf38.pdf. Accessed July 22, 2018.

20. Akintobi T, Hoffman L, McAllister C, et al. Assessing the oral health needs of African American men in low-income, urban communities. *Am J Mens Health.* 2018;12(2):326–337.

21. Stapleton S, Finlayson T, Ohmit A, Hunte H. Correlates of past year dental health visits: findings from the Indiana Black men's health study. *J Public Health Dent.* 2015;76(2):157–165.

22. Vujicic M, Buchmueller T, Klein R. Dental care presents the highest level of financial barriers, compared to other types of healthcare services. *Health Aff (Millwood).* 2016;35(12): 2176–2182.

23. Gupta N, Vujicic M, Yarbrough C, Harrison B. Disparities in untreated caries among children and adults in the US, 2011–2014. *BMC Oral Health.* 2018;18(1):30.

24. American Dental Association, Health Policy Institute. Oral health and well-being in the United States. Available at: https://www.ada.org/~/media/ADA/Science%20and%20Research/HPI/OralHealthWell-Being-StateFacts/US-Oral-Health-Well-Being.pdf?la=en. Accessed July 25, 2018.

25. Bureau of Labor Statistics. Table A-2. Employment status of the civilian population by race, sex, and age. 2018. Available at: https://www.bls.gov/news.release/empsit.t02.htm. Accessed July 22, 2018.

26. Bureau of Labor Statistics. Usual weekly earnings of wage and salary workers, second quarter 2018. Available at: https://www.bls.gov/news.release/pdf/wkyeng.pdf. Accessed July 22, 2018.

27. Semega J, Fontenot K, Kollar M. Income and poverty in the United States: 2016. Current Population Reports. US Census Bureau. 2017. Available at: https://www.census.gov/content/dam/Census/library/publications/2017/demo/P60-259.pdf. Accessed July 22, 2018.

28. Dettling L, Hsu J, Jacobs L, Moore K, Thompson J, Llanes E. Recent trends in wealth-holding by race and ethnicity: evidence from the Survey of Consumer Finances. Board of Governers of the Federal Reserve System. September 27, 2017. Available at: https://www.federalreserve.gov/econres/notes/feds-notes/recent-trends-in-wealth-holding-by-race-and-ethnicity-evidence-from-the-survey-of-consumer-finances-20170927.htm. Accessed July 23, 2018.

29. Centers for Medicare and Medicaid Services. Dental care. Available at: https://www.medicaid.gov/medicaid/benefits/dental/index.html. Accessed July 25, 2018.

30. Centers for Medicare and Medicaid Services. Your Medicare coverage, dental services. Available at: https://www.medicare.gov/coverage/dental-services.html. Accessed July 25, 2018.

31. Nasseh K, Vujicic M. The impact of the Affordable Care Act's Medicaid Expansion on dental care use through 2016. *J Public Health Dent.* 2017;77(4):290–294.

32. Singhal A, Damiano P, Sabik L. Medicaid adult dental benefits increase use of dental care, but impact of expansion on dental services use was mixed. *Health Aff (Millwood).* 2017;36(4):723–732.

33. Garfield R, Damico A, Orgera K. The coverage gap: uninsured poor adults in states that do not expand Medicaid. Henry J. Kaiser Family Foundation. 2018. Available at: https://www.kff.org/medicaid/issue-brief/the-coverage-gap-uninsured-poor-adults-in-states-that-do-not-expand-medicaid. Accessed July 22, 2018.

34. Voinea-Griffin A, Solomon E. Dentist shortage: an analysis of dentists, practices, and populations in the underserved areas. *J Public Health Dent.* 2016;76(4):314–319.

35. Mertz E, Calvo J, Wides C, Gates P. The Black dentist workforce in the United States. *J Public Health Dent.* 2017;77(2):136–147.

36. National Center for Education Statistics. Table 219.70. Percentage of high school dropouts among persons 16 to 24 years old (status dropout rate), by sex and race/ethnicity: selected years, 1960 through 2015. 2017. Available at: https://nces.ed.gov/programs/digest/d16/tables/dt16_219.70.asp?current=yes. Accessed July 23, 2018.

37. National Center for Education Statistics. Table 219.46. Public high school 4-year adjusted cohort graduation rate (ACGR), by selected student characteristics and state: 2010–11 through 2015–16. 2017. Available at: https://nces.ed.gov/programs/digest/d17/tables/dt17_219.46.asp. Accessed July 25, 2018.

38. Warnakulasuriya S, Dietrich, T, Bornstein M, et al. Oral health risks of tobacco use and effects of cessation. *Int Dent J.* 2010;60(1):7–30.

39. Centers for Disease Control and Prevention, National Center for Health Statistics. National Health and Nutrition Examination Survey questionnaire (or Examination Protocol, or Laboratory Protocol). US Department of Health and Human Services. 2017–2018. Available at: https://wwwn.cdc.gov/nchs/data/nhanes/2017-2018/questionnaires/OHQ_J.pdf. Accessed July 25, 2018.

40. Centers for Disease Control and Prevention, National Center for Health Statistics. National Health Interview Survey Questionnaire. US Department of Health and Human Services. 2017.

Available at: ftp://ftp.cdc.gov/pub/Health_Statistics/NCHS/Survey_Questionnaires/NHIS/2017/english/qadult.pdf. Accessed July 25, 2018.

41. Centers for Disease Control and Prevention. Behavioral Risk Factor Surveillance System Survey Questionnaire. US Department of Health and Human Services. 2018. Available at: https://www.cdc.gov/brfss/questionnaires/pdf-ques/2018_BRFSS_English_Questionnaire.pdf. Accessed July 25, 2018.

42. Centers for Disease Control and Prevention. Oral health data. National Oral Health Surveillance System. Available at: https://www.cdc.gov/oralhealthdata/overview/nohss.html. Accessed July 25, 2018.

43. Office of Disease Prevention and Health Promotion. Oral health. 2018. Available at: https://www.healthypeople.gov/2020/topics-objectives/topic/oral-health/objectives. Accessed July 25, 2018.

44. Jackson J, Tucker M, Bowman P. Conceptual and methodological problems in survey research on Black Americans. In: Liu WT, ed. *Methodological Problems in Minority Research*. Chicago, IL: Pacific/Asian American Mental Health Research Center; 1982.

45. Williams D, Lavizzo-Mourey R, Warren R. The concept of race and health status in America. *Public Health Rep.* 1994;109(1):26–41.

46. Boardman J. Health pessimism among Black and White adults: the role of interpersonal and institutional maltreatment. *Soc Sci Med.* 2004;59(12):2523–2633.

47. Bilheimer L, Klein R. Data measurement issues in the analysis of health disparities. *Health Serv Res.* 2010;45(5):1489–1507.

48. Braveman P, Cubbin C, Egerter S, et al. Socioeconomic status in health research: one size does not fit all. *JAMA.* 2005;294(22):2879–2888.

49. Badger E, Miller C, Pearce A, Quealy K. Extensive data shows punishing reach of racism for Black boys. *New York Times.* March 19, 2018. Available at: https://www.nytimes.com/interactive/2018/03/19/upshot/race-class-white-and-black-men.html. Accessed July 25, 2018.

50. The Sentencing Project. Report of The Sentencing Project to the United Nations Human Rights Committee regarding racial disparities in the United States criminal justice system. 2013. Available at: http://sentencingproject.org/wp-content/uploads/2015/12/Race-and-Justice-Shadow-Report-ICCPR.pdf. Accessed July 23, 2018.

51. US Census Bureau. QuickFacts. Available at: https://www.census.gov/quickfacts/fact/table/US/PST045217. Accessed July 25, 2018.

52. Federal Bureau of Prisons. Inmate statistics, inmate race. 2018. Available at: https://www.bop.gov/about/statistics/statistics_inmate_race.jsp. Accessed July 25, 2018.

53. Federal Bureau of Prisons. Inmate statistics, inmate gender. 2018. Available at: https://www.bop.gov/about/statistics/statistics_inmate_gender.jsp. Accessed July 25, 2018.

54. Chetty R, Hendren N, Jones M, Porter S. The equality of opportunity project: race and economic opportunity in the United States. Executive summary. 2018. Available at: http://www.equality-of-opportunity.org/assets/documents/race_summary.pdf. Accessed July 23, 2018.

55. Makrides N, Shulman J. The oral health needs of the incarcerated population: steps toward equal access. *Am J Public Health*. 2017;107(suppl 1):S46–S47.

56. Braveman P, Kumanyika S, Fielding J, et al. Health disparities and health equity: the issue is justice. *Am J Public Health*. 2011;101(suppl 1):S149–S155.

57. Sanders A, Spencer A. Social inequality: social inequality in perceived oral health among adults in Australia. *Aust N Z J Public Health*. 2004;28(2):159–166.

58. Finlayson T, Williams D, Siefert K, Jackson J, Nowjack-Raymer R. Oral health disparities and psychosocial correlates of self-rated oral health in the national survey of American life. *Am J Public Health*. 2010;100(suppl 1):S246–S255.

59. Borrell L, Taylor G, Borgnakke W, Woolfolk M, Nyquist L. Perception of general and oral health in White and African American adults: assessing the effect of neighborhood socioeconomic conditions. *Community Dent Oral Epidemiol*. 2004;32(5):363–373.

60. Turrell G, Sanders A, Slade G, Spencer A, Marcenes W. The independent contribution of neighborhood disadvantage and individual-level socioeconomic position to self-reported oral health: a multilevel analysis. *Community Dent Oral Epidemiol*. 2007;35(3):195–206.

61. Sabbah W, Tsakos G, Watt R. The effects of income and education on ethnic differences in oral health: a study of US adults. *J Epidemiol Community Health*. 2009;63(7):516–520.

11

Oral Cavity and Pharyngeal Cancer in Black Men: Epidemiological Trends, Inequities, and Policy and Practice Implications

Darien Weatherspoon, DDS, MPH

HEAD AND NECK SQUAMOUS CELL CARCINOMA DEFINED

Head and neck squamous cell carcinoma is a comprehensive term that is generally used to describe squamous cell carcinomas found in the oral cavity, pharynx, larynx, nasal cavity, and paranasal sinuses.[1] Oral cavity and pharyngeal cancer usually refers to the subset of head and neck cancers that are identified by *International Classification of Diseases for Oncology, Third Edition (ICD-O-3)* codes C00.0–C14.8.[2] These diagnostic codes identify malignancies located in the oral cavity and the pharynx regions.

The pharynx can be subdivided into the oropharynx, nasopharynx, and hypopharynx anatomic regions. The oral cavity anatomic subsites include the lips, labial mucosa, buccal mucosa, gingiva, anterior two thirds of the tongue, hard palate, floor of the mouth, and retromolar pad.[1] The oropharynx anatomic subsites include the posterior one third (base) of the tongue, lingual and palatine tonsils, soft palate, and posterior pharyngeal wall.[1] This chapter will generally use the term "oral cancer" to refer to combined oral cavity and oropharynx squamous cell carcinomas.

Using a targeted literature review to identify relevant articles, this chapter will describe oral cancer incidence and survival trends and related disparities and inequities observed among Black men. To conclude, factors associated with the observed disparities will be reviewed, and potential multilevel solutions to reduce or eliminate inequities and improve oral cancer outcomes in Black men will be proposed.

RISK FACTORS FOR ORAL CANCER

The American Cancer Society estimates that oral cancer is currently the eighth most common type of cancer in men in the United States and that there will be approximately 51,540 new cases diagnosed and 10,030 deaths resulting from these cancers in 2018 in the United States.[3] The morbidity associated with oral cancers can have a negative impact on quality of life and well-being, as these cancers can produce many symptoms, including pain in the mouth or throat, difficulty breathing, difficulty speaking, difficulty swallowing, difficulty chewing food, and problems with denture function.[4]

It is important to understand that risk factors for oral cancers can vary depending on the exact location of the malignancies within the head and neck region.[5,6] Tobacco and alcohol are commonly identified major risk factors for cancers in the oral cavity, and these two risk factors have been shown to act synergistically when both are present.[6] Diet, socioeconomic status, and periodontal disease are other risk factors that have been found to be associated with cancers in the oral cavity region.[5,7-9]

Human papillomavirus (HPV) is an established etiological factor for cancers in the oropharynx.[10-13] The Centers for Disease Control and Prevention (CDC) estimates that HPV is associated with 70% of oropharyngeal cancers, with HPV type-16 being the specific oncogenic HPV type associated with 60% of malignancies in this region.[14] Sexual behaviors, such as oral sex, can transmit HPV and have been identified as risk factors for oral HPV infection.[5,13] Tobacco, alcohol, and diet have also been found to be associated with malignancies in oropharynx region.[5,13] In addition to common head and neck cancer risk factors such as tobacco and alcohol, Epstein-Barr virus infection can increase the risk for cancers in the nasopharynx, and ultraviolet light exposure is a major risk factor for cancers of the lip.[4]

At the population level, an overall decline in the incidence of cancers in the oral cavity region has been observed over time.[10,11] This decline in oral cavity cancer incidence has mirrored decreases in overall tobacco use and alcohol consumption in the United States over time.[10,11] By contrast, a rise in the incidence of oropharynx cancers has been observed over time, and there has been a significant increase in the prevalence of HPV-positive oropharyngeal cancers observed over time.[10,11]

INCIDENCE OF ORAL CANCER

Historical racial/ethnic and gender disparities and distinct epidemiological trends have been observed for oral cancer incidence and survival rates in the United States.[15] In a comparison of the incidence of oral cancer by gender, men have been found to have greater than two times the incidence rate of oral cancer compared with women.[16] Black men have historically demonstrated the greatest oral cancer burden and poorest outcomes among racial–gender groups in the United States.[15]

Historically, Black men have displayed higher incidence rates for oral cancers than their racial/ethnic–gender counterparts.[15,17,18] A study that used Surveillance, Epidemiology, and End Results (SEER) 9 registry data from 1977 to 1991 found that Black men had an age-adjusted incidence rate of 23.2 per 100,000 for total oral cavity and pharynx cancer compared with a rate of 12.3 per 100,000 observed in White men during the same time period.[17] However, distinct incidence trends for oral cancers by race/ethnicity have been observed over time that have altered previously observed disparities.[10,11,16,17] SEER 9 trend data from 1992 to 2007 from the same study found that although Black men still displayed a higher incidence rate for total oral cavity and pharynx cancer than White men (15.7 per 100,000 vs. 11.1 per 100,000), Black men displayed a substantial decline in incidence from the previous time period (1977–1991), thereby decreasing the disparity in incidence between Black and White men over time.[17]

A study that used SEER 18 data from 2000 to 2010 found a similar declining trend for oral cancer incidence in Black men and also found that White men had the highest oral cancer incidence rate of all racial/ethnic–gender groups during the 2000–2010 time period.[19] In contrast to declining incidence trends for both oral cavity and oropharyngeal cancer observed in Black men over time, epidemiological studies have found a significant increase in the incidence of HPV-related oropharyngeal cancers in White men since the 1990s.[5,10,17,19–21] From 2008 to 2012, White men were found to have the highest incidence of HPV-associated oropharyngeal cancer of all racial/ethnic–gender groups.[14]

Recent SEER 18 data from 2015 (the most recent data available at the time of chapter preparation) available through the National Cancer Institute's SEER Fast Stats program, indicate that White men have a higher age-adjusted incidence rate for oral cavity and pharynx cancer than Black men (18 per 100,000 vs. 13 per 100,000).[22] Table 11-1 displays age-adjusted incidence rates for oral cavity and pharynx cancer obtained from SEER's Fast Stats from 2000 to 2015 by race and gender.[22]

ORAL CANCER SURVIVAL TRENDS

Racial/ethnic disparities have also been historically observed for oral cancer survival rates in the United States.[15] Survival is a cancer statistic that describes a patient's prognosis after receiving a cancer diagnosis. It is the proportion of people who are alive for a given time period after receiving a cancer diagnosis and is commonly expressed as a 5-year relative survival rate.[24]

SEER survival data for oral cancer from the mid-1970s through the early 1990s indicated that the overall 5-year relative survival rates remained at around 50% for all races and genders combined.[15] During this time period, Black men displayed the poorest survival of all race–gender groups, with 5-year relative survival rates of close to 30%.[15] More recent SEER data from 2008 to 2014 indicate that the overall 5-year relative survival rate for oral cancer has improved over time to about 68%; however, Black men still display the poorest rate (approximately 49%) among all race–gender groups.[25] Table 11-2 displays 5-year relative survival rates from 2008 to 2014 by race and gender from SEER Cancer Statistics Review, 1975–2015.[25] Data from the SEER Cancer Statistics Review from 2008 to 2014 also show that Black men have a lower percentage of oral cancers diagnosed at the earliest (localized) stage than other race–gender groups and, when stratified by stage at diagnosis, still display poorer outcomes than their counterparts at all stages.[25]

Table 11-1. Age-Adjusted Surveillance, Epidemiology, and End Results (SEER) Incidence Rates for Oral Cavity and Pharynx Cancer by Race and Gender, 2000–2015 (SEER 18)

Year	White		Black	
	Male	Female	Male	Female
2000	16.3381	6.3460	19.5350	5.2315
2001	16.1669	6.5344	18.5034	6.1400
2002	16.3174	6.4219	18.8084	5.3998
2003	16.0591	6.0375	18.3128	6.3385
2004	16.3772	6.2491	17.4217	5.6214
2005	16.2231	6.1403	14.9801	6.0891
2006	16.2764	6.3224	15.5135	5.7484
2007	16.9344	6.2628	15.9575	6.1021
2008	17.0284	6.5141	15.0729	5.0229
2009	17.4237	6.6081	15.0982	5.5936
2010	17.0260	6.3948	14.4936	5.4593
2011	17.7952	6.4852	14.4212	5.0113
2012	17.4083	6.4217	14.5768	5.0323
2013	18.1917	6.4286	13.6116	5.0100
2014	18.1956	6.5355	14.1658	5.2220
2015	18.1496	6.4407	13.1223	5.3129

Source: Based on data obtained from the National Cancer Institute's SEER Fast Stats.[22]
Note: Cancer site = oral cavity and pharynx; data type = SEER incidence; statistic type = age-adjusted rates; incidence source = SEER 18 areas subsite = all oral cavity and pharynx; year range = 2000–2015 (SEER 18). Cancer sites include invasive cases only unless otherwise noted. Rates are per 100,000 and are age-adjusted to the 2000 US Standard Population (19 age groups — Census P25-1130).[23]

An examination of survival statistics for individuals diagnosed with HPV-associated oropharyngeal cancers, which tend to display higher survival rates because of the better response of HPV-positive cancers to chemotherapy and radiation treatment, reveals that Black men show poorer survival outcomes than their counterparts.[27–29] Smaller, regional studies have found the same racial disparity, with Black men displaying poorer oral cancer survival than other race–gender groups.[30]

ADDRESSING INEQUITIES AND IMPROVING ORAL CANCER OUTCOMES IN BLACK MEN

The current epidemiological trends described earlier in this chapter indicate that there has been some progress made in reducing disparities and inequities observed for oral cancer statistics between Black men and their counterparts. On the one hand, the observed incidence trends for oral cancer show that the rate of new (incident) cancer cases in Black men have declined over time.[5,16,17,19] In fact, the declining incidence rates for these cancers in Black men, in combination with the increasing incidence of HPV-associated oropharyngeal cancers observed in White men, has resulted in White

Table 11-2. Oral Cavity and Pharynx Cancer (Invasive) 5-Year Relative Survival by Race and Gender, 2008–2014

All Races			Whites			Blacks		
Total	Male	Female	Total	Male	Female	Total	Male	Female
67.9	67.1	69.7	69.7	69.3	70.9	49.6	48.5	52.0

Source: Based on data from Table 20.10 in Surveillance, Epidemiology, and End Results (SEER) Cancer Statistics Review, 1975-2015.[24]

Note: SEER 9 areas. Based on follow-up of patients into 2015. Expected survival rates are derived from the US Annual Life Tables.[26]

men displaying higher overall oral cancer incidence rates than Black men in recent years, which is a reverse in the disparity observed from the 1970s through the mid-2000s.[5,19,22] However, Black men who do receive an oral cancer diagnosis continue to display poorer survival than their counterparts, and this disparity has not improved over time.[25]

Lack of access to care has been identified as a factor associated with poorer oral cancer survival in Black men compared with White men.[5,27] It has been well documented that, as a group, racial/ethnic minorities have greater barriers to accessing quality oral health care and lower dental utilization than Whites.[31–33] Regular dental visits provide an opportunity for patients to receive oral cancer examinations and oral health education from a dental provider, which is important for oral cancer prevention and early detection.[5,34–36] Lower access to quality oral health care could help explain why Black men have a substantially lower percentage of oral cancers diagnosed at the earliest (localized) stage than other race–gender groups.[5,25] Early diagnosis is important because individuals with oral cancers diagnosed at the earliest (localized) stage display substantially higher survival than those with cancers diagnosed at later stages.[37]

As the incidence of HPV-associated oropharyngeal cancers rises in this country, racial differences in the prevalence of HPV-positive cancers could also help to explain observed racial disparities in oral cancer survival.[12,27,38] Previous analyses have found Whites to have a higher proportion of HPV-positive malignancies than Blacks, which could contribute to the racial disparities in survival as HPV-positive cancers have been found to respond better to radiation and chemotherapy.[12,38,39] Other inequities that have been previously mentioned as factors associated with disparities in oral cancer survival include lower socioeconomic status, a greater number of comorbidities among Blacks, racial differences in treatment, and biological and genetic factors.[25,40–42]

Poor oral cancer survival observed in Blacks, and particularly Black men, is a public health problem that must be addressed by using multilevel approaches to achieve health equity. The poor survival outcomes currently seen for Black men who r cancer diagnosis point to the importance of primary prevention efforts to cancer presentation. Public health programs aimed at reducing tobacco an are important for primary prevention and have likely contributed to the reduced racial disparities in oral cancer incidence observed over time.[5,10,11]

Policies that promote improving access to quality health care for vulnerable and underserved groups, including racial/ethnic minorities, will also be important to ensure that Black men have equal access to appropriate primary and secondary oral cancer preventive services from health care providers, such as regular oral cancer screening examinations and oral cancer education, including appropriate counseling on American Academy of Pediatrics and CDC recommendations for HPV vaccination.[5,43] Policies that expand access to public health insurance programs, increase Medicaid oral health benefits for adults, and promote evidence-based oral health workforce and service delivery models are warranted.[5,44]

Greater interprofessional collaboration between dental and medical providers could help to enhance risk reduction, early cancer detection, and patient care coordination for underserved populations, which could ultimately help to reduce racial disparities in oral cancer survival.[5] Dental and medical providers are likely to see patients that share common risk factors for oral cancers and other systemic conditions, such as tobacco use, alcohol use, and HPV infection.

Finally, more research is warranted to further identify specific factors associated with poor oral cancer survival among Black men to inform effective, evidence-based interventions to reduce these inequities. Specifically, research should consider examining biological and genetic factors, in addition to the full range of social determinants that could help to explain racial disparities in survival.[27,28,40,41]

CONCLUSIONS

Although progress has been made in reducing the number of incident oral cancer cases in Black men over time, oral cancer survival has not improved much in this population. Policy, practice, and research solutions will be necessary to reduce and eliminate disparities in oral cancer survival that have persisted among Black men to date.

REFERENCES

1. Cleveland JL, Junger ML, Saraiya M, Markowitz LE, Dunne EF, Epstein JB. The connection between human papillomavirus and oropharyngeal squamous cell carcinomas in the United States: implications for dentistry. *J Am Dent Assoc.* 2011;142(8):915–924.

2. National Cancer Institute. *ICD-O-3 site codes.* Available at: https://training.seer.cancer.gov/head-neck/abstract-code-stage/codes.html. Accessed July 23, 2018.

3. American Cancer Society. Cancer facts & figures 2018. Atlanta, GA: American Cancer Society; 2018.

4. Centers for Disease Control and Prevention. Head and neck cancers. 2018. Available at: https://www.cdc.gov/cancer/headneck/index.htm. Accessed July 23, 2018.

5. LeHew CW, Weatherspoon DJ, Peterson CE, et al. The health system and policy implications of changing epidemiology for oral cavity and oropharyngeal cancers in the United States from 1995 to 2016. *Epidemiol Rev.* 2017;39(1):132–147.

6. Rettig EM, D'Souza G. Epidemiology of head and neck cancer. *Surg Oncol Clin North Am.* 2015;24(3):379–396.

7. Conway DI, Petticrew M, Marlborough H, Berthiller J, Hashibe M, Macpherson LM. Socio-economic inequalities and oral cancer risk: a systematic review and meta-analysis of case-control studies. *Int J Cancer.* 2008;122(12):2811–2819.

8. Xu J, Yang XX, Wu YG, Li XY, Bai B. Meat consumption and risk of oral cavity and oropharynx cancer: a meta-analysis of observational studies. *PloS One.* 2014;9(4):e95048.

9. Yao QW, Zhou DS, Peng HJ, Ji P, Liu DS. Association of periodontal disease with oral cancer: a meta-analysis. *Tumour Biol.* 2014;35(7):7073–7077.

10. Chaturvedi AK, Engels EA, Anderson WF, Gillison ML. Incidence trends for human papillomavirus-related and -unrelated oral squamous cell carcinomas in the United States. *J Clin Oncol.* 2008;26(4):612–619.

11. Chaturvedi AK, Engels EA, Pfeiffer RM, et al. Human papillomavirus and rising oropharyngeal cancer incidence in the United States. *J Clin Oncol.* 2011;29(32):4294–4301.

12. D'Souza G, Kreimer AR, Viscidi R, et al. Case–control study of human papillomavirus and oropharyngeal cancer. *N Engl J Med.* 2007;356(19):1944–1956.

13. Centers for Disease Control and Prevention. HPV and oropharyngeal cancer. 2018. Available at: https://www.cdc.gov/cancer/hpv/basic_info/hpv_oropharyngeal.htm. Accessed July 23, 2018.

14. Viens LJ, Henley SJ, Watson M, et al. Human papillomavirus-associated cancers—United States, 2008–2012. *MMWR Morb Mortal Wkly Rep.* 2016;65(26):661–666.

15. Swango PA. Cancers of the oral cavity and pharynx in the United States: an epidemiologic overview. *J Public Health Dent.* 1996;56(6):309–318.

16. Brown LM, Check DP, Devesa SS. Oral cavity and pharynx cancer incidence trends by subsite in the United States: changing gender patterns. *J Oncol.* 2012;2012:649498.

17. Brown LM, Check DP, Devesa SS. Oropharyngeal cancer incidence trends: diminishing racial disparities. *Cancer Causes Control.* 2011;22(5):753–763.

18. Shiboski CH, Shiboski SC, Silverman S Jr. Trends in oral cancer rates in the United States, 1973–1996. *Community Dent Oral Epidemiol.* 2000;28(4):249–256.

19. Weatherspoon DJ, Chattopadhyay A, Boroumand S, Garcia I. Oral cavity and oropharyngeal cancer incidence trends and disparities in the United States: 2000–2010. *Cancer Epidemiol.* 2015;39(4):497–504.

20. Colevas AD. Population-based evaluation of incidence trends in oropharyngeal cancer focusing on socioeconomic status, sex, and race/ethnicity. *Head Neck*. 2014;36(1):34–42.

21. McGorray SP, Guo Y, Logan H. Trends in incidence of oral and pharyngeal carcinoma in Florida: 1981–2008. *J Public Health Dent*. 2012;72(1):68–74.

22. National Cancer Institute. Fast Stats: An interactive tool for access to SEER cancer statistics. Surveillance Research Program, National Cancer Institute. Available at: https://seer.cancer.gov/faststats. Accessed July 23, 2018.

23. National Cancer Institute. Standard populations - 19 age groups. Available at: https://seer.cancer.gov/stdpopulations/stdpop.19ages.html. Accessed November 6, 2018.

24. National Cancer Institute. SEER Cancer Statistics Review (CSR) 1975–2015. Available at: https://seer.cancer.gov/csr/1975_2015. Accessed November 6, 2018.

25. Noone AM, Howlader N, Krapcho M, et al. SEER cancer statistics review, 1975–2015. National Cancer Institute. 2018. Available at: https://seer.cancer.gov/csr/1975_2015. Accessed July 23, 2018.

26. National Center for Health Statistics, Centers for Disease Control and Prevention. Life tables. Available at: https://www.cdc.gov/nchs/products/life_tables.htm. Accessed November 6, 2018.

27. Osazuwa-Peters N, Massa ST, Christopher KM, Walker RJ, Varvares MA. Race and sex disparities in long-term survival of oral and oropharyngeal cancer in the United States. *J Cancer Res Clin Oncol*. 2016;142(2):521–528.

28. Osazuwa-Peters N, Massa ST, Simpson MC, Adjei Boakye E, Varvares MA. Survival of human papillomavirus-associated cancers: filling in the gaps. *Cancer*. 2018;124(1):18–20.

29. Saba NF, Goodman M, Ward K, et al. Gender and ethnic disparities in incidence and survival of squamous cell carcinoma of the oral tongue, base of tongue, and tonsils: a Surveillance, Epidemiology and End Results program-based analysis. *Oncology*. 2011;81(1):12–20.

30. Kolker JL, Ismail AI, Sohn W, Ramaswami N. Trends in the incidence, mortality, and survival rates of oral and pharyngeal cancer in a high-risk area in Michigan, USA. *Community Dent Oral Epidemiol*. 2007;35(6):489–499.

31. Bentley LP. Disparities in children's oral health and access to care. *J Calif Dent Assoc*. 2007;35(9):618–623.

32. Flores G, Tomany-Korman SC. Racial and ethnic disparities in medical and dental health, access to care, and use of services in US children. *Pediatrics*. 2008;121(2):e286–e298.

33. US Department of Health and Human Services. Oral health in America: a report of the Surgeon General. Rockville, MD: National Institute of Dental and Craniofacial Research, National Institutes of Health; 2000.

34. Johnson S, McDonald JT, Corsten M. Oral cancer screening and socioeconomic status. *J Otolaryngol Head Neck Surg*. 2012;41(2):102–107.

35. Ling H, Gadalla S, Israel E, et al. Oral cancer exams among cigarette smokers in Maryland. *Cancer Detect Prev.* 2006;30(6):499–506.

36. Macek MD, Reid BC, Yellowitz JA. Oral cancer examinations among adults at high risk: findings from the 1998 National Health Interview Survey. *J Public Health Dent.* 2003;63(2):119–125.

37. National Cancer Institute. Cancer stat facts: oral cavity and pharynx cancer. Available at: https://seer.cancer.gov/statfacts/html/oralcav.html. Accessed July 23, 2018.

38. Settle K, Posner MR, Schumaker LM, et al. Racial survival disparity in head and neck cancer results from low prevalence of human papillomavirus infection in Black oropharyngeal cancer patients. *Cancer Prev Research (Phila).* 2009;2(9):776–781.

39. Dayyani F, Etzel CJ, Liu M, Ho CH, Lippman SM, Tsao AS. Meta-analysis of the impact of human papillomavirus (HPV) on cancer risk and overall survival in head and neck squamous cell carcinomas (HNSCC). *Head Neck Oncol.* 2010;2:15.

40. Hayes DN, Peng G, Pennella E, et al. An exploratory subgroup analysis of race and gender in squamous cancer of the head and neck: inferior outcomes for African American males in the LORHAN database. *Oral Oncol.* 2014;50(6):605–610.

41. Ramakodi MP, Devarajan K, Blackman E, et al. Integrative genomic analysis identifies ancestry-related expression quantitative trait loci on DNA polymerase beta and supports the association of genetic ancestry with survival disparities in head and neck squamous cell carcinoma. *Cancer.* 2017;123(5):849–860.

42. Tomar SL, Loree M, Logan H. Racial differences in oral and pharyngeal cancer treatment and survival in Florida. *Cancer Causes Control.* 2004;15(6):601–609.

43. American Academy of Pediatric Dentistry. Policy on human papilloma virus vaccinations. 2017. Available at: http://www.aapd.org/media/Policies_Guidelines/P_HPV_Vaccinations.pdf. Accessed July 23, 2018.

44. Institute of Medicine. *Improving Access to Oral Health Care for Vulnerable and Underserved Populations.* Washington, DC: The National Academies Press; 2011.

12

Implementation of Dental Care Early in HIV Diagnosis Provides an Opportunity to Significantly Reduce Health Disparities in Individuals Living With HIV/AIDS

Jennifer Webster-Cyriaque, DDS, PhD, Janet H. Southerland, DDS, PhD, MPH, Kathy Ramsey, BA, RHIA, Jo-Ann Blake, MPH, RDH, Flavia Teles, DDS, DMSc, Sarah Lowman, MPH, Beatrice Williams, BA, Camden Bay, PhD, William Seaman, PhD, and Sarah Tomlinson, DDS

Overall, HIV incidence and undiagnosed HIV infection declined during 2010 to 2014 in the United States. However, regional outcomes demonstrate that southern states accounted for half of new and undiagnosed infections in 2014.[1] While overall incidence of HIV decreased during that period, its shift from a terminal to chronic illness resulted in an aging population of people living with HIV/AIDS, challenging public programs and health care organizations to meet the comprehensive health needs of HIV-infected individuals. One significantly underserved area for this population is oral health care.

Racial disparity is reflected in both HIV and oral health status. In 2016, 43% of persons living with HIV infection were Black, and 44% of all new HIV diagnoses were in Blacks.[2] HIV-positive Blacks demonstrate higher morbidity and mortality than their White counterparts.[3,4] HIV-positive Blacks also showed 40% higher virologic failure risk than Whites (unexplained by confounders).[5] Of HIV-positive Blacks, 40.8% achieved viral suppression compared with 56.3% of Whites.[3] Non-Hispanic Black and Latino/Hispanic people living with HIV/AIDS and people experiencing severe HIV symptoms are less likely to receive oral health care services than other HIV-positive individuals.[6] This observation suggests that this subset of the population may be particularly vulnerable to oral health issues and may be missing out on the potential benefits of early dental intervention.

The southeastern United States remains an epicenter for the HIV epidemic.[1] In the context of North Carolina, racial and ethnic disparities exist within the population of HIV-positive individuals in dental utilization patterns, perceived oral health needs, and oral manifestations of HIV/AIDS.[7]

Compared with HIV-positive Whites, HIV-positive Blacks were significantly more likely to have loose teeth, need extractions, and be episodic dental care utilizers.[7] These findings are particularly significant in the context of the shifting demographics[8] of HIV/AIDS in the United States, where the number of HIV-positive non-Hispanic Blacks and Latinos/Hispanics is projected to grow steadily over the next few decades.[9]

HIV-positive individuals for whom the virus is not well controlled often experience oral malignancies and manifestations that may have an impact on their ability to eat and communicate, resulting in malnutrition, discomfort, and social stigma.[10] In fact, oral manifestations of HIV/AIDS have been a useful indicator of HIV progression, and the oral cavity provides significant diagnostic utility with widespread use of the oral HIV test. Among the most common oral manifestations of HIV/AIDS is oral candidiasis. In a study by Bodhade et al., the presence of oral candidiasis was significantly correlated with a reduced CD4 cell count of less than 200 cells per milliliter.[11] Long-term highly active antiretroviral therapy (HAART) treatment is associated with improved oral health outcomes, including decreased prevalence of oral candidiasis.[12] Yet, oral health remains a challenge in the era of HAART. Periodontal disease prevalence in the HIV-positive population remains well above the 47% prevalence in the general population of adults in the United States. In the HAART era, HIV-associated salivary gland disease and medica-tion-induced xerostomia remain a challenge, both leading to increased burden of dental disease.[13]

Human papillomavirus (HPV)–associated disease, which includes oral malignancies and oral warts, has increased among HIV-infected populations in the HAART era. Previous studies have shown that HAART did not reconstitute effective immune control of HPV in the oral cavity of HIV-infected patients and that HAART initiation was fol-lowed by increased oral HPV DNA detection.[14] Hence, the prevalence of HPV-associated oral malignancies is likely to continue to increase in the modern ART era. In keeping with this, HPV-associated cancers are shown to occur more often among people with HIV and AIDS than in the general population.[15,16] While the relationship between HIV/AIDS and virus-mediated oral mucosal lesions and malignancies is well established, new evidence suggests that systemic health and social outcomes improved with early oral health intervention for HIV-positive individuals.[13]

Self-reported oral health status is worse than systemic health status among HIV-positive individuals, and access to oral health care remains a significant unmet need for this population.[17] Nearly half of HIV-positive individuals reported unmet dental needs since their HIV diagnosis.[18] Race/ethnicity, education, health insurance, and poverty level were significant ($P < .05$) predictors of unmet dental need. In the large Houston/Harris County study, those reporting unmet needs were likely to have a historical HIV diagnosis and were diagnosed HIV-positive for more than one year.[18] In newly diagnosed HIV-positive persons, during the first 12 months after an HIV/AIDS diagnosis, oral health often suffers, with increased unmet oral health needs occurring during each additional year after diagnosis.[13,19] While increased dental needs among historically diagnosed patients may relate to older age in this group compared with newly diagnosed patients,[13,20] access-to-care issues or factors related to HIV infection and immune suppression may also account for increased needs. There is a case to be made for early dental intervention in HIV.

COMPARISON STUDY AND THE CASE FOR EARLY DENTAL INTERVENTION IN THE HIV-POSITIVE POPULATION

A comparison study of the oral disease burden and dental needs of those newly diagnosed with HIV compared with those with historical HIV diagnosis was conducted.[13] Oral health problems were assessed in persons with historical HIV diagnosis and in newly diagnosed individuals with baseline data from the Special Projects of National Significance (SPNS) Oral Health Initiative Study (n = 2,178). These data were collected before care (2007–2009) and the cumulative service utilization data that were collected throughout the 24-month study period were adjusted for age, study site, language, income, last dental care visit, and dental insurance.[13]

Participants with historical HIV diagnosis were more likely to report oral problems than were newly HIV-diagnosed participants (odds ratio [OR] = 2.10). Historically diagnosed participants were more likely to require oral surgery (OR = 1.52), restorative treatment (OR = 1.35), endodontic treatment (OR = 1.63), and more than 10 oral clinic visits over the 24-month study period (OR = 2.02). The crude cumulative two-year risk of requiring prosthetic (risk difference [RD] = 0.21) and endodontic (RD = 0.11) treatment was higher among historically diagnosed participants compared with newly diagnosed participants, despite no significance after adjustment.[13]

Poor oral health outcomes were exacerbated among those who were not on HAART. Historically diagnosed participants who were not on HAART maintained the significant increase in likelihood of self-reporting poor oral health outcomes compared with newly diagnosed individuals. These outcomes included any oral problems (OR = 2.72; 95% confidence interval [CI] = 1.17, 6.34), toothaches (OR = 2.70; 95% CI = 1.57, 4.64), tooth decay or cavities (OR = 2.28; 95% CI = 1.35, 3.87), and dental sensitivity (OR = 1.74; 95% CI = 1.02 to 2.95).[13]

Setting and Design for the Comparison Study

This group was part of a prospective multicenter longitudinal study for the SPNS Oral Demonstration Project (n = 2,178). There were 196 participants enrolled in the University of North Carolina at Chapel Hill (UNC) site study. Participants aged 18 years and older who were HIV-positive and who were out of dental care for at least 12 months were eligible. Participants were referred from infectious disease specialists and community health care centers. Approval was obtained from the institutional review boards of UNC and the Evaluation Center for HIV and Oral Health at Boston University. Participants were examined and treated at the UNC Hospital Dental Clinic. The multisite centers maintained human participants' approval for the overall and individual studies.

At baseline, participants received a comprehensive examination and treatment plan. Participants were seen at least every 6 months for dental prophylaxis and/or debridement, and information was collected including caries, oral mucosal lesions, missing teeth, and periodontal metrics including probing depths, bleeding on probing, and clinical attachment level. Baseline, 12-month, and 24-month assessments were included in this analysis. At these time points, whole unstimulated saliva was collected. Comprehensive dental care for the 196 participants included dental prophylaxis at least every 6 months, scaling and root planing, oral hygiene instruction, extractions, and restorative and prosthetic dental treatment. In addition, interviews were conducted at baseline and every 6 months that collected the following data: sociodemographic characteristics, mode of HIV transmission, past substance and tobacco use, barriers to accessing oral health care since testing HIV-positive, and oral health care habits. The Oral Health Impact Profile (OHIP) and 8-item Short Form Health Survey (SF-8) instruments were completed. Interviews were conducted in both English and Spanish, and all participants gave informed consent to participate. Baseline data collection occurred from January 2008 to August 2011. Interviewers participated in a standardized training module.

Interview and sample data were entered into a Web-based database hosted by the multisite coordinating center, where the data were merged into a single multisite database. All examiners performing oral examinations and measures were calibrated to a gold standard with kappa score greater than 0.9. CD4 counts, and HIV viral load were recorded.

Periodontal measures were also obtained and recorded. In a subset of 27 participants, saliva samples were collected for the microbiome analysis. Isolation of total DNA from salivary samples was carried out using the Qiagen Blood and Tissue Kit according to manufacturer's instruction (Qiagen, Venlo, The Netherlands). Fragmented and tagged DNA was amplified by using a limited-cycle polymerase chain-reaction program. The DNA library pool was loaded on the HiSeq 2000 reagent cartridge and on the HiSeq 2000 instrument (Illumina, San Diego, CA). Microbial profiles from the oral specimens were assessed with Microbe Analyst marker data profiling (http://www.microbiomeanalyst.ca).[21]

DISCUSSION OF RESULTS

The UNC SPNS site substudy was designed to specifically assess differences between newly diagnosed and historically diagnosed participants with HIV. The UNC initiative utilized multiple concepts central to the Chronic Care Model, a proactive, planned, and population-based approach to chronic illness such as HIV. The team included infectious disease experts, dentists, a dental case manager/hygienist, and community partners.[22] Electronic medical records were accessible to both treating physicians and dentists, and self-management support for patients was provided through aggressive patient education.

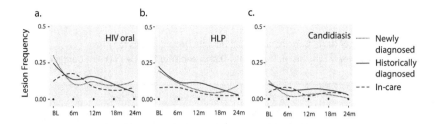

Note: BL = baseline; HLP = hairy leukoplakia. (a) HIV-associated lesions (including aphthous ulcer, hairy leukoplakia, HIV-related salivary gland disease, Kaposi's sarcoma, and candidiasis); (b) frequency of hairy leukoplakia; (c) frequency of candidiasis in newly diagnosed (dotted line), historically diagnosed (solid line), and in the in-care group (line with dashes) at baseline and 6, 12, 18, and 24 months.

Figure 12-1. Frequency of Mucosal Lesion Burden Decreases With Dental Care as Demonstrated by Loess Plots

The majority of participants were male (76.19%) and Black[3] and the mean age was 45 years (Table 12-1). All participants were provided comprehensive dental care that included oral hygiene instruction, scaling and root planing, dental prophylaxis at least every 6 months, extractions, and restorative and prosthetic dental treatment. Those with historical HIV diagnosis had fewer teeth and higher oral disease burden than the newly diagnosed group at baseline. The newly diagnosed group had a median number of 28 teeth (SD ±12.17) compared with 24 (SD ±8.96) teeth in the historically diagnosed group (Kruskal–Wallis $P < .001$). The new group had a mean number of 8.95 (SD ±12.23) decayed coronal surfaces, compared with 18.43 (SD ±29.39) in the historically diagnosed group (Kruskal–Wallis $P < .001$). The new group had a mean number of 1.93 (SD ±5.64) decayed root surfaces, compared with 8.36 (SD ±18.25) in the historically diagnosed group (Kruskal–Wallis $P < .001$). These differences in caries burden and missing teeth could contribute to lowered function and diminished nutrition.

Dental care was associated with decreased HIV-related oral mucosal lesion burden over time (Figure 12-1a). Here, HIV-related oral lesions included oral candidiasis, oral hairy leukoplakia, HIV-associated salivary gland disease, tonsil enlargement, oral Kaposi's sarcoma, and HPV-associated oral warts. Oral examination every 6 months over a 24-month period detected the highest HIV-related oral mucosal lesion burden detected at baseline in the newly diagnosed group (32%). Tonsil enlargement and cervical lymphadenopathy were more frequently detected in the newly diagnosed group. At baseline, overall lesion frequency was detected in 25% of the historically diagnosed participants without dental care and 12.5% in HIV-positive participants who had been receiving dental care.

Receiving dental care was associated with a decrease in oral mucosal lesi   ˙   ˙˙ to 12.5% or less in all groups by 24 months. The trends were also similar when frequent lesions were examinined separately—hairy leukoplakia and candi 12-1b and 12-1c).[1]

Table 12-1. University of North Carolina at Chapel Hill Site Demographics for Three
HIV-Positive Groups: Newly Diagnosed, Historically Diagnosed Who Had Been Out of Dental Care,
and In-Care Group

	Within 12 Months of HIV Diagnosis, Out of Dental Care at Baseline	HIV Diagnosis > 1 Year, Out of Dental Care at Baseline	HIV Diagnosis > 1 Year, in Dental Care at Baseline	All
	n = 63	n = 68	n = 65	n = 196
Age				
Mean years	35	44	47	42
Gender				
Male	48 (32.65%)	54 (36.73%)	45 (30.61%)	147 (75%)
Female	15 (31.25%)	14 (29.17%)	19 (39.58%)	48 (24%)
Transgender	0 (0.00%)	0 (0.00%)	1 (100.00%)	1 (0.5%)
Race/ethnicity				
American Indian or Alaska Native	0 (0.00%)	1 (100.00%)	0 (0.00%)	1 (0.5%)
Asian	0 (0.00%)	0 (0.00%)	1 (100.00%)	1 (0.5%)
Black or African American (not Hispanic)	34 (30.09%)	44 (38.94%)	35 (30.97%)	113 (57.65%)
Hispanic	9 (60.00%)	2 (13.33%)	4 (26.67%)	15 (7.65%)
White (not Hispanic)	19 (30.30%)	20 (31.82%)	24 (37.88%)	63 (32.14%)
American Indian or Alaska Native and White	1 (50.00%)	0 (0.00%)	1 (50.00%)	2 (1.02%)
Black or African American (not Hispanic) and White	0 (0.00%)	1 (100.00%)	0 (0.00%)	1 (0.5%)
Income				
Mean	1.65	1.49	1.52	1.55
Monthly	> $0 but < $1700	> $0 but < $1700	> $0 but < $1700	> $0 but < $1700
CD4, mean cells/µL				
v1 (n = 193)	485.19	462.25	510.19	485.39
v3 (n = 113)	607.21	569.15	609.14	594.13
v5 (n = 89)	738.30	690.45	648.62	691.34
HIV viral load, mean copies/mL				
v1 (n = 191)	3203.67	473.63	176.50	649.18
v3 (n = 110)	88.26	149.26	96.67	110.71
v5 (n = 88)	67.13	109.02	108.96	93.94
Education				
Mean	> High school	> High school	> High school	> High school

Note: Age, gender, race/ethnicity, income, and education levels are shown for each of the three groups. Income
categories were 0: $0; 1: > $0 but < $850; 2: $851–$1700; and 3: > $1700.

Education categories were 1: 0–11 years (less than high school); 1: 12 years (high school), 3: ≥ 13 years (more than
high school). HIV metrics are also shown at baseline (V1), 12 months (V3), and 24 months (V5). HIV viral load in
copies/mL (geomean) and mean number of CD4 cells/µL are shown for each visit.

HIV Outcomes: The Periodontal Disease Burden and the Microbiome

Periodontal Disease Burden

A high prevalence of severe periodontal disease in the UNC HIV cohort was detected across all income levels and across all ages.[23] An equivalent number of HIV-positive smokers and nonsmokers had severe periodontal disease. At baseline, gender differences were not detected, and severe periodontal disease was detected in 63% of men and in 63% of women with HIV infection. Similar percentages of men and women also were detected in the moderate disease category.

Interestingly, at baseline, periodontal measures and metrics associated with gingival inflammation were better in the newly diagnosed group than in the historically diagnosed group. The percentage of participants with extent gingival index scores greater than 1 and extent bleeding-on-probing (BOP) scores were lower in the new group compared with the historical group (gingival index = 74.03 [SD ±30.09] vs. 90.89 [SD ±18.60]; $P < .001$; and BOP = 53.17 [SD ±25.03] vs. 74.47 [SD ±21.83]; $P < .001$, respectively). In the newly diagnosed group at baseline, extent mean attachment loss of greater than or equal to 4 and BOP was 2.45 (SD ±8.53) while those in the historical diagnosis group had a mean extent attachment loss of greater than or equal to 4 and BOP of 8.04 (SD ±14.41; Kruskal–Wallis $P < .001$).

Regardless of HAART status, more than 80% of participants had moderate/severe disease. Severe periodontal disease was detected in 55% of those with undetectable viral loads and 75% of participants on short-term HAART.[22] Dental care provided significant impact with at least 50% of participants demonstrating at least one category of periodontal improvement. With care, in those on long-term HAART who were suppressed, a statistically significant improvement in periodontal status was detected (n = 28; $P = .026$).[23]

Racial differences may compound poor outcomes in the vulnerable HIV population. Severe periodontal disease is more often detected in Blacks compared with Whites (adjusted prevalence ratio [aPR] = 1.82; 95% CI = 1.44, 2.31).[24] Assessment of periodontal disease burden in a representative national sample in research by the National Health and Nutrition Examination Survey 2009–2012 detected 59.1% periodontal disease prevalence in Blacks compared with 40.8% prevalence in Whites.[25] Blacks were seven times more likely than Whites to have periodontal disease sites with severe inflammatory disease.[26]

Within the UNC cohort, severe periodontal disease was detected in 70% of HIV-positive non-Hispanic Blacks and 50% of non-Hispanic Whites.[23] The racial differences may have been associated with differences in the microbiome of non-Hispanic Blacks compared with Whites. Recent genome-wide association study results showed preferential colonization of red or orange complex periodontal disease pathogens, including *Porphyromonas gingivalis* and *Fusobacterium nucleatum* in Blacks.[27,28] Blacks were up to sixfold more likely to harbor detectable *P. gingivalis* in diseased sites,[26] with fourfold higher mean antibody concentrations for *P. gingivalis* capsular serotype K2.[29] This pathogenic bacterial profile considerably contributes to disproportionate periodontal inflammation and subsequent disease progression in Blacks.

Racial Differences in the Oral Microbiome of HIV-Positive Participants

Racial differences in the oral microbiome have been reported. In HIV-negative individuals, being Black was significantly associated with a less-diverse oral microbiome, numerically dominated by a small number of bacterial species.[30] In this study, the salivary microbiome was assessed over a two-year period in HIV-positive participants. In this UNC SPNS of 27 participants, a more diverse, more pathogenic genus-level profile was detected in Blacks compared with Whites with clear 1-effect-size differences detected in linear discriminant analysis. *Fusobacterium, Bacteroides, Porphyromonas,* and *Bergeyella* (*P* = .001) were

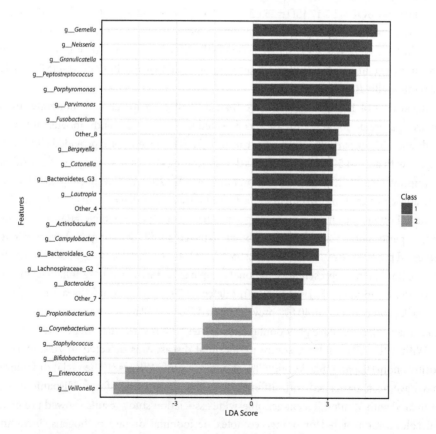

Note: g = genus; LDA = linear discriminant analysis.

Figure 12-2. Racial Differences in the Oral Microbiome in HIV-Positive Patients

associated with higher effect sizes in the Black group whereas larger effect sizes for *Bifidobacteria* ($P = .001$) and *Veillonella* were detected in the White group. This pathogenic profile in HIV-positive Black participants was associated with higher alpha diversity; however, with standard dental treatment, racial differences in bacterial diversity resolved with periodontal disease improvement at 24 months (Figure 12-2). These data suggest that, in the context of periodontal disease, HIV-positive Blacks have a more aggressive oral microbiome with higher pathogen composition than their White counterparts. Importantly, standard dental care was associated with resolution of these differences. Given the role of the microbiome in HIV, these observations can be very important.

Racial disparities have been associated with persistent immune activation and inflammation, strong independent predictors of morbidity and mortality in HIV, both of which are worse in HIV-positive Blacks than Whites.[31,32] The systemic inflammation and reduced CD4 T-cells that allow poor outcomes in HIV are thought to originate from the HIV-positive gut where circulating microbiome-driven bacterial end products (e.g., lipopolysaccharides [LPS], metabolites, short-chain fatty acids) cause persistent T-cell activation and increased chronic inflammation.[33,34] Periodontal disease mirrors the microbiome-driven process in the HIV-positive gut with enhanced microbial dysbiosis and increased proinflammatory cytokines. Translocation of microbial products is common to both immune activation in chronic HIV infection and to periodontal disease.[32,35,36] Oral bacterial LPS, fimbriae, and short-chain fatty acids are among the periodontal bacterial end products that mediate inflammation.[37–42]

Improvement in HIV Outcomes Associated With Dental Care

Comprehensive dental care was associated with improved systemic HIV outcomes over the course of the study. Mean increases in CD4 counts (cells per milliliter [cells/µL]) detected at 12 months were 75.91 cells/µL for the newly diagnosed and 75.84 cells/µL for the historically diagnosed groups. This, however, did not take HAART status into account. In the historically diagnosed group, those who had been on HAART for over 12 months and were virologically suppressed at baseline demonstrated improved periodontal status that was associated with improved CD4 ($P = .044$). In the long-term HAART-suppressed group, univariate analysis at 24 months detected a statistically significant association between improved periodontal status and increased CD4 counts ($P = .01$).[23] A recent Brazilian study determined that detectable HIV viral load was associated with elevated levels of known periodontal pathogens, such as *Prevotella nigrescens*, *Tannerella forsythia*, and *Eikenella corrodens*.[43] In this UNC SPNS study, statistically significant decreases in HIV viral load were detected in the long-term HAART group that was not suppressed at baseline. Of interest, in the group of participants that were on long-term HAART and not suppressed at baseline, univariate analysis detected highly statistically significant drops in viral load at both 12 months ($P < .001$) and 24 months ($P = .005$).[23]

een improved HIV outcomes and oral care is likely related to decreased processes in the body as a result of decreased bacterial load in the oral cavity, ntal interventions have been shown to reduce systemic inflammation, as previously demonstrated in the context of atherosclerotic vascular disease. Here, we posit that the oral microbiome contributes to microbial translocation and associated inflammation within the context of HIV. Demonstration of statistically significant improvement in periodontal disease with a clear relationship to CD4 improvement in those who were virologically suppressed suggests a role for improved local oral inflammation.

Impact of Oral Health on Quality of Life in HIV-Positive Individuals

Quality of life (QOL) was assessed, in terms of both oral health and overall health, by using well-validated instruments in the UNC SPNS population. Oral health QOL has been assessed with the OHIP.[44] At baseline (n = 188), the historically diagnosed group (n = 67) demonstrated the worst oral health QOL with a mean score of 5.81 (SD ±4.21), compared with those newly diagnosed with HIV (n = 61) whose mean OHIP score was 4.56 (SD ±3.94). Those who were receiving dental care (n = 60) demonstrated the best mean score at 4.07 (SD ±4.12).

To estimate overall health-related QOL, QOL has been previously assessed with Short Form instruments, including use of the SF-8. Previous studies suggest that the Short Form is a reliable and valid measure of health status for diverse groups of people infected with HIV.[45] We assessed QOL in 84 participants at five time points in during the UNC SPNS project. Study baseline interviews were conducted that collected the following data: mode of HIV transmission, sociodemographic characteristics, past substance and tobacco oral health care habits, SF-8, and barriers to accessing oral health care since testing HIV-positive.

Significant changes in self-perceived wellness were detected by 12 months in the newly diagnosed group and by 24 months in both the historically diagnosed group and the in-dental-care group (Figure 12-3). After 12 months of dental care, the newly diagnosed group showed the greatest improvement in their self-perceived overall QOL (P = .02). At 24 months, the historically diagnosed group showed the greatest improvement in their self-perceived overall QOL (P = .006). Improvements in mental health associated with the dental intervention were greater than those in physical health with an average change of 3.7 in the mental health composite score compared with a change of 1.7 in the physical heath composite score. Following 24 months of dental intervention, those who had been out of care (both the newly and historically diagnosed groups) demonstrated statistically significant improvements in mental health wellness (P = .006 and P = .008 respectively) and achieved mental health composite scores that were comparable with the national norm.

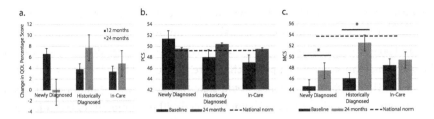

Note: (a) The mean change in quality of life (QOL) for the newly diagnosed, historically diagnosed, and in-care groups at 12 months were 6.6%, 3.8%, and 3.3%, respectively (P = .02, .13, and .15, respectively). The mean changes in QOL for the three groups at 24 months were 0.4%, 7.7%, and 4.8%, respectively (P = .95, .006, and .06, respectively). (b) Physical health component (PCS) scores were assessed at baseline (dark gray) and met the national norm (dotted line) at 24 months (light gray). PCS scores for the newly diagnosed, historically diagnosed, and in-care groups were 49.5, 50.3, and 49.4, respectively. Changes were not statistically significant. (c) Mental health composite score (MCS) were assessed at baseline (dark gray) and at 24 months (light gray) when scores approached the national norm (dotted line). MCS scores for the new, historical, and in-care groups were 47.5, 52.5, and 49.4, respectively. The change from baseline for the newly and historically diagnosed groups were statistically significant via student t test (P = .006; P = .008).

Figure 12-3. The Effect of Comprehensive Dental Care on Quality of Life in Newly Diagnosed and in Those With Long-Term HIV Based on the 8-Item Short Form Survey

The positive change in the QOL scores in the both the historical and in-care groups suggests that the study's dental intervention has a positive impact in QOL for those with long-term HIV diagnosis. Comprehensive dental care in HIV-positive individuals was associated with an increase in self-perceived overall health. Dental intervention has an impact on both oral health and overall wellness in this population.

CONCLUSIONS

Sadly, of all unmet needs, dental care remains among the top unmet needs for persons infected with HIV. Oral health in HIV is the least federally funded health care need related to HIV-positive individuals.[46] In this population, the need for dental care is at least twice as prevalent as the need for medical care.[19,47] Twenty-three percent of participants reported dental care as an unmet need in 2014.[48] Among men who had sex with men with newly diagnosed HIV, young non-Hispanic Black or Hispanic/Latino men had the lowest levels of HAART use and viral suppression and had substantial unmet needs for ancillary services that included dental care.[43] Analysis of the HIV Cost and Services Utilization Study determined that non-Hispanic Blacks, Hispanics, those exposed to HIV through drug use or heterosexual sexual contact, and those in poor physical health were less likely to have a dental visit.[6]

People living with HIV experience major problems related to disparities in oral health and often do not have access to oral health care. Improving access to preventive and restorative dental care has been shown to improve oral health outcomes and has the potential to help reduce age and racial/ethnic disparities in HIV-related health outcomes.[48] We have shown earlier that dental intervention would decrease the burden of oral hard and soft tissue infections, improve the microbial balance, improve oral health QOL and overall QOL, and potentially improve HIV outcomes. On the basis of the evidence, there is a compelling argument in support of a policy change related to oral health care for individuals living with HIV/AIDS. Such a policy would state that dental care should be included in HIV care guidelines and required to be implemented within 12 months of HIV diagnosis.

This health care policy change will require simultaneous updates in the HIV care continuum, in the membership of the provider team, and in the culture of care such that broader collaboration is supported and rapidly adopted. All contributors, including medical providers, dentists, and patients must play a role if this policy change is to be relevant. Dentists will need to establish themselves as oral health service providers willing to enter the HIV-positive care arena. Medical providers must want to lessen the impact of poor oral health on their patients' overall health. And HIV-positive individuals must value oral health's role in their health and well-being.

Not only should medicine and dentistry collaborate to improve the overall health of HIV-positive individuals, but the 2000 Report of the US Surgeon General on Oral Health has also suggested that all health care providers address oral health.[49] This unifying message has been underscored by the Institute of Medicine and by the Health Resources and Services Administration.[50,51] In today's age of health care transformation, providers are offering patient-centered, team-based care, yet dental providers are often on the periphery. Thought leaders and policymakers should acknowledge oral health's intimate relationship to overall health and outline a framework for medical–dental collaboration.

Best practices for medical teams treating HIV-positive individuals exist. In 2011, Gardner et al. observed that full benefit from HAART was achieved with knowledge of HIV-positive status, engagement in regular HIV care, and receipt of and adherence to effective HAART.[52] As a practice, the HIV care continuum consists of diagnosis, linkage to care, retention in care, prescription of HAART, and suppression of HIV. In 2014, in the United States, 85% of those infected with HIV had been diagnosed and 49% were virally suppressed.[53] However, even among those who are suppressed, we show that dental care can make a difference. Linkage to dental care as a critical ancillary health need is important and may be easily added to the existing paradigm of health care. It has been demonstrated that factors significantly associated with dental care visits for those with HIV were frequent physician visits and dental care referrals.[54]

By including dentists as members of the caregiver team, providers can improve patient outcomes by improving oral health, overall health, and well-being. Medical providers can include oral health services, such as dental assessments, patient education, and referrals to dental providers. Dental professionals contribute to the continuum of care by screening and making referrals to medical care, providing clinical dental treatment to improve oral health, providing nutritional counseling, and addressing dental pain issues. There are tangible opportunities for implementation in federally qualified health centers where dental and medical programs are physically co-located. These environments could constitute a patient-centered medical–dental home.[55] Leveraging the current medical and dental Ryan White programs for early dental intervention will help decrease cost, decrease disease burden, and ultimately improve health in our HIV/AIDS population.

With current efforts in health care to improve quality and health outcomes and decrease costs, now is the time to bring dentists more centrally and uniformly onto the caregiver team for HIV-positive individuals. Inclusion of oral health care in national HIV guidelines is needed.

In New York in 2010, in response to a lack of standardization in oral health care for people living with HIV/AIDS, the New York State Department of Health, AIDS Institute, Office of the Medical Director, hosted a forum to bring in oral health experts from across the nation. The following tasks were outlined:

- "Develop best practices in oral health & HIV"
- "Update [New York State's] oral health guidelines"
- "Develop guidelines on the role of dentists in prevention"[56]

The North Carolina Department of Health and Human Services, Division of Public Health, and its Oral Health Section plan to convene a task force in 2019 charged with addressing improvement of oral health for individuals who are living with HIV. Membership to the task force will include lead administrators and educators from both medical and dental schools, community providers, and health policy influencers. The overarching goal of the task force will be to develop a collaborative practice framework supporting the assurance that HIV-positive individuals have access to oral health services. Such a framework, if used as a best practice, could redefine the culture of health care while addressing persistent oral health disparities faced by HIV-positive patients in general and the deeper oral health disparities that HIV-positive minorities face.

The need is great. The International Advisory Panel on HIV Care Continuum Optimization released guidelines in 2015 for improved care for adults and adolescents with HIV.[57] Of the 36 recommendations offered, none addressed oral health or suggested a referral to an oral health care home. Now is the time for focused, evidence-based collaboration across disciplines to advance a broad health care agenda for people living with HIV/AIDS that includes the provision of oral health care services.

ACKNOWLEDGMENTS

We acknowledge the National Dental Association Foundation for its continued assistance in combatting oral health care disparities. This study was supported by grant H97HA07519 from the Health Resources and Services Administration (HRSA), US Department of Health and Human Services. This grant was funded through the HRSA HIV/AIDS Bureau's Special Projects of National Significance program.

REFERENCES

1. Satcher Johnson A, Song R, Hall HI. Estimated HIV incidence, prevalence, and undiagnosed infections in US states and Washington, DC, 2010–2014. *J Acquir Immune Defic Syndr.* 2017;76(2):116–122.

2. Centers for Disease Control and Prevention. HIV among African Americans. 2018. Available at: https://www.cdc.gov/hiv/group/racialethnic/africanamericans/index.html. Accessed November 12, 2018.

3. Crepaz N, Dong X, Wang X, Hernandez A, Hall H. Racial and ethnic disparities in sustained viral suppression and transmission risk potential among persons receiving HIV care—United States, 2014. *MMWR Morb Mortal Wkly Rep.* 2018;67:113–118.

4. Alcendor DJ. Evaluation of health disparity in bacterial vaginosis and the implications for HIV-1 acquisition in African American women. *Am J Reprod Immunol.* 2016;76(2):99–107.

5. Ribaudo HJ, Smith KY, Robbins GK, et al. Racial differences in response to antiretroviral therapy for HIV infection: an AIDS Clinical Trials Group (ACTG) study analysis. *Clin Infect Dis.* 2013;57(11):1607–1617.

6. Dobalian A, Andersen RM, Stein JA, Hays RD, Cunningham WE, Marcus M. The impact of HIV on oral health and subsequent use of dental services. *J Public Health Dent.* 2003;63(2):78–85.

7. Patton LL, Strauss RP, McKaig RG, Porter DR, Eron JJ. Perceived oral health status, unmet needs, and barriers to dental care among HIV/AIDS patients in a North Carolina cohort: impacts of race. *J Public Health Dent.* 2003;63(2):86–91.

8. Liu G, Sharma M, Tan N, Barnabas RV. HIV-positive women have higher risk of human papilloma virus infection, precancerous lesions, and cervical cancer. *AIDS.* 2018;32(6):795–808.

9. Hood JE, Golden MR, Hughes JP, et al. Projected demographic composition of the United States population of people living with diagnosed HIV. *AIDS Care.* 2017;29(12):1543–1550.

10. Coulter ID, Heslin KC, Marcus M, et al. Associations of self-reported oral health with physical and mental health in a nationally representative sample of HIV persons receiving medical care. *Qual Life Res.* 2002;11(1):57–70.

11. Bodhade AS, Ganvir SM, Hazarey VK. Oral manifestations of HIV infection and their correlation with CD4 count. *J Oral Sci.* 2011;53(2):203–211.

12. Satyakiran G, Bavle R, Alexander G, Rao S, Venugopal R, Hosthor S. A relationship between CD4 count and oral manifestations of human immunodeficiency virus–infected patients on highly active antiretroviral therapy in urban population. *J Oral Maxillofac Pathol.* 2016;20(3):419–426.

13. Burger-Calderon R, Smith JS, Ramsey KJ, Webster-Cyriaque J. The association between the history of HIV diagnosis and oral health. *J Dent Res.* 2016;95(12):1366–1374.

14. Shiboski CH, Lee A, Chen H, et al. Human papillomavirus infection in the oral cavity of HIV patients is not reduced by initiating antiretroviral therapy. *AIDS.* 2016;30(10): 1573–1582.

15. Jemal A, Simard EP, Dorell C, et al. Report to the nation on the status of cancer, 1975–2009, featuring the burden and trends in human papillomavirus (HPV)–associated cancers and HPV vaccination coverage levels. *J Natl Cancer Inst.* 2013;105(3):175–201.

16. Chaturvedi AK, Engels EA, Pfeiffer RM, et al. Human papillomavirus and rising oropharyngeal cancer incidence in the United States. *J Clin Oncol.* 2011;29(32):4294–4301.

17. Fox JE, Tobias CR, Bachman SS, Reznik DA, Rajabiun S, Verdecias N. Increasing access to oral health care for people living with HIV/AIDS in the US: baseline evaluation results of the Innovations in Oral Health Care Initiative. *Public Health Rep.* 2012;127(2 suppl): 5–16.

18. Mgbere O, Tabassam F, Barahmani N, Wang J, Arafat R. Determinants of met and unmet dental care needs among HIV patients receiving medical care in Houston/Harris County, 2009–2013. Paper presented at: Council of State and Territorial Epidemiologists. Annual Conference; June 4–8, 2017; Boise, ID.

19. Jeanty Y, Cardenas G, Fox JE, et al. Correlates of unmet dental care need among HIV-positive people since being diagnosed with HIV. *Public Health Rep.* 2012;127(suppl 2):17–24.

20. Burger-Calderon R, Ramsey KJ, Dolittle-Hall JM, et al. Distinct BK polyomavirus non-coding control region (NCCR) variants in oral fluids of HIV-associated salivary gland disease patients. *Virology.* 2016;493(suppl C):255–266.

21. Dhariwal A, Chong J, Habib S, King I, Agellon LB, Xia J. MicrobiomeAnalyst: a web-based tool for comprehensive statistical, visual and meta-analysis of microbiome data. *Nucleic Acids Res.* 2017;45(W1):W180–W188.

22. Southerland JH, Webster-Cyriaque J, Bednarsh H, Mouton CP. Interprofessional collaborative practice models in chronic disease management. *Dent Clin North Am.* 2016;60(4):789–809.

23. Valentine J, Sanders AE, Saladyanant T, et al. Impact of periodontal intervention on local inflammation, periodontitis and HIV outcomes. *Oral Dis.* 2016;22(suppl 1):87–97.

24. Eke PI, Wei L, Thornton-Evans GO, et al. Risk indicators for periodontitis in US adults: NHANES 2009 to 2012. *J Periodontol.* 2016;87(10):1174–1185.

25. Eke PI, Dye BA, Wei L, et al. Update on prevalence of periodontitis in adults in the United States: NHANES 2009 to 2012. *J Periodontol.* 2015;86(5):611–622.

26. Beck JD, Koch GG, Zambón JJ, Genco RJ, Tudor GE. Evaluation of oral bacteria as risk indicators for periodontitis in older adults. *J Periodontol.* 1992;63(2):93–99.

27. Divaris K, Monda KL, North KE, et al. Genome-wide association study of periodontal pathogen colonization. *J Dent Res.* 2012;91(7 suppl):S21–S28.

28. Socransky SS, Haffajee AD, Cugini MA, Smith C, Kent RL. Microbial complexes in subgingival plaque. *J Clin Periodontol.* 1998;25(2):134–144.

29. Califano JV, Schifferle RE, Gunsolley JC, Best AM, Schenkein HA, Tew JG. Antibody reactive with *Porphyromonas gingivalis* serotypes K1-6 in adult and generalized early-onset periodontitis. *J Periodontol.* 1999;70(7):730–735.

30. Mason MR, Nagaraja HN, Camerlengo T, Joshi V, Kumar PS. Deep sequencing identifies ethnicity-specific bacterial signatures in the oral microbiome. *PLoS ONE.* 2013;8(10): e77287.

31. Douek DC. Immune activation, HIV persistence, and the cure. *Top Antivir Med.* 2013;21(4): 128–132.

32. Hunt PW. HIV and inflammation: mechanisms and consequences. *Curr HIV/AIDS Rep.* 2012;9(2):139–147.

33. Raab-Traub N. Novel mechanisms of EBV-induced oncogenesis. *Curr Opin Virol.* 2012;2(4): 453–458.

34. Webster-Cyriaque J, Middeldorp J, Raab-Traub N. Hairy leukoplakia: an unusual combination of transforming and permissive Epstein-Barr virus infections. *J Virol.* 2000;74(16): 7610–7618.

35. Lederman MM, Funderburg NT, Sekaly RP, Klatt NR, Hunt PW. Residual immune dysregulation syndrome in treated HIV infection. *Adv Immunol.* 2013;119:51–83.

36. Salas JT, Chang TL. Microbiome in human immunodeficiency virus infection. *Clin Lab Med.* 2014;34(4):733–745.

37. Assinger A, Laky M, Badrnya S, Esfandeyari A, Volf I. Periodontopathogens induce expression of CD40L on human platelets via TLR2 and TLR4. *Thromb Res.* 2012;130(3):e73–e78.

38. Clark RB, Cervantes JL, Maciejewski MW, et al. Serine lipids of *Porphyromonas gingivalis* are human and mouse toll-like receptor 2 ligands. *Infect Immun.* 2013;81(9):3479–3489.

39. Cueno ME, Ochiai K. Re-discovering periodontal butyric acid: new insights on an old metabolite. *Microb Pathog.* 2015;94:48–53.

40. Fleetwood AJ, O'Brien-Simpson NM, Veith PD, et al. *Porphyromonas gingivalis*–derived RgpA-Kgp complex activates the macrophage urokinase plasminogen activator system: implications for periodontitis. *J Biol Chem.* 2015;290(26):16031–16042.

41. Fujita Y, Nakayama M, Naito M, et al. Hemoglobin receptor protein from *Porphyromonas gingivalis* induces interleukin-8 production in human gingival epithelial cells through stimulation of the mitogen-activated protein kinase and NF-κB signal transduction pathways. *Infect Immun.* 2014;82(1):202–211.

42. Takahashi N. Microbial ecosystem in the oral cavity: metabolic diversity in an ecological niche and its relationship with oral diseases. *Int Congr Ser.* 2005;1284:103–112.

43. Singh S, Bradley H, Hu X, Skarbinski J, Hall HI, Lansky A. Men living with diagnosed HIV who have sex with men: progress along the continuum of HIV care—United States, 2010. *MMWR Morb Mortal Wkly Rep*. 2014;63(38):829–833.

44. John MT, Slade GD, Szentpétery A, Setz JM. Oral health–related quality of life in patients treated with fixed, removable, and complete dentures 1 month and 6 to 12 months after treatment. *Int J Prosthodont*. 2004;17(5):503–511.

45. Delate T, Coons SJ. The discriminative ability of the 12-item Short Form Health Survey (SF-12) in a sample of persons infected with HIV. *Clin Ther*. 2000;22(9):1112–1120.

46. Benjamin RM. Oral health care for people living with HIV/AIDS. *Public Health Rep*. 2012;127(suppl 2):1–2.

47. Lennon CA, White AC, Finitsis D, et al. Service priorities and unmet service needs among people living with HIV/AIDS: results from a nationwide interview of HIV/AIDS housing organizations. *AIDS Care*. 2013;25(9):1083–1091.

48. DeGroote N, Korhonen L, Shouse R, Valleroy L, Bradley H. Unmet needs ancillary services among men who have sex with men and who are receiving HIV medical care—United States, 2013–2014. *MMWR Morb Mortal Wkly Rep*. 2016;65(37):1004–1007.

49. US Department of Health and Human Services. Oral health in America: a report of the Surgeon General. 2000. Available at: https://profiles.nlm.nih.gov/ps/access/NNBBJT.pdf. Accessed November 26, 2018.

50. Institute of Medicine. Advancing Oral Health in America. Washington, DC: National Academies Press; 2011.

51. Health Resources and Services Administration. Oral health: people with HIV/AIDS. Available at: http://www.hrsa.gov/publichealth/clinical/orgalhealth/hivaids.html. Accessed June 30, 2011.

52. Gardner EM, McLees MP, Steiner JF, Del Rio C, Burman WJ. The spectrum of engagement in HIV care and its relevance to test-and-treat strategies for prevention of HIV infection. *Clin Infect Dis*. 2011;52(6):793–800.

53. Centers for Disease Control and Prevention. HIV continuum of care, US, 2014, overall and by age, race/ethnicity, transmission route and sex. 2017. Available at: https://www.cdc.gov/nchhstp/newsroom/2017/HIV-Continuum-of-Care.html. Accessed October 22, 2018.

54. Metsch LR, Pereyra M, Messinger S, et al. Effects of a brief case management intervention linking people with HIV to oral health care: Project SMILE. *Am J Public Health*. 2015;105(1):77–84.

55. Advisory Committee on Training in Primary Care Medicine and Dentistry. Coming home; the patient-centered medical–dental home in primary care training. Seventh annual report to the secretary of the US Department of Health and Human Services and Congress. 2008. Available at: http://hrsa.gov/advisorycommittees/bhpradvisory/actpcmd/Reports/seventhreport.pdf. Accessed October 20, 2018.

56. New York State Department of Health AIDS Institute, Office of the Medical Director. Priorities in HIV and Oral Health: Report of a National Oral Health Forum. Available at: https://www.health.ny.gov/diseases/aids/providers/reports/docs/oral_health.pdf. Accessed November 26, 2018.

57. The International Advisory Panel on HIV Care Continuum Optimization. IAPAC guidelines for optimizing the HIV care continuum for adults and adolescents. *J Int Assoc Provid AIDS Care.* 2015;14(suppl 1):S3–S34.

13

Oral Health Disparities and Inequities in Asian Americans and Pacific Islanders*

Huong Le, DDS, Sherry Hirota, Julia Liou, MPH, Tiffany Sitlin, Curtis Le, and Thu Quach, PhD, MPH

Oral health does not just affect the mouth, but can also have a significant impact on one's overall health. Poor oral health can affect chronic diseases and be affected by these health conditions. Toothaches, caries, missing teeth, and periodontal diseases can cause considerable pain and low self-esteem, which can affect quality of life. Poor oral health has a disproportionate impact on racial/ethnic minority populations, limited-English-proficient populations, and low-income populations.[1] Risk factors for poor oral health include lack of dental insurance and access to dental care.[2]

Asian Americans and Pacific Islanders are the fastest-growing population in the nation,[3] yet remain the most understudied. Much of the data on this ethnically diverse population are aggregated, leading to hidden health disparities within some of the ethnic groups. Despite the limited disaggregated data, some evidence of oral health disparities among Asian Americans and Pacific Islanders exists. In California, 44% of low-income Asian Americans and Pacific Islander (AAPI) preschoolers had developed early childhood caries, one of the highest rates among all ethnic/racial groups.[4] AAPI children were also significantly more likely than White children to have teeth in suboptimal condition.[5] Absent of such data, dental providers serving the AAPI population are a valuable resource for identifying and addressing oral health disparities.

Drawing upon the experiences of a federally qualified health center (FQHC) serving Asian Americans and Pacific Islanders, this editorial highlights oral health disparities faced by Asian Americans and Pacific Islanders, and how FQHCs can play a major role in addressing them.

ACCESS TO DENTAL CARE AT A FEDERALLY QUALIFIED HEALTH CENTER

For medically underserved populations, including Medicaid enrollees, FQHCs have become the mainstay of US safety nets. A vast majority of the 24 million FQHC patients are disproportionately low-income, limited-English-proficient, racial/ethnic minorities

---

*This is a modified version of the article that appeared in the *American Journal of Public Health*. See: Le H, Hirota S, Liou J, Sitlin T, Le C, Quach T. Oral health disparities and inequities in Asian Americans and Pacific Islanders. *Am J Public Health*. 2017;107(suppl 1):S34–S35.

and tend to suffer from poorer health compared with the general population.[6] The presence of dental programs in FQHCs addresses a number of barriers to access and quality dental care, including affordability, and cultural and linguistic competency, as well as enhances the opportunity to provide whole-person care.

Founded in 1974, Asian Health Services (AHS) is an FQHC in Oakland, California, serving 27,000 patients. Asian Health Services provides comprehensive primary care, behavioral health services, and dental care in English and 12 Asian languages. Nearly 70% of AHS patients are limited-English-proficient. Asian Health Services opened its first dental clinic in 2003, and now has two dental clinics and three school-based sites, serving nearly 6,000 patients, of its 27,000 primary care patients.

Having had little to no dental care in their native country, many AAPI immigrants and refugees come to the United States with poor oral health and in need of critical dental care. Figure 13-1 shows some of the dental outcomes among AHS dental patients, taken from its dental electronic health records. In the fiscal year 2015–2016, 51.7% of AHS's patients had untreated tooth decay compared with the national average of 18.9%.[8] Similarly, 61.1% of AHS's dental patients aged between 20 and 64 years had a missing tooth compared with the national average of 51.8%. These results highlight some of the oral health disparities among Asian Americans and Pacific Islanders that often go unidentified because of the limited data.

Affordable and Patient-Centered Dental Care

Access to oral health care for low-income populations is a major challenge because many private dental providers do not accept Medicaid coverage, which is the primary payer source of low-income populations. Federally qualified health centers rely on Medicaid as a primary funding source for providing dental services to its low-income patients. Because the provision of adult dental services is optional in the Medicare/Medicaid Act, a state is not obligated to offer adult dental services in its Medicaid scope. This can leave Medicaid patients vulnerable as dental services can be cut in a budget deficit year. Thus, it is important that dental services become part of the mandatory benefits in Medicaid.

Rooted in the patient-centered care concept, the idea of colocation and coordination of medical and dental care on-site is to increase access to and utilization of dental care for low-income and underserved patients. Integration of care, for primary care, dental, and behavioral health, enhances the opportunity to provide whole-person care. One of AHS's school-based clinic sites provides primary care, mental health care, and dental care.

Building a Workforce Pipeline

A shortage of culturally and linguistically competent dental providers contributes to major problems with access to care. Recognizing the need for workforce development, AHS has participated since 2003 in a national dental pipeline effort, in which it has

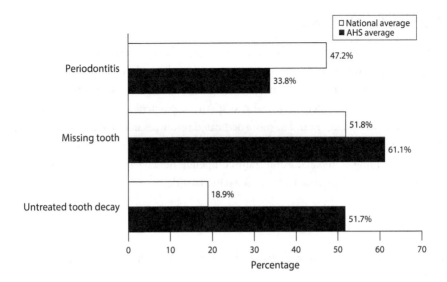

Note: Periodontitis is among those who are aged 30 years and older; national average from Eke et al.[7] Missing tooth is among those who are aged 20–64 years who have lost their permanent teeth; national average from Dye et al.[8] National average for untreated tooth decay from Dye et al.[8]

Figure 13-1. Dental Outcomes of Asian Health Services (AHS) Patients (n = 5620): United States, Fiscal Year 2015–2016

developed sustainable partnerships with dental schools to invest in future dental providers. Through it, AHS has attracted a number of dental students and residents interested in working in the AAPI community. Under the mentorship of bilingual and bicultural providers and staff, these individuals are given opportunities to obtain on-the-job cultural competency training, ultimately building a pipeline for a culturally competent workforce. The financial benefit of this pipeline has been evidenced by the significant contribution it has made to clinic productivity and finances.[9]

Social Determinants of Health

Social factors can affect oral health, which can have a reciprocal effect on such factors. For example, an adult with no dental care to fix his or her missing teeth may suffer discrimination in employment, thus impacting the family's income.[1] As such, FQHCs provide an array of enabling services (i.e., nonclinical services that increase access to health care and improve health outcomes) to address these social determinants of health, including interpretation services, health education, and health coverage assistance. In addition, AHS takes an active role in promoting public policies (e.g., promoting tobacco and soda taxation) aimed at addressing social inequities that can have an impact on oral and overall health.

RECOMMENDATIONS

Dental care is integral to overall heath and should be integrated with primary care. Federally qualified health centers can play a major role as they provide culturally and linguistically competent care, advocate the right to such services, and provide critical data that illuminate hidden oral health disparities, particularly for the understudied AAPI population. There should be more dedicated resources invested in starting up dental clinics within FQHCs serving Asian Americans and Pacific Islanders, as well as recruiting, training, and placing culturally competent dental care providers at FQHCs to serve underserved Asian Americans and Pacific Islanders.

ACKNOWLEDGMENTS

We would like to thank Masa Tsutsumi for his data collection and Khanh Nguyen for editing.

REFERENCES

1. Cantu R. Taking a bite out of oral health inequities: promoting equitable oral health policies for communities of color. California Pan-Ethnic Health Network. 2016. Available at: http://cpehn.org/blog/201601/taking-bite-out-oral-health-inequities. Accessed October 20, 2016.

2. Manski RJ. Public programs, insurance, and dental access. *Dent Clin North Am.* 2009;53(3): 485–503.

3. The Asian Population: 2010. Washington, DC: US Census Bureau; 2012.

4. Weintraub JA, Ramos-Gomez F, JueB, et al. Fluoride varnish efficacy in preventing early childhood caries. *J Dent Res.* 2006;85(2):172–176.

5. Flores G, Lin H. Trends in racial/ethnic disparities in medial and oral health, access to care, and use of services in US children: has anything changed over the years? *Int J Equity Health.* 2013;12:10.

6. National Association of Community Health Centers. United States health center fact sheet. 2016. Available at: http://nachc.org/wp-content/uploads/2015/06/Americas-Health-Centers-March-2016.pdf. Accessed October 5, 2016.

7. Eke PI, Dye BA, Wei L, et al. Prevalence of periodontitis in adults in the United States: 2009 and 2010. *J Dental Res.* 2012;91(10):914–920.

8. Dye BA, Thornton-Evans G, Li X, Iafolla TJ. Dental caries and tooth loss in adults in the United States, 2011–2012. Centers for Disease Control and Prevention. 2015. NCHS Data Brief No. 197. Available at: http://www.cdc.gov/nchs/products/databriefs/db197.htm. Accessed October 15, 2016.

9. Le H, McGowan TL, Bailit HL. Community-based dental education and community clinic finances. *J Dent Educ.* 2011;75(10):S48–S53.

14

Improving Access to Oral Health Services Among Uninsured and Underserved Populations: FirstHealth Dental Care Centers*

Sharon Nicholson Harrell, DDS, MPH, FAGD, FICD, Marguerite Ro, DrPH, and Lisa Gaarde Hartsock, MPH

In 1998, as part of the W.K. Kellogg Foundation Community Voices Initiative, FirstHealth of the Carolinas, a regional health care network, took up the challenge of eliminating long-standing rural disparities in access to oral health services by opening the first of three pediatric dental care centers serving Hoke, Montgomery, and Moore counties in North Carolina. Since the opening of these dental public health practices in private settings, a plethora of factors have changed. Shifts in demographics and insured status, demand for services, and economic backing have all contributed to an altered landscape for the FirstHealth model.

Ensuring access to oral health services is crucial in efforts to eliminate oral health disparities. However, from a business perspective, stand-alone dental care delivery models that focus primarily on safety-net populations may not be sustainable. Here we describe how FirstHealth has continued to address disparities in access to oral health services among rural low-income children while adjusting to the changing fiscal environment.

DISPARITIES

A local oral health task force in North Carolina identified oral health care as the primary unmet need among low-income children in the state's Sandhills region. Inadequate access to oral health care results in preventable oral disease and conditions. In general, dental provider shortages in rural areas are well documented. In the case of low-income and minority populations, this issue is compounded by a lack of dentists who accept Medicaid and, with recent increases in racial/ethnic diversity, the need for more culturally and linguistically responsive care.[1]

---

*This is a modified version of the article that appeared in the *American Journal of Public Health*. See: Harrell SN, Ro M, Hartsock LG. Improving access to oral health services among uninsured and underserved populations: FirstHealth dental care centers. *Am J Public Health*. 2017;107(suppl 1):S48–S49.

Table 14-1. Comparison of the Percentages of Kindergarten Children With Untreated Tooth Decay Before and After Introduction of FirstHealth Dental Care Centers: Three North Carolina Counties and the State as a Whole, 1997–1998 and 2013–2014

	Children With Decayed Teeth, %	
Area	1997–1998	2013–2014
Hoke County	33	11
Montgomery County	38	21
Moore County	23	17[a]
State overall	23	13

Source: Data were derived from the North Carolina Department of Health and Human Services.[3]
[a]The latest data for Moore County are for 2009–2010.

In the late 1990s, private practice offices in the region were at capacity owing to the large number of retirees in the area and the fact that few dentists accepted Medicaid. Furthermore, there were only 47 practicing pediatric dentists in North Carolina.[2] In the three counties of Hoke, Montgomery, and Moore, there were 12 000 medically underserved children without access to dental care. FirstHealth took the innovative step of building dental care centers under the auspices of a hospital system, and these centers provide comprehensive dental care to underserved children up to the age of 21 years.

The most significant racial/ethnic demographic shift in Hoke, Montgomery, and Moore counties has been the increase in the Hispanic population (between 2000 and 2015, the Hispanic populations in these counties increased by 5.2%, 5.1%, and 2.4%, respectively). The FirstHealth clinic populations reflect the same shift observed in the general population. Over the past 12 years, the growth in Hispanic patients has outpaced that of all other racial groups. The percentage of Caucasians in the clinic populations has decreased from 38% to 21%, the percentage of African Americans has decreased from 42% to 34%, and the percentage of Hispanics has more than doubled, from 16% to 34%.

FirstHealth's response has been swift and deliberate, providing bilingual staff members in each office and translating all clinic materials into Spanish. Although the technical aspects of interpretation and translation are paramount, even more important are the cultural sensitivity efforts made to meet the needs of the Spanish-speaking population and to increase dental health literacy.

Results since the dental centers' inception have been significant in terms of pediatric oral health status. The data in Table 14-1 show the percentage of kindergartners with decayed teeth in the 1997–1998 school year, before the centers opened, as compared with the latest data for children in the region.[3]

FINANCING

In response to the evolving fiscal environment, FirstHealth has made explicit efforts to improve enrollment and retention of patients eligible for Medicaid or other public coverage. Also, it has sought supplemental financial support to offset "loss leader" services (e.g., a dental service for which reimbursement does not cover the expense of delivering the service).

Medicaid is a crucial component in the financing and sustainability of the dental care centers. FirstHealth has made concerted efforts to help the families and individuals eligible for the program apply for Medicaid or Health Choice (Children's Health Insurance Program). The number of insured patients has increased dramatically since the centers opened, with an insured rate of 72% across the three centers in 1998 as compared with the current rate of 96%.

Even with the increases in coverage, the dental care centers are at high risk for being loss leaders as a result of shifting Medicaid reimbursement rates. Over the past 12 years, there have been notable changes in Medicaid reimbursement.

In 2000, plaintiffs (low-income Medicaid children in North Carolina) brought a lawsuit against the North Carolina Department of Health and Human Services challenging the adequacy of dental reimbursement rates and the state's efforts to ensure access to dental care. As part of the settlement of the *Antrican v. Bruton* case in 2003, the Division of Medical Assistance increased the reimbursement rates for a selected list of dental procedures commonly provided to children.[4] Although the increase in Medicaid reimbursement did not influence the payor mix, the centers had a positive bottom line in the full year after the increase for the first time since their inception. In the following years, Medicaid reimbursement has fluctuated, with sharp decreases in the last seven years. Since 2009, although operating costs have stabilized as a result of stream-lining, Medicaid reimbursements have decreased by 9.52%.[5]

Being part of a larger system has been critical to the sustainability of the dental care centers, as FirstHealth has financial mechanisms in place to offset loss leader services (albeit fewer such mechanisms than in the early 2000s owing to recent increases in charity care across the system as a whole). A "stand-alone" clinic would not be able to shift any debt at all.

The Foundation of FirstHealth has also played a vital and significant role, first by supplementing capital support and second by providing an annual disbursement that serves as a buffer between Medicaid reimbursements and program operating expenses. The annual disbursement offsets almost 40% of the net income loss. In addition, the Foundation of FirstHealth has established a dental care endowment that will allow the centers to use interest to offset any additional losses when a target amount is reached.

Financially maintaining an existing successful dental public health program becomes more difficult each year. To sustain the dental care centers, FirstHealth is exploring options that include diversifying the payor mix. Although commercial insurance is not broadly accepted, the clinics have opened the practices to the children of FirstHealth employees. The dental care centers' service population remains 99% Medicaid, Health Choice, and uninsured, low-income self-pay, and thus the threat of patients losing services owing to their finances continues.

CONCLUSIONS

With nearly two decades of delivering care, FirstHealth's experiences can provide lessons for other communities addressing oral health needs. Most important, FirstHealth has demonstrated the role that a health care system can play in addressing oral health disparities. By adding pediatric dental care centers, FirstHealth has expanded access to oral health services among at-risk children, and it continues its efforts to ensure culturally and linguistically appropriate care for an increasingly diverse population.

FirstHealth also demonstrates how a large health system can be part of the dental safety net and respond to an ever-evolving fiscal environment. Dental care staff continue to help many uninsured families enroll in Medicaid so that they can receive much-needed care. In addition, FirstHealth continues to seek other sources of funding to address evolving changes in Medicaid reimbursement.

The dental care centers' membership in a large health system has been a major component in ensuring their financial sustainability. FirstHealth has an undaunted commitment to improving the oral health of children and will continue to pilot, model, and seek strategies that lead to oral health equity regardless of place, income, or race/ethnicity.

REFERENCES

1. Bayne A, Knudson A, Garg A, Kassahun M. Promising practices to improve access to oral health care in rural communities. Available at: http://www.norc.org/PDFs/Walsh%20Center/Oral_Rural%20Evaluation%20Issue%20Brief-6pg_mm.pdf. Accessed March 14, 2017.

2. North Carolina Institute of Medicine Task Force on Dental Care Access. *Report to the North Carolina General Assembly and to the Secretary of the North Carolina Department of Health and Human Services*. Morrisville, NC: North Carolina Institute of Medicine; 1999.

3. North Carolina Department of Health and Human Services. North Carolina oral health. Available at: https://www2.ncdhhs.gov/dph/oralhealth. Accessed March 14, 2017.

4. North Carolina Institute of Medicine Task Force on Dental Care Access. 2003 update: report to the North Carolina General Assembly and to the secretary of the North Carolina Department of Health and Human Services. Available at: http://www.nciom.org/wp-content/uploads/2003/01/dentalupdate03.pdf. Accessed March 14, 2017.

5. Baker D. *Documentation of Medicaid Rate Changes*. Raleigh, NC: North Carolina Department of Health and Human Services; 2016.

15

Oral Health Care Receipt and Self-Rated Oral Health for Diverse Asian American Subgroups in New York City*

Molly Jung, MPH, Simona C. Kwon, DrPH, Neile Edens, PhD,
Mary E. Northridge, PhD, MPH, Chau Trinh-Shevrin, DrPH, and
Stella S. Yi, PhD, MPH

Asian Americans are the fastest growing immigrant group in the United States.[1] Yet, evidence-based programs and policies to promote health are not possible, because they often are not represented in research. In recent data from New York City, Asian American adults compared with other racial/ethnic groups were most likely to report not having seen a dentist in the past year.[2,3] Similarly, Asian American children were most likely to never have had a dental visit[4] and to have a high prevalence of dental caries.[5] Asian Americans in previous studies have been represented predominantly by Chinese Americans or in aggregate.[2-6] Whether results disaggregated by Asian American subgroup show different findings is unknown. Our objectives were to identify determinants of receipt of annual oral health examinations and self-rated oral health in a diverse sample of Asian Americans.

METHODS

We conducted a cross-sectional analysis of data from the Community Health Resources and Needs Assessment at the NYU School of Medicine Center for the Study of Asian American Health. This in-person community-based survey of low-income, self-identifying adults of Asian descent was conducted in the New York City metropolitan region from 2013 to 2016 and was administered in the participant's preferred language.

Oral Health Outcomes

To assess receipt of an annual oral health examination, participants were asked, "When was the last time, if ever, you received a check-up for oral/dental health?" Responses included the following: in the past 12 months, 1 to 2 years ago, 2 to 3 years ago, 3 or more

*This is a modified version of the article that appeared in the *American Journal of Public Health*. See: Jung M, Kwon SC, Edens N, Northridge ME, Trinh-Shevrin C, Yi SS. Oral health care receipt and self-rated oral health for diverse Asian American subgroups in New York City. *Am J Public Health*. 2017;107(suppl 1):S94–S96.

years ago, and never. Receipt of an oral health examination was categorized into a binary variable (in the past 12 months vs. other responses). Self-rated condition of the mouth and teeth was evaluated by the following question: "How would you describe the condition of your mouth and teeth?" Responses included the following: very good, good, fair, and poor. Self-rated condition of the mouth and teeth was categorized into a binary variable (poor vs. other responses).

Determinants

The following potential determinants of oral health care that were identified a priori were included in the analysis: age (18–44, 45–64, or ≥65 years), gender, residence (each of the 5 New York City boroughs and other, which included neighboring areas in New Jersey), ethnic group (South Asian [Asian Indian, Bangladeshi, Pakistani, Himalayan, Sri Lankan], East Asian [Chinese, Korean, Japanese], Southeast Asian [Filipino, Vietnamese, Cambodian], and Arab), nativity (US-born or foreign-born), English fluency (very well, well, not well, or not at all), education (< high school, high school/some college, or college), currently working, income (< $25,000, $25,000–$55,000, > $55,000, or missing), self-rated health (excellent, very good, good, fair, and poor), and dental insurance (public, private, or none).

Statistical Analysis

We used frequencies to assess the distributions of nonreceipt of annual oral health examinations and self-rated oral health by potential determinants. We used multivariable logistic regression models to estimate odds ratios and 95% confidence intervals (CI) to assess the associations between the potential determinants and the receipt of oral health care and self-rated oral health. All tests were considered statistically significant at $P < .05$. Analyses were performed in Stata version 14.0 (StataCorp LP, College Station, TX).

RESULTS

The analytic sample was composed of 1,288 of the initial 1,537 participants (we excluded people missing oral health data, n = 123; missing covariate data, n = 126). Half of the study participants were aged between 18 and 44 years (49%); 57% were women. The largest ethnic group represented was South Asian (42%), followed by East Asian (31%), Southeast Asian (19%), and Arab (8%). Participants were mostly foreign-born (90%) and had various levels of English fluency (31% reported speaking English very well, whereas 7% reported not speaking English at all). The participants were highly educated (40% college educated), yet the household income level was low (26% earned more than $55,000). Forty percent reported not working, and 16% reported no dental insurance.

The prevalence of nonreceipt of annual oral health examinations was 41.5% and was higher in younger than in older adults and in men than in women. Participants lacking receipt of annual oral health examinations were more likely to live in the Bronx (Table 15-1), be of Southeast Asian background, have poorer English fluency, have lower educational attainment, self-report moderate health, and lack dental insurance. In multivariable analyses, ethnic group was not associated with an increased prevalence of nonreceipt of annual oral health examinations. Lacking dental insurance compared with having private dental insurance was associated with a nearly 3-fold prevalence of nonreceipt of oral health care, and not possessing English fluency compared with being very fluent in English was associated with a 2-fold increase in nonreceipt of oral health care.

Despite the high prevalence of lack of oral health care, only 13.2% of the participants self-rated their oral health as poor. Poor self-rated oral health was higher in those who lacked access to oral health care (15.8% vs. 11.4%; $P = .02$) and was reported more frequently in older versus younger age groups, women versus men, and East Asian versus Southeast Asian. Furthermore, poor self-rated oral health was more prevalent in adults with lower versus higher English fluency, lower versus higher income, poor versus excellent general health, and public or no dental insurance versus private dental insurance. In multivariable analyses, self-reported oral health was statistically significantly poorer for adults who were younger versus older, who had poor general health versus excellent health, and who did not have insurance versus did have dental insurance. When controlling for these factors, gender, ethnic background, English fluency, working status, and income were not associated with poor self-rated oral health.

DISCUSSION

Nonreceipt of annual oral health examinations was common in our sample of mostly immigrant Asian Americans living in the New York City metropolitan region. These findings are consistent with the results of a previous study of oral health care use among diverse immigrants living in the city, including adults born in China, the Dominican Republic, Haiti, India, Puerto Rico, and other Caribbean islands, where Chinese-born immigrants were the least likely to report having seen a dentist in the past year.[2] In a related study, dental insurance and a regular source of dental care were associated with higher oral health care use.[6]

We found that adults who self-reported poor general health were more likely to self-report poor oral health, but it did not fully explain the variation. Our results suggest that self-rated oral health may capture a different set of perceived health attributes that may be of interest to providers. Self-rated general health items have been shown to be valid and reliable predictors of mortality and morbidity.[7]

Our study had several limitations. We used self-report to assess receipt of oral health examinations, which may be subject to reporting bias. These results were from a

Table 15-1. Distribution and Multivariable Associations Between Determinants of Oral Health and Nonreceipt of an Annual Oral Health Examination and Poor Self-Rated Oral Health in Asian Americans: New York City, 2013–2016

	Annual Oral Health Examination		Self-Rated Status of Mouth and Teeth	
	Prevalence of Nonreceipt (n = 1288), %	OR (95% CI) of Nonreceipt vs. Receipt[a]	Prevalence of Poor Self-Reported Status (n = 1268), %	OR (95% CI) of Poor vs. Not Poor Status[a]
Age, y				
18–44	44.2	1.71 (1.12, 2.62)	7.5	0.53 (0.30, 0.94)
45–64	39.8	1.06 (0.70, 1.61)	15.9	0.83 (0.50, 1.40)
≥65	36.6	1 (Ref)	25.6	1 (Ref)
Gender				
Female	38.7	1 (Ref)	14.6	1 (Ref)
Male	45.1	1.35 (1.05, 1.74)	11.5	0.85 (0.58, 1.24)
Place of residence				
Bronx	71.4	3.11 (1.57, 6.16)	19.2	2.43 (0.92, 6.40)
Brooklyn	37.9	1.15 (0.65, 2.03)	10.1	0.72 (0.33, 1.61)
Manhattan	28.3	1 (Ref)	14.6	1 (Ref)
Queens	39.2	1.02 (0.59, 1.77)	15.0	1.13 (0.54, 2.36)
Staten Island	28.4	0.72 (0.33, 1.57)	3.1	0.36 (0.07, 1.92)
New Jersey	33.6	0.98 (0.52, 1.86)	8.9	0.83 (0.32, 2.12)
Ethnic group				
South Asian	42.0	1.48 (0.89, 2.47)	11.2	0.98 (0.39, 2.47)
East Asian	33.1	1.06 (0.61, 1.85)	19.2	1.58 (0.62, 4.02)
Southeast Asian	57.3	1.65 (0.90, 3.02)	11.9	0.54 (0.18, 1.61)
Arab	29.4	1 (Ref)	7.0	1 (Ref)
English fluency				
Very well	36.9	1 (Ref)	5.7	1 (Ref)
Well	36.0	0.90 (0.64, 1.25)	10.0	1.16 (0.64, 2.08)
Not well	50.3	1.62 (1.05, 2.49)	19.9	1.31 (0.67, 2.58)
Not at all	54.7	2.26 (1.21, 4.23)	36.6	2.08 (0.91, 4.72)
Education				
< high school	51.7	1.20 (0.81, 1.78)	23.3	1.30 (0.73, 2.30)
High school equivalent/some college	41.8	1.01 (0.75, 1.37)	12.2	1.21 (0.74, 1.99)
College graduate	34.3	1 (Ref)	7.4	1 (Ref)

(Continued)

Table 15-1. (Continued)

	Annual Oral Health Examination		Self-Rated Status of Mouth and Teeth	
	Prevalence of Nonreceipt (n = 1288), %	OR (95% CI) of Nonreceipt vs. Receipt[a]	Prevalence of Poor Self-Reported Status (n = 1268), %	OR (95% CI) of Poor vs. Not Poor Status[a]
Working	40.6	1 (Ref)	9.5	1 (Ref)
Not working	42.8	0.98 (0.73, 1.33)	18.9	0.94 (0.60, 1.46)
Income, $				
< 25 000	46.0	1.17 (0.86, 1.60)	18.9	1.10 (0.72, 1.68)
25 000–55 000	46.1	1.45 (1.06, 1.97)	9.5	0.96 (0.59, 1.59)
> 55 000	29.8	1 (Ref)	9.1	1 (Ref)
Self-reported overall health				
status				
Excellent	28.7	1 (Ref)	5.7	1 (Ref)
Very good	37.1	1.58 (1.02, 2.45)	7.4	1.13 (0.50, 2.53)
Good	44.0	1.90 (1.25, 2.87)	8.9	1.11 (0.53, 2.35)
Poor	39.7	1.28 (0.68, 2.40)	44.7	6.50 (2.80, 15.11)
Insurance status				
Public	41.1	1.14 (0.82, 1.59)	16.0	1.42 (0.80, 2.51)
Private	30.6	1 (Ref)	6.2	1 (Ref)
No insurance	63.3	2.96 (1.99, 4.41)	16.9	2.13 (1.14, 3.99)

Note: CI = confidence interval; OR = odds ratio. ORs and 95% CIs were estimated with multivariable logistic regression models.
[a]Models included all of the covariates listed in the table.

community-based sample, and generalizability to Asian Americans outside of the New York metropolitan region may be limited.

This study adds to the scarce evidence base on oral health care use and self-rated oral health among low-income Asian Americans from diverse backgrounds. New models of community-based oral health promotion by community educators[6] and team-based integrated care coordinated by dental hygienists[7] may provide access to culturally tailored, cost-effective oral health care for immigrant Asian American populations.

PUBLIC HEALTH IMPLICATIONS

In our analysis of diverse, low-income, primarily foreign-born Asian Americans living in the New York metropolitan region, English proficiency, dental insurance status, and self-rated health were determinants of receipt of oral health care. Culturally tailored messages to promote dental insurance sign-up to Asian American immigrants are key to providing improved oral health care access and ultimately improved oral health.

ACKNOWLEDGMENTS

Molly Jung was supported by the National Institutes of Health (NIH)/National Heart, Lung, and Blood Institute (training grant T32 HL007024). Mary E. Northridge was supported in part by NIH, National Institute of Dental and Craniofacial Research, and Office of Behavioral and Social Sciences Research (grant R01-DE023072). This research was supported in part by NIH (P60MD000538), National Institute on Minority Health and Health Disparities (U48DP005008), Centers for Disease Control and Prevention (CDC; U58DP005621), and National Center for Advancing Translational Sciences/NIH (UL1TR001445).

The contents of this publication are solely the responsibility of the authors and do not necessarily represent the official views of the National Institutes of Health and Centers for Disease Control and Prevention.

REFERENCES

1. Cohn D. Future immigration will change the face of America by 2065. Pew Research Center. October 5, 2015. Available at: http://www.pewresearch.org/fact-tank/2015/10/05/future-immigration-will-change-the-face-of-america-by-2065. Accessed October 26, 2016.

2. Cruz GD, Chen Y, Salazar CR, Le Geros RZ. The association of immigration and acculturation attributes with oral health among immigrants in New York City. *Am J Public Health.* 2009; 99(suppl 2):S474–S480.

3. New York City Department of Health and Mental Hygiene. EpiQuery: NYC Interactive Health Data: Last Dental Cleaning by Race/Ethnicity (Age-Adjusted), NYC Community Health Survey 2014. Available at: https://a816-healthpsi.nyc.gov/epiquery/CHS/CHSXIndex.html. Accessed October 26, 2016.

4. New York City Department of Health and Mental Hygiene. EpiQuery: NYC Interactive Health Data: Dental Visits by Race/Ethnicity, Child Community Health Survey 2009. Available at: https://a816-healthpsi.nyc.gov/epiquery/Child/CCHSIndex.html. Accessed October 26, 2016.

5. Chinn CH, Cruz GD, Chan A. Caries experience among Chinese-American children in Manhattan Chinatown. *N Y State Dent J.* 2011;77(4):43–47.

6. Cruz GD, Chen Y, Salazar CR, Karloopia R, LeGeros RZ. Determinants of oral health care utilization among diverse groups of immigrants in New York City. *J Am Dent Assoc.* 2010; 141(7):871–878.

7. Jylhä M. What is self-rated health and why does it predict mortality? Towards a unified conceptual model. *Soc Sci Med.* 2009;69(3):307–316.

III. DENTAL THERAPY

16

A Workforce Strategy for Reducing Oral Health Disparities: Dental Therapists*

Jane Koppelman, MPA, and Rebecca Singer-Cohen, MPP

It has been more than 17 years since the first surgeon general report on oral health spotlighted "a silent epidemic" of oral disease that was affecting our most vulnerable citizens: racial/ethnic minority groups, poor children, people with disabilities, and the elderly. Today, oral health disparities by race/ethnicity persist and are well documented. Rates of tooth decay, periodontal disease, oral cancers, and edentulism are far higher and dental care utilization rates considerably lower for racial/ethnic minorities than for Whites in this nation.[1,2]

A particularly thorny factor that contributes to oral health disparities is an oral health workforce that provides insufficient access to care for the underserved, which disproportionately comprises racial/ethnic minorities. The workforce shortage is a double-barreled problem. Although there is debate among researchers on the adequacy of the aggregate supply of dentists for the US population,[3] data demonstrate that a poorly distributed workforce leaves thousands of areas of the country with a shortage of dentists, many of them rural and inner-city regions.

In 2017, more than 56 million people lived in areas of the country that the federal government designated as having a lack of dentists.[4] The Health Resources and Services Administration projects that by 2025 the shortage of dentists in pockets around the country will double (from 7,000 to 15,600), even accounting for an expected increase in the number of new dentists in the work force.[5] As a result, access to care is constrained for people in these communities regardless of income or insurance coverage.

Perhaps more consequential for racial/ethnic minorities is that more than 60% of dentists in 2016 did not accept Medicaid or other public insurance.[6] In 2015 Medicaid and other forms of public insurance covered more than 11 million (26%) Blacks and more than 18 million (~32%) Hispanics, with children disproportionately represented.[7-9]

---

*This is a modified version of the article that appeared in the *American Journal of Public Health*. See: Koppelman J, Singer-Cohen R. A workforce strategy for reducing oral health disparities: dental therapists. *Am J Public Health*. 2017;107(S1):S13–S17. Figures A and B are available as supplements to the online version of the *AJPH* article at http://www.ajph.org.

(Although state coverage of an adult dental benefit in Medicaid is optional and coverage levels are highly variable across the nation, Medicaid dental benefits are mandatory for children.) Minorities are also disproportionately represented among those who have no dental insurance.

Recently, federally qualified health centers—the nation's dental safety net providers with more than 10,000 delivery sites across the country—have seen a surge in demand for dental care. Between 2006 and 2012, according to an American Dental Association analysis, although the total number of dental visits declined nationally, dental visits to federally qualified health centers rose by 74%.[10] These centers do not deny care to low-income patients because they have Medicaid; they also provide free or low-cost care to the low-income uninsured. Yet they do not meet the demand for care, serving only one third of low-income uninsured patients and one in six Medicaid beneficiaries nationally.[11,12]

The shortcomings of the dental care delivery system are apparent, and the public health crisis is persistent. Increasingly, states are considering authorizing midlevel dental providers (often called "dental therapists") as a strategy to expand access to care for the underserved. Akin to physician assistants in medicine, dental therapists are oral health practitioners who work under the supervision of a dentist to provide routine preventive and restorative care. Primarily, what distinguishes dental therapists from dental hygienists is their ability to prepare and fill cavities using a hand drill and perform nonsurgical extractions.

For the tens of millions of people in this nation with untreated tooth decay, many will need a traditional filling that under current law only dentists are allowed to provide. Without care, dental decay can worsen to cause infection and abscesses, which in rare instances have caused death. Research finds that untreated decay is the chief reason for dental-related hospital emergency department visits.[13] In 2015 such visits cost the US health care system $2 billion.[14]

Dentists hire and supervise dental therapists to expand routine care to more patients, grow their practices, offer evening and weekend hours, and expand care locations to underserved at-risk populations in community settings such as Title 1 schools and nursing homes. The scope of practice of a dental therapist is about one quarter that of a general dentist.[*] In the United States they currently practice in Minnesota and serve Native American tribes across Alaska and in parts of Washington and Oregon. They have been authorized in Vermont, Maine, and Arizona, and in the case of Washington, to

---

[*]We determined this on the basis of Pew Charitable Trusts analysis that used 2016 American Dental Association Codes on Dental Procedures and Nomenclature, American Dental Association Commission on Dental Accreditation 2015 Accreditation Standards for Dental Therapy Programs, and North Dakota administrative codes 20-01 through 20-05 (via the North Dakota Board of Dental Examiners), which are current as of April 1, 2015. This number reflects the proposed scope of a dental therapist in House Bill 1256, introduced in North Dakota on January 9, 2017, and is consistent with statute and legislative proposals in other states.

serve Native Americans only. About a dozen state houses around the country are actively considering them.

We have chronicled the growth of dental therapy in the United States, how it is being used to expand care access, and its potential to diversify the oral health workforce and provide an economically sustainable source of employment for people of color interested in the health professions.

EVOLUTION OF DENTAL THERAPY

The dental therapy model began nearly 100 years ago in New Zealand as a public health intervention using government-employed therapists working in public schools to treat high rates of dental decay among children. Dental therapists now practice in 54 countries. Today dental therapists in several nations—Great Britain, New Zealand, Australia, Canada, the Netherlands, and the United States—treat people of all ages and work in public clinics as well as private practices.[15]

Dental therapists were first employed in the United States in 2004 as a way to combat tremendous oral health disease rates among Alaska Natives, who have two to four times the rates of untreated caries as do other US persons, depending on their age.[16-18] Dental health aide therapists (DHATs) have been deployed to be an ongoing presence in rural Alaska Native villages that previously would be visited just a few times a year by a dentist. They deliver care while a supervising dentist is in a more centrally located office providing clinical guidance. As of June 2018, 34 DHATs practice in Alaska, and they have provided care to more than 40,000 Alaska Natives in more than 80 communities. DHATs are authorized by the Indian Health Service Act as a part of Alaska's Community Health Aide Program, an initiative that trains Alaska Natives in a variety of health auxiliary occupations.

In 2009, Minnesota became the first state to pass a dental practice act that authorizes dental therapists. The law was passed in response to dental shortages in most of the state's counties—many of them rural. As of April 2018, 86 dental therapists work in public clinics and private practices to treat more of the states' underserved people.

Private practices are using dental therapists to serve more patients on Medicaid. Nationally, as the average Medicaid reimbursement for dental care is about half that of commercial fees,[19] it is not surprising that dentists report low payment as a chief reason for not serving patients on Medicaid or other public insurance.[20] Dental therapists command lower salaries than do dentists (on average dental therapists make 33% to 50% less than dentists),[21] and for practices that employ them, dental therapists lower the cost of delivering care to patients. This makes accepting Medicaid's discounted payment rates more feasible for a dental practice.

In the public sector, Minnesota public clinics and federally qualified health centers are using dental therapists as a cost-effective way to increase capacity to serve more patients on Medicaid and offer free or low-cost care to more low-income uninsured patients.

GROWING STATE AND TRIBAL INTEREST

More recently, Maine in 2014, Vermont in 2016, and Arizona in 2018 authorized dental therapists. These states are in the early stages of implementing their laws. About a dozen state legislatures are considering similar proposals, including those of Florida, Kansas, Massachusetts, Michigan, New Mexico, Ohio, Washington, and Wisconsin (Supplemental Figure A).

There has also been substantial interest in the model among Native American tribes. In early 2016 the Washington State Swinomish tribe brought an Alaska-trained DHAT to work at its clinic. Tribal leaders took this action although the Indian Health Care Improvement Act, which Congress amended in 2010, forbids DHATs from operating in Indian Country outside Alaska unless permitted by state law.[22] In 2017, the Washington legislature authorized dental therapists to serve Native Americans and be reimbursed by Medicaid. In Oregon, two tribal groups—the Coquille Indian Tribe and the Confederated Tribes of Coos, Lower Umpqua, and Siuslaw Indians—launched dental therapy programs under state pilot authority. And in June 2016 the Indian Health Service invited comments on a draft policy statement that would allow dental therapists to practice in Indian Health Service facilities across the nation.[23]

EMERGING RESEARCH ON THE BUSINESS CASE

Research on the effectiveness of dental therapists that is often cited includes a synthesis of 1,100 studies and reports of dental therapists globally and a 2010 evaluation of the Alaskan DHAT program.[24,25] Both studies found that dental therapists provide safe and effective care at a level of quality comparable to that of dentists. In 2013, the American Dental Association published a review of studies that found that dental teams employing dental therapists reduce untreated caries rates more than do dentist-only teams.[26] In Minnesota, the first evaluation of dental therapists jointly conducted by the state health department and the board of dentistry was released in 2014. Among its findings was that therapists were practicing safely, allowing clinics to expand capacity to treat more underserved patients and reducing wait and travel times for care, with reports of high patient satisfaction.[27]

Numerous studies have also tracked the economic impact on practices—both public and private—that employ dental therapists. The Minnesota state evaluation found that two thirds of clinics employing dental therapists reported considerable personnel cost savings. One clinic saved $62,000 annually, and others estimated annual savings to be $35,000 to $50,000 per dental therapist over hiring a dentist.[27]

A 2012 economic assessment of DHATs practicing in Alaska found that, after accounting for the costs of their employment (including a dental assistant's salary), dental therapists brought in an average of $127,000 in net collected revenues for their practices (written report, Alaskan Native Tribal Health Corporation, January 11, 2012).

The Pew Charitable Trusts in 2014 released two case studies of a rural private pract. and an urban community health center that employed dental therapists. One private practice accrued an additional $24,000 in profits after the dental therapist's first year (after accounting for the therapist employment costs), while also increasing by more than 200 the number of Medicaid patients served.[28] This is notable because Minnesota has one of the lowest Medicaid reimbursement rates in the nation.[19] The increased revenue was accomplished in part by allowing the dentist to delegate routine restorative care to a lower-cost provider, which freed his time to perform more complex and costly procedures.

First-year findings from a Minnesota community health center employing a dental therapist demonstrated that the Medicaid revenue the dental therapist generated exceeded the cost of her employment by more than $30,000. This estimate did not account for additional income from nearly 600 visits she conducted that were not billed to Medicaid.[29]

CULTURAL DIVERSITY IN THE DENTAL WORKFORCE

Because people of color have the highest burden of dental disease in this country, it is concerning that there is little racial/ethnic diversity in the oral health professions. In 2015, Blacks constituted 13% of the country but only 3% of dentists.[30] Hispanics that year constituted 18% of the population but just 9% of dentists.[31] In 2015, the 863 Black, Hispanic or Latino, and Native Americans enrolled in dental school constituted less than 2% of the estimated nearly 54,000 minority dentists needed to achieve parity in the delivery system.[32] Ratios are out of balance for dental hygienists as well. In 2015, the proportion of Black and Hispanic dental hygienists was 4% and 5%, respectively.[33] These ratios do not bode well for a nation where by 2044, the US Census Bureau projects, more than half of all persons living in the United States will belong to a minority group[34] (Supplemental Figure B). Research finds that racial/ethnic diversity among health professionals is linked to improved access to care, greater patient choice and satisfaction, and better patient—provider communication for racial/ethnic minority patients.[35] In view of this research and the severe under representation of minorities in the oral health workforce, some experts hold that workforce diversity is an "essential component" of systematic efforts to reduce oral health disparities by race.[32]

Advocates for dental therapy see an opportunity for people of color to take advantage of a new field of employment—in addition to, not as a replacement for, dentistry. Dental therapy has been found to be an economically sustainable profession. Starting salaries for dental therapists in Alaska in 2013 were about $70,000 per year after a two-year full-time post—high school program and an additional four-month preceptorship.[36] In Minnesota, data show that dental therapist hourly wages ranged approximately from $35 to $45.[21,29,30]

cost of educational requirements cannot be ignored in discussions racially/ethnically diverse dental therapy workforce. Educational ⸝ been a point of contention in state legislative debates to date. Currently, requirements range from a two-year full-time requirement, as the DHAT model calls for, to masters-level training, as required for the Minnesota advanced dental therapist. Interestingly, while their scopes of practice are essentially the same, DHAT students in Alaska earn an associate's degree, while the Minnesota statute requires that dental therapists have at least a bachelor's degree.[37]

Higher costs associated with longer educational requirements will create entry barriers for people with modest resources—barriers that will disproportionately affect people of color. Dental therapists carrying a higher educational debt load may also be dissuaded from practicing in communities of color, where there are higher concentrations of Medicaid and uninsured patients. Studies find that minority dentists leave school with more debt than do their nonminority peers. Moreover, a recent survey found, unsurprisingly, that although more than half of minority dentists reported that serving patients of their own racial/ethnic group contributed to their job satisfaction, earning potential was their top priority in determining where they practiced.[32]

FUTURE DYNAMICS

With numbers of dental therapists approaching 100 and increased state and tribal interest, the dental therapy profession in the United States appears to be gaining momentum. Recent events and trends in the health care marketplace may accelerate state adoption of this model and increase market demand for dental therapists, respectively.

State legislative debates on dental therapy have been contentious, with state- and national-level dental societies voicing strong opposition. Among their chief arguments are that dental therapists are ill prepared to provide fillings and extractions and that dentists with empty chair time can address the care access need with proper outreach strategies (although this latter argument does not account for low dentist participation in Medicaid or the existence of dental shortage areas).[38,39] The Commission on Dental Accreditation's 2015 implementation of guidelines for dental therapy training programs may help to change the tenor of these legislative debates and offer assurance to policymakers of the safety of dental therapy. The Commission on Dental Accreditation is the sole agency authorized by the US Department of Education to accredit dental education training programs in the United States.

The standards the commission has set provide new and established dental therapy programs with guidelines to ensure quality and consistency and to protect public safety.[40]

In addition, Medicaid and large health systems are increasingly moving to accountable care systems that adopt bench marks for utilization and outcomes and offer financial rewards (and penalties) on the basis of provider or system performance in meeting them.

Dentistry is slowly being integrated into these systems, as evidenced by Oregon's Medicaid program, and held to accountability standards; for example, California now requires health plans on its exchange to have accountability standards. Lower-cost providers who can expand access to quality care may become more attractive.[37]

Furthermore, although the 115th Congress is considering repealing parts of the Affordable Care Act, with health care expenditures approaching 18% of gross domestic product, public and private payers of dental care will likely face continuing pressure to adopt efficiencies to lower health care costs. Because dental therapists command a substantially lower salary than do dentists, employing them is a cost-effective way to keep patients healthy and out of hospital emergency departments.

CONCLUSIONS

Disparities in oral health disease rates and access to care persist despite growing national attention. A shortage of providers in thousands of US communities and for those who are publicly insured is well documented. Growing evidence shows that private and public practices can employ dental therapists to treat traditionally underserved populations—those on Medicaid, the uninsured, and those living in dentist shortage areas.

The employment of dental therapists also holds promise for creating a more culturally diverse oral health workforce and creating sustainable jobs for people of color who may not have considered a career in the oral health field. State and federal policymakers should consider how dental therapists can be used to improve public health in a market that is increasingly being held to cost, quality, and accessibility standards.

REFERENCES

1. Centers for Disease Control and Prevention. Disparities in oral health. Available at: http://www.cdc.gov/OralHealth/oral_health_disparities/index.htm. Accessed November 18, 2016.

2. Dye BA, Thornton-Evans G, Li X, Iafolla T. Dental caries and tooth loss in adults in the United States, 2011–2012. NCHS data brief 197. Hyattsville, MD: National Center for Health Statistics; 2015.

3. Vujicic M. Interpreting HRSA's latest dentist workforce projections. Chicago, IL: American Dental Association Health Policy Institute; 2015.

4. Health Resources and Services Administration. Designated health professional shortage areas statistics, fourth quarter of fiscal year 2018. Designated HPSA quarterly summary, as of September 30, 2018. Available at: https://ersrs.hrsa.gov/ReportServer?/HGDW_Reports/BCD_HPSA/BCD_HPSA_SCR50_Qtr_Smry&rs:Format=PDF. Accessed October 31, 2018.

5. Health Resources and Services Administration. National and state-level projections of dentists and dental hygienists in the US (2012–2025). Available at: http://bhw.hrsa.gov/health-workforce-analysis/research/projections. Accessed November 18, 2016.

6. American Dental Association, Health Policy Institute. Characteristics of private dental practices: selected 2016 results from the survey of dental practice. Available at: https://www. ada.org/en/science-research/health-policy-institute/data-center/dental-practice. Accessed October 31, 2018.

7. US Census Bureau. Population estimates program (PEP). Available at: https://www.census. gov/popest. Accessed December 27, 2016.

8. US Census Bureau. 2010 census of population: P94-171 redistricting data file. Available at: http://factfinder.census.gov. Accessed December 27, 2016.

9. Kaiser Family Foundation. Total number of residents. Available at: http://kff.org/other/ state-indicator/total-residents/?currentTimeframe=0. Accessed December 27, 2016.

10. Vujicic M. Where have all the dental care visits gone? *J Am Dent Assoc.* 2015;146(6):412–414.

11. National Association of Community Health Centers. Health centers and the uninsured: improving access to care and health outcomes. 2014. Available at: http://www.nachc.org/ wp-content/uploads/2015/11/Uninsured-FS-0514.pdf. Accessed November 18, 2016.

12. National Association of Community Health Centers. Community health center chart book. 2018. Available at: http://www.nachc.org/wp-content/uploads/2018/06/Chartbook_FINAL_6.20.18. pdf. Accessed October 31, 2018.

13. Allareddy V, Rampa S, Lee MK, Nalliah RP. Hospital-based emergency department visits involving dental conditions: profile and predictors of poor outcomes and resource utilization. *J Am Dent Assoc.* 2014;145(4):331–337.

14. American Dental Association. Health Policy Institute. Emergency Department Visits for Dental Conditions—A Snapshot. Available https://www.ada.org/~/media/ADA/Science%20 and%20Research/HPI/Files/HPIgraphic_0218_2.pdf?la=pdf. Accessed October 31, 2018.

15. Nash DA, Friedman JW, Mathu-Muju KR, et al. A review of the global literature on dental therapists. *Community Dent Oral Epidemiol.* 2014;42(1):1–10.

16. Dye BA, Thornton-Evans G, Li X, Iafolla TJ. Dental caries sealant prevalence in children and adolescents in the United States, 2011–2012. NCHS Data Brief No. 191. National Center for Health Statistics. March 2015. Available at: http://www.cdc.gov/nchs/data/databriefs/db191.pdf. Accessed November 18, 2016.

17. Phipps KR, Ricks TL, Blahut P. The oral health of 13–15 year old American Indian and Alaska Native children compared to the general US population and *Healthy People 2020* targets. Indian Health Service Data Brief. May 2014. Available at: https://www.ihs.gov/DOH/ documents/surveillance/Data%20Brief%20IHS%20Adolescent%2005-05-2014.pdf. Accessed November 18, 2016.

18. Dye BA, Li X, Thornton-Evans G. Oral health disparities as determined by selected *Healthy People 2020* oral health objectives for the United States, 2009–2010. NCHS Data Brief No. 104. National Center for Health Statistics. August 2012. Available at: http://www.cdc.gov/ nchs/data/databriefs/db104.pdf. Accessed November 18, 2016.

19. Gupta N, Yarbrough C, Vujicic M, Blatz A, Harrison B. Medicaid fee-for-service reimbursement rates for child and adult dental care services for all states, 2016. Available at:https://www.ada.org/~/media/ADA/Science%20and%20Research/HPI/Files/HPIBrief_0417_1.pdf. Accessed October 31, 2018.

20. Efforts under way to improve children's access to dental services, but sustained attention needed to address ongoing concerns. GAO 11-96. Washington, DC: US Government Accountability Office; 2010.

21. Minnesota Department of Health, Minnesota Department of Human Services, and Health Reform Minnesota. Dental therapy toolkit: a resource for potential employers. 2017. Available at: http://www.health.state.mn.us/divs/orhpc/workforce/emerging/dt/2017dttool.pdf. Accessed October 31, 2018.

22. Heisler EJ, Walke R. Indian Health Care Improvement Act provisions in the Patient Protection and Affordable Care Act. PL 111-148. Washington, DC: Congressional Research Service; 2010.

23. Lee TH. Indian country leads health revolution sweeping US. Indian Country Today. July 6, 2016. Available at: https://newsmaven.io/indiancountrytoday/archive/indian-country-leads-health-revolution-sweeping-us-le0WaGNjwkaEHmUqqEDPrw. Accessed November 18, 2016.

24. Nash DA, Friedman JW, Mathu-Muju KR, et al. A review of the global literature on dental therapists. *Community Dent Oral Epidemiol.* 2014;42(1):1–10.

25. Weterhall S, Bader JD, Burrus BB, Lee JY, Shugars DA. *Evaluation of the Dental Therapist Workforce Model in Alaska.* Research Triangle Park, NC: RTI International; 2010.

26. Wright JT, Graham F, Hayes C, et al. A systematic review of oral health outcomes produced by dental teams incorporating midlevel providers. *J Am Dent Assoc.* 2013;144(1):75–91.

27. Minnesota Department of Health, Minnesota Board of Dentistry. Early impacts of dental therapists in Minnesota: report to the Minnesota legislature. Available at: https://mn.gov/boards/assets/2014DentalTherapistReport_tcm21-45970.pdf. Accessed November 18, 2016.

28. Pew Charitable Trusts. Expanding the dental team: studies of two private practices. 2014. Available at: http://www.pewtrusts.org/en/research-and-analysis/reports/2014/02/12/expanding-the-dental-team. Accessed November 18, 2016.

29. Pew Charitable Trusts. Expanding the dental team: increasing access to care in public settings. 2014. Available at: https://www.pewtrusts.org/~/media/assets/2014/06/27/expanding_dental_case_studies_report.pdf. Accessed November 18, 2016.

30. US Census Bureau. Quick facts V2015 data. Population estimates program. Available at: https://www.census.gov/quickfacts/table/PST045215/00#headnote-js-b. Accessed November 16, 2016.

31. US Bureau of Labor Statistics. Household data: annual averages. Employed persons by detailed occupation, sex, race, and Hispanic or Latino ethnicity. Available at: http://www.bls.gov/cps/cpsaat11.pdf. Accessed November 18, 2016.

32. Mertz EA, Wides CD, Kottek AM, Calvo JM, Gates PE. Underrepresented minority dentists: quantifying their numbers and characterizing the communities they serve. *Health Aff (Millwood)*. 2016;35(12):2190–2199.

33. Andersen RM, Carreon DC, Davidson PL, Nakazono TT, Shahedi S, Gutierrez JJ. Who will serve? Assessing recruitment of underrepresented minority and low income dental students to increase access to dental care. *J Dent Ed*. 2010;74(6):579–592.

34. Colby SL, Ortman JM. Projections of the size and composition of the US population: 2014–2060. Current Population Reports P25-1143. Washington, DC: US Census Bureau; 2014.

35. Smedley BD, Butler AS, Bristow LR. *In the Nation's Compelling Interest: Ensuring Diversity in the Health Care Workforce*. Washington, DC: National Academies Press; 2004.

36. Pew Charitable Trusts. Growing the dental workforce: the critical role of community colleges and workforce investment boards. 2013. Available at: http://www.pewtrusts.org/~/media/legacy/uploadedfiles/pcs_assets/2013/pewdentalworkforcepdf.pdf. Accessed November 18, 2016.

37. Koppelman J, Vitzhum K, Simon L. Expanding where dental therapists can practice could increase Americans' access to cost-efficient care. *Health Aff (Millwood)*. 2016;35(12):2200–2207.

38. Vermont State Dental Society. Position statement: dental therapists. 2016. Available at: http://legislature.vermont.gov/assets/Documents/2016/WorkGroups/House%20Human%20Services/Bills/S.20/Testimony/S.20~Jamie%20Feehan~Vermont%20Dental%20Society%20Position%20on%20S.20~1-20-2016.pdf. Accessed October 18, 2016.

39. Brown C. Therapists and advocacy. Paper presented at: the National Leadership Conference of the American Student Dental Association; November 2, 2012; Chicago, IL.

40. Commission on Dental Accreditation. Accreditation standards for dental therapy education programs. 2015. Available at: http://www.ada.org/~/media/CODA/Files/dt.pdf?la=en. Accessed October 17, 2016.

17

The Dental Health Aide Therapist Program in Alaska: An Example for the 21st Century*

Dane Lenaker, DMD, MPH

In 2009, I stepped off a plane in Bethel, Alaska, to begin my career as a dentist for the Yukon Kuskokwim Health Corporation (YKHC), a regional medical hub for more than 26,000 Alaska Natives in 48 remote villages. Although I knew of Alaska's dire need for dentists, I was unprepared for what awaited me.

Within a few days, I had treated three children from outlying villages who needed their decayed and abscessed front teeth removed. All were younger than three years. All were strapped to papoose boards for protective stabilization.

These were not isolated cases. A 2008 investigation of oral disease in Alaska Native children found that

> Among children aged 4–5 years and 12–15 years who were evaluated, 87% and 91%, respectively, had dental caries, compared with 35% and 51% of U.S. children in those age groups. Among children from the Alaska villages, those aged 4–5 years had a mean of 7.5 dental caries, and those aged 12–15 years had a mean of 5.0, compared with 1.6 and 1.8 dental cares in same-aged U.S. children.[1(p. 1275)]

I had walked into an epidemic of oral disease. Fortunately, a solution was already in the works—one with the potential to change everything.

At that time, YKHC was in the early stages of implementing the Dental Health Aide Therapist (DHAT) program, which was established by the Alaska Native Tribal Health Consortium (ANTHC), a nonprofit tribal health organization, to expand oral health care access. After repeated failures to recruit and retain dentists, ANTHC adopted the DHAT model, which was developed nearly a century ago in New Zealand to improve the oral health of underserved schoolchildren.

DHATs—also known as dental therapists—are midlevel dental care providers, similar to physician assistants in medical care. They work as part of a dentist-led team under general supervision to provide preventive and restorative services within a defined scope

*This is a modified version of the article that appeared in the *American Journal of Public Health*. See: Lenaker D. The dental health aide therapist program in Alaska: an example for the 21st century. *Am J Public Health*. 2017;107(suppl 1):S24–S25.

of practice. Under this model, DHATs function as extensions of their dentist supervisors, working in underserved communities to provide routine services that prevent and treat oral disease.

INTRODUCING A NEW MIDLEVEL APPROACH

More than 50 countries have adopted the New Zealand model. A comprehensive review of the DHAT experience worldwide, covering more than 1000 studies and reports, found that DHATs have successfully expanded access to safe, effective oral health care.[2]

In the DHAT model, ANTHC saw an opportunity to reverse Alaska's oral disease epidemic. For the first time, Alaska implemented a team-based approach to oral health care that expanded access in rural, underserved villages by adding a specially trained midlevel provider to complement and extend the reach of dentists. Alaska's DHAT program also marked the introduction of dental therapists to practice in the United States.

Here's how the DHAT training program works. Alaska students are recruited by their tribal communities. They complete a rigorous education program that is the equivalent of three academic years delivered in two calendar years. Next, they complete preceptorships with dentists. They are then certified to work offsite under general supervision, consulting with their supervising dentists via telemedicine or phone and referring treatment services outside their scope to dentists.

DHATs practice in underserved communities like those where they grew up. They understand these communities' customs and needs and have the trust of community members. They are adept at providing culturally competent care, which is part of their training, and serve as role models to younger community members.

The first class of Alaska DHAT students trained in New Zealand and began practicing in Alaska in 2006. By 2009, ANTHC was training DHATs through a new University of Washington School of Medicine program grounded on the New Zealand model.

From 2006 to 2013, the DHATs and their dentist supervisors in the Yukon Delta focused on treating dental emergencies and reducing the large backlog of untreated oral disease. There was no systematic approach.

PROGRESS FROM A TEAM-BASED APPROACH

That changed starting in 2013, when YKHC implemented a population-based oral health strategy for examining and providing sealants and needed care to all children in the region. YKHC assigned dentist–DHAT teams to specific subregions; I led the team for the Aniak subregion. Under this strategy, dentist–DHAT teams triaged patients with dental emergencies while (1) working to reduce the needs of patients at moderate and high risk for caries, and (2) maintaining the health of patients with lower risk or good oral health.

Between 2009 and 2014, we significantly shifted our services from emergent to preventive care. In 2009, emergency care accounted for 38% of dental services provided by YKHC; by 2014, that proportion had fallen to 24%.[3] During that same period, the proportion of preventive services increased from 28% to more than 40%.[3]

The number of pediatric patients who received annual, comprehensive, nonurgent examinations almost tripled, from 976 in 2013 to 2770 in 2016. Our clinical data showed that the numbers of examinations and completed treatments were significantly higher in communities served by DHATs than in those not served by DHATs.

DHATS HELP EXPAND TREATMENT REACH

For example, in the village of Russian Mission, my team examined 64% of all children aged zero to five years during 2015 and treated 75% of those children. We examined 100% of children aged six to eight years and treated 85%. The DHATs attended to routine pediatric needs, performed uncomplicated extractions, and taught prevention to children in school, while I focused on complicated extractions and other, more difficult cases.

By comparison, in Quinhagak, a village 140 miles south of Russian Mission that did not have DHATs, 23% of children aged zero to five years received oral health examinations during 2015, and 29% of those children received full treatment of problems identified. Forty-three percent of children aged six to eight years were examined, of whom 40% were treated.

By 2015, we started seeing significant improvements in our ability to keep healthy patients cavity free. For example, in Emmonak, a small town on the Bering Sea, we had a report of a Head Start class with no new cavities. In rural Alaska, that is a small miracle.

Prior to DHATs, many tribal communities had never had a full-time dental provider. They relied instead on itinerant dentists. Patients with dental emergencies had to fly to Bethel. For a parent and child, airfare to Bethel could cost $1000 or more.

Even with incentives like loan repayments, YKHC struggled to retain practicing dentists in remote tribal areas, but certified DHATs tend to stay in their communities, providing continuity of care that helps maintain good oral health. Today, because of DHATs, 45,000 Alaska Natives have regular access to care.[4]

DHATs also make economic sense. In 2011 alone, DHATs generated 76 jobs in Alaska and $9 million worth of economic activity. They saved $40,000 a year in patient travel costs.[5]

ATTENTION NEEDED TO INTEGRATE DHATS INTO TEAMS

There are challenges to onboarding DHATs to dental teams. Many dentists are unfamiliar with how to work with DHATs, and new dentists may find themselves paired with DHATs who have more clinical experience in the field. This can make for a difficult dynamic.

Communities interested in employing DHATs should recruit experienced dentists with a public health mission to lead a DHAT program and support preceptorships between DHATs and dentists. They should also collect and track data on per-encounter performance to secure dentist buy-in, enhance team communication, and improve quality.

Interest in DHATs is growing. Since the launch of Alaska's DHAT program, Minnesota, Maine, Vermont, and Washington have passed laws allowing midlevel dental providers to practice, and other states are considering similar legislation. In addition, tribal communities in the Pacific Northwest employ DHATs.

There's good reason for this interest. The team-based approach to treatment under the DHAT model supports care that is high quality, timely, patient centered, coordinated, and efficient.[6,7] That certainly was my experience working in the Alaska Native villages. I believe that, together, DHATs and dentists can bring high-quality dental care to communities where oral health needs are not being met.

REFERENCES

1. Centers for Disease Control and Prevention. Dental caries in rural Alaska Native children—Alaska, 2008. *MMWR Morb Mortal Wkly Rep.* 2011;60(37): 1275–1278.

2. Nash DA, Friedman JW, Mathu-Muju KR, et al. A review of the global literature on dental therapists. *Community Dent Oral Epidemiol.* 2014;42(1):1–10.

3. Lenaker D. Workforce innovation: dental health aide therapists (DHATs). 2016. Available at: http://www.nnoha.org/resources/5607-2/workforce-innovation-to-increase-access-to-dental-care. Accessed December 14, 2016.

4. Shoffstall-Cone S, Williard M. Alaska Dental Health Aide Program. *Int J Circumpolar Health.* 2013;72:21198.

5. Williard ME. Alaska tribal health system: oral health. Available at: http://dhss.alaska.gov/ahcc/Documents/meetings/201303/AlaskaTribalHealth-OralHealth-Williard.pdf. Accessed December 13, 2016.

6. Minnesota Department of Health; Minnesota Board of Dentistry. Early impacts of dental therapists in Minnesota. 2014. Available at: http://www.health.state.mn.us/divs/orhpc/workforce/dt/dtlegisrpt.pdf. Accessed December 13, 2016.

7. Wetterhall S, Bader JD, Burrus BB, Lee JY, Shugars DA. *Evaluation of the Dental Health Aide Therapist Workforce Model in Alaska. Final report.* Research Triangle Park, NC: RTI International; 2010.

18

How Dental Therapists Can Address the Social and Racial Disparities in Access to Care*

Albert K. Yee, MD, MPH, Kristen McGlaston, MS, and Robert Restuccia, MPA

There is mounting evidence linking poor oral health to poor overall health outcomes, in addition to significant economic impacts through higher health care costs, lost productivity, and lost wages.[1] Yet, oral health care is still treated as separate from the rest of health care. There are myriad systemic barriers to accessing dental services, particularly among the vulnerable, the underserved, and communities of color. An alternative model of dental care delivery that could address racial and social disparities in access to care is dental therapy.

A RACE AND SOCIAL JUSTICE ISSUE

Access to oral health care is an overlooked race and social justice issue, with the inability to access dental services affecting the vulnerable, the underserved, and communities of color at disproportionate rates. In 2010, the Government Accountability Office reported that the most frequent barrier children enrolled in Medicaid faced in obtaining dental care was finding a dentist who would accept Medicaid payment.[2] In 2015, the National Health and Examination Nutrition Survey found that Hispanic (46%) and non-Hispanic Black (44%) children younger than eight years are more likely to have cavities than non-Hispanic White children (31%).[3] The barriers these communities face in accessing care are complex and broad reaching—from social, structural, and cultural, to economic and geographic. It is imperative that we not only look for comprehensive solutions, but also consider the disproportionate burden these communities face when tailoring solutions to address them.

SHORTAGE OF DENTAL PROVIDERS

Currently, there are not enough providers to meet the demands of the general population, with the shortage projected to worsen. A 2015 Department of Health and Human Services—Health Resources and Services Administration report found that by 2025, the

*This is a modified version of the article that appeared in the *American Journal of Public Health*. See: Yee A, McGlaston K, Restuccia R. How dental therapists can address the social and racial disparities in access to care. *Am J Public Health*. 2017;107(suppl 1):S28–S29.

supply of dentists is expected to grow by 11,800 full-time equivalents (FTEs), whereas the demand is projected to grow by 20,400 FTEs. Combined with the existing shortages in dental health professional shortage areas, there is a projected national shortage of approximately 15,600 FTE dentists in 2025.[4] There is an even greater shortage of providers who accept Medicaid and are adequately trained for serving the underserved, particularly in the areas where they live.[5] Dental therapists could immediately address these workforce shortages and disparities in access to care.

AN ALTERNATIVE DENTAL CARE DELIVERY MODEL

Dental therapists are early intervention and prevention dental professionals who are trained to provide a limited scope of services under the supervision of a dentist and are specifically designed to work in underserved areas. Working worldwide since the 1920s, dental therapists have been part of the US dental team for over a decade now. They work in Alaska, Minnesota, and the Swinomish Indian Tribal Community, and were also recently authorized in Vermont and Maine.

Traditionally, the education pathway for dental therapists was developed so that community members become dental therapists through accessible and achievable training programs and can return to their communities to provide care under the general supervision of a dentist in a few years. Long-term evidence and experience have shown that dental therapists can be trained in just two years, which lowers cost and debt burden barriers and increases access to dental therapy education for students, especially those from poor and underserved communities.[3] Additionally, as a result of their training, dental therapists are able to deliver patient-centered care because they understand the history, culture, and language of their patients and provide continuity of care in communities that face recruitment and retention challenges. These factors are critical in building the community's health care delivery capacity and improving oral health outcomes.

In addition to addressing workforce shortages, dental therapists are able to relieve the financial burden that dental practices shoulder as a result of limited resources for oral health care for vulnerable and underserved populations. Because dental therapists are less expensive to hire, dental practices can provide care for more patients on Medicaid even with lower reimbursement rates and still be profitable. According to a 2014 report from the Minnesota Department of Health and Board of Dentistry to the state legislature evaluating the impacts of dental therapists in Minnesota, dental therapists served 6338 new patients over a 13-month period, 84% of whom were public program enrollees or from underserved communities. Additionally, the report found that benefits attributable to dental therapists included direct costs savings (estimated between $35,000 and $62,000) and a reduction in wait time for patients, which made it possible for clinics to see more underserved patients.[6] These findings are supported by Community Catalyst's Economic Viability of Dental Therapists report and case studies conducted by Pew, which demonstrated cost-effective benefits for a variety of practices, even when the majority of patients were low-income and Medicaid populations (in Alaska and Minnesota, their salaries account for less than 30% of the revenue they generate).[7] These components would benefit all underserved populations, particularly racial and ethnic minorities, and are critical in addressing the systemic barriers that prevent them from achieving and maintaining access to oral health services.

FUTURE DIRECTIONS

Over a dozen states are pursuing midlevel providers to improve access to care. In 2015, the Commission on Dental Accreditation (CODA), the entity that oversees dentists' education, approved core educational standards for dental therapists and allowed advanced standing for hygienists to become joint dental hygiene–therapy providers. Prior to the CODA standards, state legislatures arbitrarily determined educational requirements, resulting in early adopter states having varying pathways to dental therapy, with most requiring the dual degree therapist–hygienist model necessitating more education time and costs. As states move forward, it is important to adopt the core CODA-approved pathway for dental therapists, as well as the dual degree pathway for advanced standing dental therapists, to ensure that the existing workforce is maximized and to create new opportunities to recruit students from rural, underserved areas and ethnically diverse communities. This core pathway was used in Alaska, resulting in the first group of dental professionals that shared the language and culture of the underserved population being served. The intentional design of the Alaska program offers insight into not just improving oral health care but successfully building a culturally competent workforce and creating employment opportunities in rural America.

It is imperative to treat access to oral health care as the race and social justice issue it is by expanding and bolstering the traditional dental delivery system to serve underserved communities. Dental therapists have been practicing in Alaska for more than ten years, resulting in more than 45,000 Alaska Natives across 81 communities gaining access to dental care.[7] With dental therapists in Alaska and Minnesota demonstrating that they are increasing access to care—especially for hard-to-reach populations—the implementation of dental therapy programs is clearly in the public interest.

Dental therapy is not a limited or temporary solution. Training a group of dental professionals that are members of, and share the language and culture of, the community that they will serve greatly improves communication, trust, patient satisfaction, and adherence to advice and treatment. It is a solution that can increase access to care for all populations and help achieve equity for those who are disparately affected by barriers to oral health services.

REFERENCES

1. Jackson SL, Vann WF, Kotch JB, Pahel BT, Lee JY. Impact of poor oral health on children's school attendance and performance. *Am J Public Health.* 2011;101(10):1900–1906.

2. US Government Accountability Office. Efforts under way to improve children's access to dental services, but sustained attention needed to address ongoing concerns. 2010. Available at: http://www.gao.gov/assets/320/312818.pdf. Accessed November 25, 2016.

3. Dye BS, Thornton-Evans G, Li X, Iafolla TJ. Dental caries and sealant prevalence in children and adolescents in the United States, 2011–2012. March 2015. Available at: https://www.cdc.gov/nchs/data/databriefs/db191.pdf. Accessed January 5, 2017.

4. National and state-level projections of dentists and dental hygienists in the US, 2012–2025. 2015. Available at: https://bhw.hrsa.gov/sites/default/files/bhw/nchwa/projections/nationalstatelevel-projectionsdentists.pdf. Accessed January 7, 2017.

5. Pew Charitable Trusts. Expanding the dental safety net: a first look at how dental therapists can help. 2012. Available at: http://www.pewtrusts.org/en/research-and-analysis/reports/2012/07/31/expanding-the-dental-safety-net. Accessed October 31, 2016.

6. Minnesota Department of Health. Early impacts of dental therapists in Minnesota: report to the Minnesota Legislature 2014. 2014. Available at: http://www.health.state.mn.us/divs/orhpc/workforce/dt/dtlegisrpt.pdf. Accessed October 31, 2016.

7. Kim FM. Economic viability of dental therapists. Community Catalyst. 2013. Available online at: http://www.communitycatalyst.org/doc-store/publications/economic-viability-dental-therapists.pdf. Accessed January 5, 2017.

19

Indian Country Leads National Movement to Knock Down Barriers to Oral Health Equity*

Chairman M. Brian Cladoosby (Spee Pots), Swinomish
Indian Tribal Community

INCIDENCE, PREVALENCE, AND RISK FACTORS FOR ORAL DISEASE IN AMERICAN INDIAN/ALASKA NATIVE COMMUNITIES

It is not an exaggeration to say that the current delivery system of dental care in the United States is failing communities of color. Black, Hispanic, Asian, and American Indian and Alaska Native (AI/AN) children are less likely to see a dentist and receive preventive treatments than White children, and people of color are more likely than Whites to suffer from untreated tooth decay. Native communities are struggling under the weight of devastating oral health disparities. Prevalence of tooth decay in AI/AN children aged two to five years is nearly three times the US average.[1] More than 70% of AI/AN children aged two to five years have a history of tooth decay experience compared with 23% of White children.[1] AI/AN adult dental patients suffer disproportionately from untreated decay, with twice the prevalence of untreated caries as the general US population and more than any other racial/ethnic group.[2] AI/AN adult dental patients are also more likely to have severe periodontal disease and more missing teeth, and they are more likely to report poor oral health than the general US population.[2]

Unfortunately, these numbers do not surprise anyone who grew up or lives in a tribal community, but they are staggering nonetheless. There is an oral health crisis in Indian Country. The reasons for poor dental health in tribal communities include factors such as geographic isolation that continues to limit available providers, economic and racial disparities, and the historical trauma of decades of inadequate health care. In response, with the end goal of achieving oral health equity, AI/AN communities are searching for innovative solutions to address the unique barriers that keep oral health care out of reach for many tribal members and to strengthen their communities.

*This is a modified version of the article that appeared in the *American Journal of Public Health*. See: Cladoosby B. Indian Country leads national movement to knock down barriers to oral health equity. *Am J Public Health*. 2017;107(suppl 1):S81–S84.

IMPROVING ORAL HEALTH IN INDIAN COUNTRY

Dental Therapy Defined

There is no one silver bullet for improving oral health in Indian Country. However, one key tool to overcome the barriers to dental care in Indian Country is the use of dental health aide therapists (hereafter, dental therapists). Notably, tribes in Alaska have been on the forefront of developing a system of village-based paraprofessionals through the Community Health Aide Program (CHAP) for the past several decades, and in 2005 they added dental therapists to that program. In Alaska, dental therapists are part of a mature system of village-based, midlevel primary care providers available through CHAP.

As part of the dental team, dental therapists advocate for the needs of patients, extend care to tribal communities, and help dentists see more patients. Under the general (off-site/indirect) supervision of dentists, dental therapists can practice in remote settings where there is need for additional provider capacity. They provide routine services such as fillings and simple extractions and free up the dentist to work at the top of his/her scope and take more challenging cases.

Dental therapists are not mini-dentists or dentist replacements; rather, they are part of a high-functioning dental team. As colleagues, dentists, hygienists, and dental therapists can provide support to one another over their entire patient population. In Alaska, dentists provide remote supervision by phone or through other technology such as teledentistry equipment. The dental team shares x-rays and intraoral photos to collaborate on patient care.

The scope of dental therapists' work[3] is intentionally limited to procedures that can provide relief from pain, basic treatment of disease, and preventive education and services. Opponents of dental therapy often suggest that dental therapists should not be trained to provide restorative services and that, rather than lack of service, lack of patient education is the real problem. However, the ability of dental therapists to address pain, infection, and the damage to teeth (fillings and extractions) is very important for patients who have experienced lack of access to dental care. Relationships between providers and patients are crucial to long-term behavior change. If a provider cannot address the immediate needs of the patient, he or she will not be in a strong position to successfully connect with the patient and build that trusting relationship. Dental therapists can bring people back into care who have stopped seeking care because of fear or lack of trust and can serve as a bridge back to a dentist to ensure patients have access to a full range of oral health services.

Preventive programs must engage the patient to effectively support long-term behavior changes. But prevention alone will not address the existing treatment needs. Therefore, dental therapists focus not only on prevention of oral diseases but also on alleviation of pain, infection relief, and basic restorative services.

DENTAL THERAPISTS IN AMERICAN INDIAN/ALASKA N COMMUNITIES

Since our first dental therapist joined the Swinomish clinic, he has, in addition to providing excellent clinical care, been visiting our preschool and Head Start programs to brush teeth and provide oral health education for our youngest citizens. This has helped our kids feel very comfortable in our clinic when they come in for their oral health checkups and treatment. The dental therapist also works closely with our oral hygiene staff on elder-specific programs such as partnering with the elder lunch delivery program. He has built a rapport with our elders by joining them for a group lunch most days. Our dentists are happier because they have been able to increase access to a higher level of dentistry and provide more functionality to our patients.

Tribal communities have long struggled to retain providers, most of whom are not AI/AN. Only 0.1% of dentists are AI/AN.[4] People should not consider it a privilege to see a provider that looks like them and understands their language, culture, history, and community; it should be the norm. In Alaska, 78% of dental therapists practice in their village/region of origin[5] and 87% are AI/AN in origin.[6] The retention rate for dental therapists in Alaska is 81% over 13 years.[5] Currently, more than 45 dental therapists serve approximately 45,000 people in 81 tribal communities in rural Alaska. In addition to expanding preventive care options to populations most in need, dental therapists are also very cost effective.[7]

Long-term improvement requires more than simply tweaking the existing broken system. Improving care and access is not just about bringing more providers to Indian Country or other underserved communities; rather, it includes fixing the current training system for health professionals as the Alaska Native Tribal Health Consortium (ANTHC) has been doing through the CHAP program. We can and should "grow our own" providers, create jobs in our communities, and establish and support an education system that breaks down barriers to training health professionals from tribal and other underrepresented communities.

Dental therapists in Alaska build community health care delivery capacity and create jobs by training community members to become dental therapists. ANTHC, in partnership with Iḷisaġvik College, administers the two calendar-year (three academic-year) training program for dental therapists. At the end of the training program, they receive an Associate of Applied Science degree in dental therapy.

Dental therapists have a proven record of success in Alaska Native communities.[8] A study published in January 2018 by the University of Washington School of Dentistry[9] found that, over 10 years, villages in the Yukon Delta in Alaska with dental therapists (compared with villages without dental therapists) experienced the following outcomes:

- Significant decrease in first four front teeth extractions for children aged younger than three years,
- 26% decrease in extractions for adults,

- 60% increase in access to preventive care for children,
- 75% increase in access to preventive care for adults, and
- 44% decrease in the need to put children under general anesthesia for full mouth rehabilitations.

At the request of legislators, the Washington State Department of Health conducted a health impact review[10] of statewide dental therapy legislation. Such reviews can inform and enhance equitable, health-aware decision-making and are used to evaluate a policy and its potential impact on the health of a population and help identify the health equity effects of proposed legislation. According to the review's findings, passing legislation to authorize dental therapists statewide had

> [the] potential to improve oral health and overall health outcomes, particularly for low-income and communities of color as well as individuals with medical disabilities or chronic conditions. These communities are disproportionately impacted by negative oral and other health impacts; therefore, improving health outcomes for these populations would likely decrease health disparities.[10]

Dental therapists are also working to improve access to care to underserved communities in Minnesota. Given their success rate, dental therapists should be available throughout the United States to address the oral health needs of their communities. As primary oral health care providers, they can be successful in any population, not only tribal communities. However, a significant legal barrier has prevented expansion in Indian Country, a barrier that was embedded in amendments of legislation intended to expand and improve access to health care for AI/AN communities and all persons in the United States. The Indian Health Care Improvement Act (IHCIA; Pub L no. 94-437) was passed in 1976 to address the health status of the AI/AN population in the United States. In 2010 the IHCIA was permanently reauthorized as part of the Affordable Care Act (Pub L No. 111-148). During that permanent reauthorization, the American Dental Association (ADA) successfully lobbied for the addition of language to the IHCIA intended to slow the expansion of dental therapists in tribal communities.

LEGAL BARRIERS TO THE EXPANDED DENTAL TEAM

The ADA is effectively protective of its market. Similar to the American Medical Association, it has unparalleled control over its own professional licensure, structure, and regulation in the delivery of health care. But, unlike medicine, in which a variety of midlevel and allied health professionals work with physicians, there is only a small cadre of providers of oral health services. The ADA has used this control over licensure and regulation to stifle competition in the industry.[11]

In 2005, the first dental therapists in Alaska were certified by the CHAP board. In February 2005, the Alaska Board of Dental Examiners asked the Alaska Department of Law to take action against dental therapists practicing dentistry without a license.

Tribes as sovereign nations have a government-to-government relationship with the United States and states do not have jurisdiction over tribes except as delegated by Congress or determined by federal courts.[12] In September 2005, the Alaska assistant attorney general wrote an opinion in favor of dental therapists citing federal preemption[13]; according to the opinion, "[t]he [Alaska] state dental licensure laws stand as an obstacle to Congress' objective to provide dental treatment to Alaska Natives by using non-dentist, non-hygienist paraprofessionals."[14] Nonetheless, in January of 2006, the Alaska Dental Society and the ADA filed a lawsuit against ANTHC, the State of Alaska, and eight dental therapists.[15] Organized dentistry lacks an understanding of barriers to dental care. While the lawsuit was pending, the president of the Alaska Dental Society stated on an e-mail list for dentists that AI/AN oral health disparities were a result of personal responsibility and that "[a]ny culture that allows such disease will soon disappear and rightfully so."[16] Unfortunately, racist and uninformed viewpoints can often enter policy discussions and create and perpetuate barriers to access.

In June 2007, the Alaska Superior Court ruled, in a comprehensive and strongly worded 21-page opinion, that the Alaska Dental Practice Act conflicted with federal law and obstructed the execution of the purpose of the federally implemented CHAP. In addition, according to the opinion, "[C]ongress' expressed purpose to create an independent statutory framework as a way to provide health care to Alaska Natives would be wholly defeated if the court were to allow a system, which has failed to serve the dental health care needs of Alaska natives, to oversee and regulate the dental health aide therapists."[15] There was no appeal.

When the IHCIA was being permanently reauthorized as part of the Affordable Care Act, the ADA lobbied to include language in the legislation that would exclude dental therapists from the nationalization of the CHAP. Because, as a result of federal preemption, the ADA had been unsuccessful in shutting down the dental therapy program in Alaska through its court action, it wanted new language in federal law that would preclude the spread of dental therapy to states outside Alaska. As part of the permanent reauthorization, the IHCIA was amended to allow for the nationalization of the CHAP program subject to certain limitations. Two such limitations are on the expansion of dental therapists without state authorization and the exclusion of certain procedures from the scope of practice of dental therapists.[17] That language seemingly left tribes at the whim of the state legislatures. Until 2017, no tribe had successfully moved state legislation that would authorize the use of dental therapists in tribal health programs. But tribes are resilient. As governments, tribes have the responsibility to provide for the health and welfare of their citizens—so Swinomish began seeking other ways to expand the dental team.

DENTAL CARE IN WASHINGTON STATE: A TURNING POINT

As chairman of the Swinomish Indian Tribal Community, this author was frustrated that the language in the IHCIA represented a clear and inappropriate disruption of the long-standing federal–tribal government-to-government-relationship. This specific and unprecedented language injected the states into the federal–tribal relationship, which is inconsistent with fundamental federal Indian law that has long recognized the federal trust responsibility and the federal nature of the government-to-government relationship with tribes.

Nonetheless, for six years, tribal leaders in the State of Washington worked with a coalition of advocates in an attempt to pass a state law that would authorize dental therapists statewide. This is not only a tribal issue in Washington State or in the United States; it is also a matter of creating jobs, strengthening communities, and providing equitable oral health care to rural and underserved communities. After many failed attempts to pass legislation authorizing the use of dental therapists either statewide or in Indian Country, in 2015, the Swinomish Tribe could no longer wait for state permission to provide much-needed dental care for its citizens. Tribal leaders have a responsibility and the inherent authority to take a stand for tribal citizens, especially the children and elders, who are suffering unnecessarily and face a health crisis. Their health and well-being could not be put on hold because of the strength of the Washington State Dental Association's lobbying machine.

THE MODERN DENTAL TEAM IN INDIAN COUNTRY

In the absence of a state regulatory structure authorizing dental therapists, the Swinomish Tribe, with the full support of the Tribal Senate and the entire community, exercised its sovereign authority and created the Swinomish Division of Licensing and a Dental Health Provider Licensing Board. This board consults with and advises the Division of Licensing concerning the licensing of all Swinomish dental providers. The Swinomish Tribe adapted the federal CHAP code as a basis for scope of practice, supervision, certification requirements, and disciplinary actions for practicing dental therapists. Since 2017, the Swinomish Tribe has extended the exercise of its licensing authority. Through evolution of the Swinomish Tribal Code, intergovernmental agreements, and amendments to other tribes' legal codes, the Swinomish Division of Licensing can and does issue licenses to a dental therapist and supervising dentist working for another tribe at that tribe's health care facility. This is an exercise of both tribes' inherent sovereignty and responsibility to care for the health of their tribal members.

It may be a first in Indian Country, but it will not be the last. Other tribes will similarly exercise their own sovereignty to license professionals in a manner that is consistent with their needs and values. The Swinomish Tribal Code requires that dental providers demonstrate cultural competence through interviews with community members and through formal education, training, or personal or professional experience that would be reasonably expected to result in cultural competency, something that is absolutely essential for successful oral health services in AI/AN communities.

At present, services provided by dental therapists in Alaska to Medicaid-eligible individuals are reimbursed by Medicaid. Tribes continue to work on setting up a framework that would allow Medicaid reimbursement for services provided by dental therapists outside Alaska. This is necessary for economic sustainability, as without Medicaid reimbursement, tribal communities with the most need will not have access to dental therapists.

NEXT STEPS AND NATIONAL MOMENTUM FOR DENTAL THERAPY IN INDIAN COUNTRY

The need for dental therapists is great across the country. There is a positive movement in some states that will have a significant impact on the ability of communities to expand access to care by bringing dental therapists to rural, underserved, and tribal communities. In 2018, the Indian Health Service (IHS) Area offices throughout the country named representatives to a newly formed Community Health Aide Program Technical Advisory Group (CHAP-TAG). This CHAP-TAG has been tasked with providing input and support on the national policy for implementing CHAP in states outside Alaska. This work is necessary to continue to clear hurdles for tribes seeking to utilize dental therapists. Creating a full tribal licensing law and establishing a board to license one provider is an expensive and onerous task and means that the tribes with the most need will be the least likely to have access to these providers. Creating area-wide infrastructure to certify dental therapists through the CHAP program will help tribes to use these providers in states that have authorized dental therapists. It will also make these providers available in federal IHS-run clinics and should provide support to the tribes as they work to build the legal infrastructure to ensure Medicaid reimbursement.

To date, five states have authorized dental therapists—Maine, Vermont, Arizona, Minnesota, and Washington. In 2017, we successfully passed tribal-specific dental therapy legislation in Washington on the foundation of the work of the previous eight years and the strong collaboration and support from all 29 tribes in Washington.[18-20] An additional 12 states are actively exploring dental therapy legislation, and Oregon has authorized a tribal dental therapy pilot project. As of the date of the publication of this book, four individuals from two Oregon tribes have completed the Alaska Dental Therapy Education Program and have returned to their communities to join dental teams, and there is a dental therapist at the Urban Indian Dental Clinic in Portland, Oregon. The dental therapy workforce in Washington, Oregon, and Idaho is growing. In addition to the dental therapist working at the Swinomish dental clinic, an experienced dental therapist has joined the Port Gamble S'Klallam Tribe's dental team and currently there are eight students in the Alaska Dental Therapy Education Program from tribes throughout Washington, Oregon, and Idaho. Two students from Swinomish will graduate in 2019 and join the Swinomish dental team.

In Washington, we are working with Skagit Valley College to replicate the Alaska Dental Therapy Education Program and create the first dental therapy education program outside Alaska that is accredited by the Commission on Dental Accreditation. This exciting project will help tribes outside Alaska train workforce from their communities to serve their communities.

CONCLUSIONS

Governments, the ADA, educators, and communities all share a responsibility to eliminate health disparities in tribal and other underserved communities. It will take a united effort to achieve oral health equity in our communities. I pray that all who read this will come to the conclusion that they need to be on the right side of history. Dental therapy programs will only grow. Instead of wasting money fighting the inevitable, I urge the ADA and all others to invest in scholarships for students who want to go to school to become dental therapists in their community.

Regardless, the Swinomish Tribe will continue this fight on all fronts—legislative, administrative, and in the clinic—to provide oral health services to our communities, which is a basic need of all youth, adults, and elders. This generation will be the last generation to suffer needlessly and the first to usher in a new era of oral health care.

ACKNOWLEDGMENTS

I would like to recognize the Swinomish Senate; our Health, Education, and Social Services Committee; and the Swinomish Dental Health Provider Licensing Board for their leadership, as well as our dental clinic team for their willingness to be trailblazers, and the entire Swinomish community for their support of this important and innovative project. I would also like to acknowledge the Northwest Portland Area Indian Health Board, the W.K. Kellogg Foundation, and The Pew Charitable Trusts for their longstanding efforts to make dental therapists available outside of Alaska and their generous support of Swinomish's work. Finally, I recognize the dedication of tribal leaders across Indian Country to improving their communities' health and health care and the Washington State legislators who advocated for recognition of this tribal solution to a tribal health challenge.

REFERENCES

1. Phipps KR, Ricks, TL. The oral health of American Indian and Alaska Native children aged 1–5 years: results of the 2014 IHS Oral Health Survey. Indian Health Service data brief. Rockville, MD: Indian Health Service; 2015.

2. Phipps KR, Ricks TL. The oral health of American Indian and Alaska Native adult dental patients: results of the 2015 IHS oral health survey. Indian Health Service data brief. Rockville, MD: Indian Health Service; 2016.

3. Community Health Aide Program Certification Board. Standards and procedures. Chapter 2, Article 30. 2018. Available at: http://www.akchap.org/resources/chap_library/CHAPCB_Documents/CHAPCB_Standards_Procedures_Amended_2018-01-25.pdf. Accessed October 31, 2018.

4. Valachociv RW. Current demographics and future trends of the dentist work force. American Dental Education Association. 2009. Available at: http://www.nationalacademies.org/hmd/~/media/Files/Activity%20Files/Workforce/oralhealthworkforce/2009-Feb-09/1%20-%20Valachovic.ashx. Accessed December 8, 2016.

5. Williard ME. Dental health aide therapists celebrate graduation and program enhancements in new partnership with Iḷisaġvik College. Alaska Native Tribal Health Consortium. 2016. Available at: http://anthc.org/dental-health-aide. Accessed October 14, 2016.

6. Williard ME. Meet our dental aide therapists. Alaska Native Tribal Health Consortium. 2016. Available at: http://anthc.org/wp-content/uploads/2016/02/DHAT_BIOS.pdf. Accessed October 14, 2016.

7. Pew Charitable Trusts. Expanding the dental team, increasing access to care in public settings. June 2014. Available at: http://www.pewtrusts.org/~/media/assets/2014/06/27/expanding_dental_case_studies_report.pdf. Accessed October 14, 2016.

8. Wetterhall S, Bader JD, Burrus BB, Lee JY, Shugars DA. Evaluation of the dental health aide therapist workforce model in Alaska. Research Triangle International. October 2010. Available at: https://www.rti.org/sites/default/files/resources/alaskadhatprogramevaluation final102510.pdf. Accessed December 8, 2016.

9. Chi DL, Lenaker D, Mancl L, Dunbar M, Babb M. Dental therapists linked to improved dental outcomes for Alaska Native communities in the Yukon-Kuskokwim Delta. *J Public Health Dent.* 2018;78(2):175–182.

10. Washington State Board of Health, Rotakhina S, Hoff C. Executive summary: Health impact review of HB 2321 concerning mid-level dental professionals. Available at: http://sboh.wa.gov/Portals/7/Doc/HealthImpactReviews/HIR-2014-08-HB2321.pdf. Accessed December 12, 2016.

11. Smith EB. Dental therapists in Alaska: addressing unmet needs and reviving competition in dental care. *Alaska Law Rev.* 2007;24(1):105–143.

12. National Congress of American Indians. Tribal nations and the United States: an introduction. Available at: http://www.ncai.org/tribalnations/introduction/Tribal_Nations_and_the_United_States_An_Introduction-web-.pdf. Accessed October 31, 2018.

13. Legal Information Institute. Preemption. Available at: https://www.law.cornell.edu/wex/preemption. Accessed October 17, 2016.

14. State of Alaska Department of Law. Memorandum to Robert E. Warren from Paul R. Lyle, RE: State licensure of federal dental health aides. September 2005: 2. Available at: http://law.alaska.gov/pdf/opinions/opinions_2005/05-020_663050152.pdf. Accessed October 17, 2016.

15. *Alaska Dental Society et al. v Alaska Native Tribal Health Consortium et al.*, No. 3AN-06-04797CI (Alaska Super Ct 2006): 19.

16. DeMarban A. Dentist's remarks called racist, misinformed. *Anchorage Daily News*. September 27, 2016. Available at: http://www.adn.com/rural-alaska/article/dentists-remarks-called-racist-misinformed-41406/2012/04/05. Accessed October 25, 2016.

17. 25 USC § 1616l (d)(2)(B), (d)(3)(A), and (b)(7)(B).

18. Hoekstra K. Washington tribe beats dental lobby, gets dental therapy. *Watchdog*. April 4, 2017. Available at: https://www.watchdog.org/national/washington-tribe-beats-dental-lobby-gets-dental-therapy/article_b34717a9-c38e-5483-8114-f7edb296063c.html. Accessed October 31, 2018.

19. Van Cleave A. Tribes planning next steps now that dental therapy bill is law. *KNKX*. February 27, 2017. Available at: http://www.knkx.org/post/tribes-planning-next-steps-now-dental-therapy-bill-law. Accessed October 31, 2018.

20. Washington State Legislature. SB 5079 - 2017-18 Concerning dental health services in tribal settings. Available at: http://apps2.leg.wa.gov/billsummary?BillNumber=5079&Year=2017&BillNumber=5079&Year=2017. Accessed October 31, 2018.

IV. DENTAL EDUCATION

National Momentum Toward a Repre Workforce and Oral Health Equity

Albert K. Yee, MD, MPH, Tera Bianchi, MSW, and Kasey Wilson, MSW

Oral health is vital to overall health, yet difficulty accessing dental care, especially care that is culturally appropriate and respectful, remains out of reach for many communities. People of color still experience greater barriers to accessing dental care and poorer oral health outcomes than their White counterparts. For example, about a third of White older adults have lost six or more teeth because of decay or gum disease compared with more than half of Black older adults.[1] In addition, American Indian children have four times more tooth decay[2] and Black and Latino children have two times more tooth decay than White children.[3] Combined with the fact that more than 62 million people across the country live in areas without an adequate supply of oral health providers,[4] these data display the need for innovative solutions to improve access to care.

A HOLISTIC APPROACH TO ACHIEVING ORAL HEALTH EQUITY

Achieving oral health equity will require a holistic approach that includes improving access to oral health services, expanding the oral health workforce, elimination of structural discrimination, and attention to the social determinants of health—the social and economic conditions where people live, work, and play (outside the health care system) that influence oral and overall health and well-being.[5] We know that social determinants such as access to transportation, income and poverty, and discrimination have an impact on oral health, so these are important areas of oral health policy change. Equally important as the equitable provision of oral health services and the equitable distribution of the social determinants of oral health is attention to the social determinants of equity: racism and other systems that inequitably allocate the social determinants of health.[6]

DENTAL THERAPISTS AS AN APPROACH TO ORAL HEALTH EQUITY IN UNDERSERVED COMMUNITIES

One solution to address these oral health disparities that has been getting a lot of recent attention is dental therapy. Practiced for more than a century in countries around the world and brought to the United States more than a decade ago by Alaska Native (AN)

_ seeking accessible and culturally respectful dental care for their communities, _ental therapy has proven safe and effective for communities in Alaska[7] and Minnesota.[8] Dental therapists are members of an enhanced dental team that improves access to care for residents in previously underserved communities by expanding the number of available providers and delivering both prevention and treatment services.

Numerous studies and reports have documented that dental therapists provide safe, competent, and appropriate care for their patients.[7-9] Most impressively, a recent study has shown that there are long-term positive health outcomes in communities served by dental teams with dental therapists.[6] Over a ten-year period, Alaska communities with access to dental therapists showed a decrease in the number of extractions and increased use of preventive services among both adults and children. Notably, this increased access to care was not associated with an increase in children needing treatment under anesthesia.[6]

On the basis of the track record of success in Alaska and Minnesota, interest in dental therapy and momentum toward spreading the profession throughout the country has grown over the last several years. In addition to Alaska and Minnesota, dental therapists are now also authorized to practice in Maine, Vermont, and Arizona, as well as on tribal lands in Washington and at tribal pilot sites in Oregon. About a dozen other states have active legislation or are actively exploring introducing legislation to authorize dental therapy as a solution to the long-term oral health needs of their communities.

Dental Therapy Training and Standards

As a model that improves access to preventive services and treatment for underserved populations, creates jobs in underserved communities, and expands a workforce that is culturally and linguistically representative of patients, dental therapy is an innovative and effective approach to oral health equity. A recent significant milestone that allows the model to maintain its focus on health equity is the Commission on Dental Accreditation's (CODA's) Standards for Dental Therapy Education Programs.[10] The same accrediting body that creates standards for dental schools and other oral health professional training programs, CODA finalized standards for dental therapy education programs in 2015, recognizing dental therapy as a legitimate oral health profession and paving the way for uniform training and accountability standards across the country.

The CODA standards reflect and are similar to the educational requirements of dental therapy academic programs around the world as well as the first dental therapy training program in the United States, which was developed by and for AN communities in 2004.[11] To replicate these successful training programs, which have graduated dental therapists that are well prepared as culturally competent providers to practice in community-based settings, the CODA standards recommend that dental therapists be trained in three academic years. This recommendation is based on decades of experience and scientific evidence and ensures enough time for dental therapists to gain the skills they need to practice safely and effectively. The CODA standards also allow individuals who already have training as dental hygienists to receive advanced standing and the opportunity to complete dental therapy training in less time. Importantly, CODA does not recommend additional training requirements that are unnecessary for patient care or safety and that add burdensome time onto training programs that unnecessarily increase costs—and educational debt—for trainees. Preexisting and newly authorized dental therapy academic programs are currently submitting and preparing to submit applications for accreditation under the CODA standards.

Beyond improved access and direct patient and population health benefits, dental therapy training based on the CODA educational standards also allows communities to address some of the social and economic determinants of oral health described previously, such as the following:

- Economic opportunities: The three-academic-year educational standards set by CODA allow communities to recruit local students to train in local educational programs. Dental therapists graduating from these programs return to work in their home communities, many of which have been underserved by the traditional oral health workforce. This fosters local job creation and economic development in underserved areas.
- Transportation: By recommending a three-year training program, the CODA standards keep the cost of dental therapy education accessible for students from diverse communities, cutting down on student debt and facilitating new dental therapy graduates to work in community-based settings and provider shortage areas. By deploying and expanding the workforce into these traditionally underserved communities, dental therapists address transportation issues many people face when trying to access oral health services.
- Discrimination: By keeping the length and cost of dental therapy education accessible, the CODA standards facilitate the recruitment of local providers who will practice in their home communities. This ensures an oral health workforce that understands the culture, language, and health beliefs and practices of their local community, reducing experiences with discrimination, enhancing effective patient–provider communication, and strengthening patient–provider relationships in oral health settings.

Growing National Momentum for Dental Therapy

Because of the demonstrated success of dental therapy where it is authorized and the model's ability to address oral health equity, dental therapy is now expanding across the country beyond Alaska and Minnesota. In recent years, Maine, Vermont, and Arizona have all passed statewide legislation to authorize dental therapists to practice. Washington State and Oregon have authorized dental therapists to practice in some capacity on tribal lands.

Maine's Dental Therapy Legislation

In 2014, Maine passed legislation that authorized dental therapists to practice across the state. Because this legislation passed before the adoption the CODA dental therapy education standards in 2015, Maine did not have the benefit of standardized training guidelines to guide their legislation or implementation. This has created some delays for developing a dental therapy education program in Maine, but the passage of this legislation represented a major milestone in the national momentum of dental therapy, as it was only the second state in the lower 48 to authorize dental therapy and the first state to successfully do so in the six years since Minnesota did in 2009.

Vermont's Dental Therapy Legislation

Building on Maine's successful passage of dental therapy legislation, Vermont authorized dental therapists to practice statewide soon thereafter in 2016. As the first state to successfully pass dental therapy legislation after the CODA standards were adopted, Vermont's law requires that dental therapists graduate from a program that is accredited by CODA. This requirement leverages the power and health equity potential of these standardized educational guidelines and sets the stage for other states to build successful models of dental therapy. Just two years after passing legislation, Vermont is on the cusp of creating only the third dental therapy education program in the country at Vermont Technical College (VTC). Vermont's dental therapy education program is being designed to serve as a regional training program where future dental therapists from Maine (and other nearby states, as this model spreads) as well as those from Vermont can receive CODA-accredited training. In July 2018, VTC received a four-year federal grant from the Health Resources and Services Administration to cover equipment, supplies, and other program start-up costs. The grant will provide $400,000 per year over four years for a total of a $1.6 million investment in the oral health of Vermonters.

Arizona's Dental Therapy Legislation

The most recent development in dental therapy's growing national momentum was the passage of statewide legislation in Arizona in 2018. Like Vermont's, Arizona's legislation requires dental therapists to be trained at a CODA-accredited educational program. The law also allows Arizona's tribal nations to send tribal community members to Alaska to be trained and return to practice in Arizona. These tribal members will not have to wait until dental therapy training programs are up and running in Arizona before they can be trained to practice on tribal lands. Arizona's legislation was significant in its recognition of and respect for tribal sovereignty and the leadership of tribal communities in the US dental therapy movement. This successful legislation was the direct result of the involvement of tribal communities and other grassroots community organizations in policy advocacy and community organizing as the dental therapy bill was progressing through the Arizona legislature.

Washington State's Dental Therapy Legislation

Since 2009, a diverse coalition of consumer advocates, tribal governments, and provider groups have supported efforts to pass statewide dental therapy legislation. While these efforts continue, in 2014, the Swinomish Indian Tribal Community (SITC), with the support of the Northwest Portland Area Indian Health Board (NPAIHB), elected to exert their tribal sovereignty rights and, in 2016, became the first tribe in the lower 48 states to start its own dental therapy program. The SITC set up a regulatory infrastructure to authorize and oversee dental therapists within their tribal health program and recruited an experienced dental therapist from Alaska to see patients under the supervision of a dentist at their health center. The SITC have since recruited additional students from their tribe who are currently being trained in the Alaska dental therapy education program and, upon graduation, will begin practicing at their health center.

The leadership of the SITC and the success of its dental therapy program led to the passage of a tribal dental therapy bill in Washington in 2017.[12] This legislation authorizes dental therapists to work in American Indian health programs on tribal lands and directs Washington State to work with the Centers on Medicare and Medicaid Services (CMS) to ensure that dental therapists are eligible for Medicaid reimbursement. In May of 2018, CMS denied Washington State's proposal that would authorize dental therapists as eligible Medicaid providers. In June, Washington State appealed the decision; this appeal is still under review. The SITC and the NPAIHB are working with a local community college to build a training program that will educate dental therapists closer to their home community.

Oregon's Dental Therapy Legislation

In 2011, Oregon passed legislation authorizing dental pilot projects to implement innovative models of oral health delivery and evaluate their impact on access, quality of care, workforce, and cost. As part of this broader project, a number of tribal nations in Oregon, together with the NPAIHB, were approved by the Oregon Health Authority—the state agency overseeing this pilot—to administer the Oregon Tribes Dental Health Aide Therapist Pilot in 2016.[13] The dental therapist pilot authorized dental therapists to practice on tribal lands in Oregon. This pilot project is based on the highly successful Alaska dental therapy program and allows Oregon tribes to send community members to Alaska to be trained.

Currently, the dental therapy pilot is operating at three tribal sites: the Coquille Indian Tribe; the Confederated Tribes of Coos, Lower Umpqua, and Siuslaw Indians (CTCLUSI); and at the Native American Rehabilitation Center of the Northwest. One CTCLUSI tribal member went to Alaska to be trained and has since returned to Oregon to practice at a dental therapy pilot site along with an experienced dental therapist from Alaska who recently joined the project. Three additional Oregon tribal members graduated from the Alaska dental therapy training program in June 2018. As part of the pilot project, a comprehensive evaluation is underway and the findings will inform and guide future efforts to institutionalize dental therapy in the state.

A Concerning Trend by State Legislatures

The preceding state examples demonstrate that the national dental therapy movement is advancing in the direction of standardization and recognizing and respecting tribal leadership and sovereignty. However, a concerning trend is emerging in which state legislatures are undermining the flexibility of the national standards and undercutting the success of the model by mandating a degree requirement (a master's degree in Maine) or that dental therapists be dually trained and credentialed as dental hygienists (in Vermont and Arizona). This is inconsistent with the standards set by CODA and the long history of the profession across the world.

As this movement continues to grow and spread to more states and tribal nations, it is important to continue the trend of legislation that requires dental therapists to graduate from a CODA-accredited program and to ensure that no additional unnecessary, burdensome, and costly educational requirements are added. Adoption of CODA's standardized educational model creates freedom for providers to move and practice across the country, ensures that the time and cost of dental therapy education remains accessible, and leaves decisions and details about curriculum and educational policy in the hands of local institutions that are based in communities.

CONCLUSIONS

As the experience with dental therapy has grown over the years, health programs that incorporate this emerging profession as part of dental teams have seen tangible benefits. These include consistent, safe, and high-quality care; improved access to both oral health treatment and prevention services (especially in traditionally underserved communities); culturally competent providers; highly satisfied patients; and some impressive long-term population health outcomes. In addition to health benefits, states and tribal nations also view the dental therapy profession as an opportunity to create new and good-paying local jobs that contribute to strengthening their respective economies. Dental therapy is spreading across the country in a growing number of states and tribal nations. Great momentum is driving additional efforts to expand this highly promising profession to address the oral health disparities that have persisted for many years among tribal communities, low-income populations, rural parts of the country, and in communities of color.

Finally, the CODA dental therapy education standards have fostered an incredible opportunity to standardize academic requirements across states and tribal nations. Having cross-jurisdictional academic consistency will ensure reliable care and service quality, greater career opportunities and mobility for providers, and good access to dental therapy training opportunities for residents from all communities. National, tribal, state, and local efforts are underway to promote the CODA standards as the foundation for dental therapy education across the country.

REFERENCES

1. Centers for Disease Control and Prevention. Oral health data by location. Oral health data. Available at: https://www.cdc.gov/oralhealthdata. Accessed October 5, 2018.

2. Phipps KR, Ricks TL. The oral health of American Indian and Alaska Native children aged 1–5 years: results of the 2014 IHS oral health survey. Indian Health Service Data Brief. Rockville, MD: Indian Health Service; 2015.

3. Dye BA, Thornton-Evans G, Li X, Iafolla, TJ. Dental caries and sealant prevalence in children and adolescents in the United States, 2011–2012. NCHS Data Brief. 2015(191):1–8.

4. Henry J. Kaiser Family Foundation. Dental care health professional shortage areas (HPSAs). State health facts. Available at: https://www.kff.org/other/state-indicator/dental-care-health-professional-shortage-areas-hpsas/?currentTimeframe=0&sortModel=%7B%22colId%22:%22Location%22,%22sort%22:%22asc%22%7D. Accessed October 5, 2018.

5. Tellez M, Zini A, Estupiñan-Day S. Social determinants and oral health: an update. Curr Oral Health Rep. 2014;1(3):148–152.

6. Jones CP, Jones CY, Perry GS, Barclay G, Jones CA. Addressing the social determinants of children's health: a cliff analogy. J Health Care Poor Underserved. 2009;20(4 suppl):1–12.

7. Chi DL, Lenaker D, Manci L, Dunbar M, Babb M. Dental therapists linked to improved dental outcomes for Alaska Native communities in the Yukon–Kuskokwim Delta. J Public Health Dent. 2018;78(2):175–182.

8. Minnesota Department of Health. Early impacts of dental therapists in Minnesota. Report to the Minnesota Legislature. 2014. Available at: http://www.health.state.mn.us/divs/orhpc/workforce/oral/dtlegisrpt.pdf. Accessed October 5, 2018.

9. Nash DA, Friedman JW, Mathu-Muju KR, et al. A review of the global literature on dental therapists. Community Dent Oral Epidemiol. 2013;42(1):1–10.

10. Commission on Dental Accreditation. Accreditation standards for dental therapy education programs. 2015. Available at: http://www.ada.org/~/media/CODA/Files/dt.ashx. Accessed October 5, 2018.

11. Alaska Native Tribal Health Consortium. Alaska dental therapy educational programs. Available at: https://anthc.org/alaska-dental-therapy-education-programs. Accessed October 5, 2018.

12. Community Catalyst. Washington becomes latest state to join dental therapy movement. 2017. Available at: https://www.communitycatalyst.org/resources/publications/document/cc_wabill_pressrelease_2-22-17.pdf. Accessed October 5, 2018.

13. Oregon Health Authority. Dental pilot project application #100, "Oregon Tribes Dental Health Aide Pilot Project" approval with addendum. 2016. Available at: https://www.oregon.gov/oha/PH/PREVENTIONWELLNESS/ORALHEALTH/DENTALPILOTPROJECTS/Documents/100-approval.pdf. Accessed October 5, 2018.

21

Dental Therapy Education in Minnesota*

Karl Self, DDS, MBA, and Colleen Brickle, RDH, EdD, RF

The Institute of Medicine stated that "Improving access to oral health care is a critical and necessary first step to improving oral health outcomes and reducing disparities."[1] Many Minnesota communities suffer from the same access-to-care challenges that have been noted nationwide.[2,3] Minnesota stakeholders have worked diligently for years to address access to care and oral health care disparities. Solutions included efforts to address low reimbursement rates and health literacy challenges, as well as implementation of school-based care services, care coordination, and expanded allied dental professionals' scopes of practice. Yet Minnesotans continued to experience difficulty accessing care, and workforce barriers remained.

In 2009, Minnesota took a bold approach to address workforce issues by authorizing dental therapy as one tool with a successful history in other parts of the world in improving access to care and reducing oral health disparities.[4] Legislation limited dental therapists to primarily practicing in settings that serve low-income, uninsured, and underserved patients or in a dental health professional shortage area and aligned educational requirements with their scope of practice. The statutes defined two levels of dental therapy practice: (1) a bachelor-prepared licensed dental therapist (DT) and (2) a certified advanced dental therapist (ADT), which requires master's-level education. A DT/ADT is required to work under the supervision of a licensed Minnesota dentist through a collaborative management agreement, which is viewed as a contract outlining protocols and standing orders.[5]

Minnesota's aim of educating a DT/ADT was to produce clinically competent oral health professionals to address access to care and reduce cost of providing care. Programs would educate students to a level of competency that mirrors what dental students receive for a defined scope of practice.

---

*This is a modified version of the article that appeared in the *American Journal of Public Health*. See: Self K, Brickle C. Dental therapy education in Minnesota. *Am J Public Health*. 2017;107(S1):S77–S80.

DENTAL THERAPY PROGRAM DEVELOPMENT AND IMPLEMENTATION

During the legislative process, the University of Minnesota, School of Dentistry (SOD), and the Minnesota State College and University System (MnSCU) indicated that they would implement programs to promote established standards of dentistry. The vision of both academic institutions was to utilize existing curriculum, faculty, and facilities to educate new dental team members. Each program developed from different philosophies yet maintained that this intraprofessional team member would allow the entire dental team to work to the top of their license to improve access.

The SOD's dental therapy program created two tracks. One track, leading to a Bachelor of Science in Dental Therapy (BSDT), was designed to admit students with roughly one year of post–high-school college education. The other track, leading to a Master of Dental Therapy (MDT), was designed for those already possessing a bachelor's degree. Both tracks were full-time, 28-month programs that prepared students to practice at the licensed DT level. Admissions criteria focused on previous academic success, volunteer experiences, community involvement, and the applicant's potential to meet the mission of the dental therapy legislation. Given the school's commitment to one standard of care required in dental education, dental therapy students took courses alongside dental and dental hygiene students.

Two MnSCU institutions—Normandale Community College, which has a strong history of dental hygiene education, and Metropolitan State University, which is known for advancing nursing education and the capacity to confer graduate degrees—began their first cohort of students in a part-time, 26-month Master of Science in Advanced Dental Therapy program. Admission requirements included a bachelor's degree, an active Minnesota dental hygiene license, restorative functions course, and recent clinical practice. The foundational competencies achieved as a licensed dental hygienist allowed for advanced standing for students and, thus, a shorter program.

Both programs have evolved since their first classes in 2009. Each program engaged in its own quality-improvement efforts. Program changes were driven by feedback from students, graduates, dentists, and other engaged stakeholders. See Table 21-1 for program comparisons.

From its inception, the MnSCU program combined the education of both dental therapy and advanced dental therapy scope-of-practice procedures (Table 21-2). After one year, the program restructured to a 20-month part-time program and added more clinical time in the summer. The decision for the part-time program was to allow dental hygienists the ability to work. According to faculty and student feedback, the rigor of the program did not lend itself to working; also, more daily lab and clinic time was needed to master the high-speed handpiece. In 2015, the program changed to a full-time 16-month program.

Table 21-1. Minnesota Dental Therapy Education Programs Comparison

Component	University of Minnesota School of Dentistry	Minnesota State College and University System
Healthcare background requirement	No previous health care background required; other prerequisites apply	Minnesota licensed dental hygienist (DH); completion of restorative functions course
Original program design	Bachelor of Science in Dental Therapy: • One year college required • 28-month full-time program • Licensed dental therapist (DT) upon graduation Master of Dental Therapy: • Baccalaureate degree required • 28-month full-time program • Licensed DT upon graduation	Master of Science in Advanced Dental Therapy: • Baccalaureate degree required • 26-month part-time program • Licensed DT upon graduation • Eligible for Advanced Dental Therapy certification • Dual licensed as DT/DH
First program modification	Master of Dental Therapy: • Baccalaureate degree required[a] • 28-month full-time program • Licensed DT upon graduation • Eligible for Advanced Dental Therapy certification[a]	Master of Science in Advanced Dental Therapy: • Baccalaureate degree required • 20-month part-time program[a] • Licensed DT upon graduation • Eligible for Advanced Dental Therapy certification • Dual licensed as DT/DH
Current program design	Bachelor of Science in Dental Hygiene/ Master of Dental Therapy: • Minimum one year of college required[a] • 32-month full-time program[a] • Licensed DT upon graduation • Eligible for Advanced Dental Therapy certification • Dual licensed as DT/DH[a]	Master of Science in Advanced Dental Therapy: • Baccalaureate degree required • 16-month full-time program[a] • Licensed DT upon graduation • Eligible for Advanced Dental Therapy certification • Dual licensed as DT/DH

[a]Program modification.

The SOD incorporated ADT standards into their curriculum in 2013 following research and conversations with safety-net dental providers and other potential employers, combined with the philosophy of a new dean. In addition, some employers and potential employers, especially out-of-state solo practitioners, voiced a desire for a DT who was also dual-licensed in dental hygiene. This direction was also supported by some graduates. In fall of 2016, the SOD program evolved into a 32-month Bachelor of Science in Dental Hygiene/MDT dual-degree program.

Now, all future DTs will have the same educational background and be eligible for the same credentials, eliminating confusion and misinformation in Minnesota and nationally. Both programs are also committed to engaging in collaborative education and exposing students to collaborative care to promote better communication, understanding, and trust for professionals to work collaboratively to enhance patient outcomes.

Table 21-2. Minnesota Dental Therapist Scope of Practice and Level of Supervision

General Supervision	Indirect Supervision	Procedures
ADT DT		Perform preliminary charting of the oral cavity, oral health instruction, and disease prevention, including nutritional counseling, dietary analysis.
ADT DT		Apply topical medications such as, but not limited to, topical fluoride and cavity varnishes in appropriate dosages.
ADT DT		Perform mechanical polishing.
ADT DT		Etch appropriate enamel surfaces, apply and adjust pit and fissure sealants.
ADT DT		Placement of temporary restorations.
ADT DT		Fabrication of soft occlusal guards and athletic mouthguards.
ADT DT		Pulp vitality testing.
ADT DT		Administer local anesthesia.
ADT DT		Administer nitrous oxide inhalation analgesia.
ADT DT		Take radiographs.
ADT DT		Application of desensitizing medication or resin.
ADT DT		Tissue conditioning and soft reline.
ADT DT		Atraumatic restorative therapy.
ADT DT		Tooth reimplantation.
ADT DT		Dressing changes.
ADT DT		Dispense and administer analgesics, anti-inflammatories, and antibiotics as permitted by the collaborative management agreement. Advanced Dental Therapist may provide, dispense and administer.
ADT	DT	Cavity preparation and restoration of primary and permanent teeth.
ADT	DT	Pulpotomies on primary teeth and indirect and direct pulp capping on primary and permanent teeth.
ADT	DT	Stabilization of re-implanted teeth.
ADT	DT	Remove sutures.
ADT	DT	Brush biopsies.
ADT	DT	Repair of defective prosthetic devices.
ADT	DT	Placement of temporary crowns and preparation and placement of preformed crowns.
ADT	DT	Provide emergency palliative treatment of dental pain.
ADT	DT	Recement permanent crowns.
ADT	DT	Extractions of primary teeth.
ADT		Extraction of periodontally diseased permanent teeth with mobility of +3 to +4 as permitted by the collaborative management agreement. Not to include unerupted, impacted, fractured, or need for sectioning.

(Continued)

Table 21-2. (Continued)

General Supervision	Indirect Supervision	Procedures
ADT		Oral evaluation and assessment of dental disease and the formation of an individualized treatment plan authorized by a collaborating dentist.
ADT		Make appropriate referrals to dentists, physicians, and other practitioners in consultation with the collaborating dentist.

Source: Adapted from Minnesota Board of Dentistry.[6]
Note: ADT = advanced dental therapist; DT = dental therapist; general supervision = the dentist has given consent for the procedures being performed during which the dentist is not required to be present in the dental office; indirect supervision = the dentist is in the office, authorizes the procedures, and remains in the office while the procedures are being performed by the licensed dental therapist.

PROGRAM OUTCOMES

Evaluation of dental therapy practice and education in Minnesota is still in its infancy. A report submitted to the Minnesota legislature detailing the early impact of dental therapy noted positive results.[7] Both education programs have been approved by the Minnesota Board of Dentistry (BOD) through 2020. The new Commission on Dental Accreditation (CODA) standards were approved for implementation in August 2015. The Minnesota BOD standards are consistent with CODA standards. Each program anticipates achieving full CODA accreditation.

Minnesota graduates must pass a clinically based competency examination to be eligible for licensure. No national dental therapy examination exists. The BOD collaborated with the Central Regional Dental Testing Services to establish a licensure examination that mirrors the examination for dentists. Because of different scopes of practice, the manikin component is different, but the restorative components evaluate the same scope of practice.

To achieve ADT certification, a graduate must have practiced for 2000 hours as a licensed DT and successfully completed the BOD's three-part certification examination. The examination includes a review of patient records, an objective structured clinical examination, and an interview with the Licensing and Credentials Committee.

While the value of dental therapy is still being debated in the United States, the integration of DTs into Minnesota's oral health workforce continues to progress. Following is the status as of June 2018:

- There were 88 licensed DTs, 52 of which were certified as an ADT.
- Thirty four of the 88 were dually licensed in dental hygiene and dental therapy.
- Ninety-seven percent of DTs seeking employment were employed.
- Forty-two percent of clinics employing a DT employed more than one.

- DTs were geographically distributed in proportion to the state's population:
  - Fifty-five percent of the state's population lives in the seven-county Greater Twin Cities metro area, where 59% of working DTs were employed.
- Forty-five percent of Minnesotans live outside the Metro area, where 41% of working DTs are employed (Figure 21-1).

DTs are working in a variety of practice types including private practices, nonprofit clinics, federally qualified health centers, educational institutions, and hospitals. In all cases, DTs and ADTs are limited to practicing in locations designed to improve access to care for underserved populations.

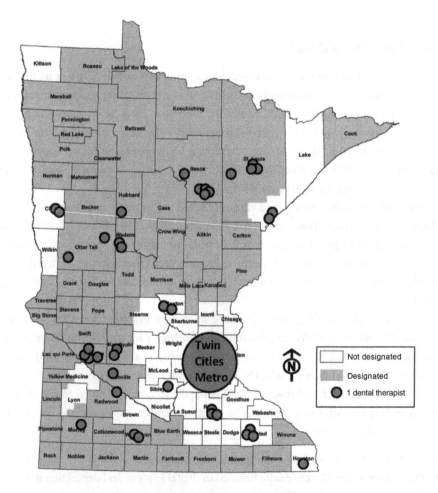

Source: Based on data from Collaborative Management Agreement documents publicly available at the Minnesota Board of Dentistry. The map is courtesy of the author (KS).

Figure 21-1. Dental Therapy Employment Sites by Dental Health Professional Shortage Areas

PUBLIC HEALTH SIGNIFICANCE

As dental therapy continues to evolve in the United States, those involved in implementing dental therapy in Minnesota believe that it is a workforce model that will assist dentistry in achieving the triple aim of health care[8]—simultaneously improving patient care experience, improving the health of populations, and reducing the cost of care. Dental therapy is authorized in four states (Minnesota, Maine, Vermont, and Arizona) and is utilized by tribal communities in Alaska, Oregon, and Washington State. Currently there are three dental therapy educational programs in the United States: two Minnesota programs and the Alaskan Health Aide Therapist program. A dental therapy educational program is under development in Vermont while Maine has yet to create a program. The American Dental Education Association estimated that eight other states were actively exploring dental therapy authorization in 2018.[9]

CONCLUSIONS

As more states elect to incorporate dental therapy into practice, the creation and approval of educational programs is an important consideration for statute implementation. Minnesota's dental therapy educational programs stand ready to assist efforts to develop and implement high-quality programs to educate the newest member of the oral health care team.

REFERENCES

1. Institute of Medicine and National Research Council. Improving access to oral health care for vulnerable and underserved populations. The National Academies Press. 2011. Available at: http://www.nationalacademies.org/hmd/Reports/2011/Improving-Access-to-Oral-Health-Care-for-Vulnerable-and-Underserved-Populations.aspx. Accessed October 1, 2016.

2. Minnesota Department of Health, Oral Health Program. The status of oral health in Minnesota, 2013. Available at: http://www.health.state.mn.us/oralhealth/pdfs/MNOralHealthStatus2013.pdf. Accessed October 4, 2016.

3. Brandt B, Ling L. Transforming the University: final report of the AHC Task Force on Health Professional Workforce. University of Minnesota. 2006. Available at: http://conservancy.umn.edu/handle/11299/5630. Accessed October 4, 2016.

4. Nash DA. A review of the global literature on dental therapists: in the context of the movement to add dental therapists to the oral health workforce in the United States. Battle Creek, MI: W.K. Kellogg Foundation; 2012.

5. Minnesota Board of Dentistry. Dental therapists and advanced dental therapists. Available at: https://mn.gov/boards/dentistry/currentlicensees/processingandapplications/dental-therapists.jsp. Accessed November 2, 2018.

6. Minnesota Board of Dentistry. Delegated duties for dental therapists and advanced dental therapists. 2016. Available at: http://mn.gov/boards/assets/DT%20Chart%20BA_tcm21-262696.pdf. Accessed November 7, 2018.

7. Minnesota Department of Health, Minnesota Board of Dentistry. Early impacts of dental therapists in Minnesota. February 2014. Available at: https://mn.gov/boards/assets/2014Dental-TherapistReport_tcm21-45970.pdf. Accessed December 19, 2016.

8. Berwick DM, Nolan TW, Whittington J. The triple aim: care, health, and cost. *Health Aff (Millwood)*. 2008;27(3):759–769.

9. American Dental Education Association. ADEA United States interactive legislative tracking map. Available at: http://www.adea.org/State-Legislative-Tracker. Accessed July 6, 2018.

22

The Dental Professional*

Terrence Batliner, DDS, MBA

On Friday afternoons, the phone usually rings steadily in my dental office. I try to stop practicing dentistry at 3PM; however, more often than not, one of the front-desk people will tell me that there is another patient in pain on the phone. Most of the people calling are covered by Medicaid, and they have been looking for dentists to see them for a while. If they are in pain or have swelling, we will see them on Friday afternoon, Saturday morning—whenever. Why? Because I am a professional and that is what professionals are supposed to do. I strongly hold this belief and, frankly, it angers me when I see colleagues who do not get it. We all should serve Medicaid patients because we are professionals.

Maybe it is my background. My mother was a Native American with little education. My father was a smart, tough World War II veteran who grew into adulthood during the New Deal. He was a die-hard liberal. They both fought alcoholism their entire lives, which sometimes made my life hell. But, through the ups and downs, I learned a couple of lessons that I do not think enough dentists ever learned.

First, I am successful because I am lucky, not because I am better than everyone else. I was lucky to have a father who pushed education, and I was lucky to grow up in a situation where I could get a good education. I could have grown up like my mother in severe poverty, being shuttled between Denver, Colorado, and Oklahoma with no one to show her how different life could be. She never graduated from high school and may never have made it to the middle class without my father.

Second, luck is fleeting. Things may be good at this moment, but as children of alcoholics know, chaos can break out at any minute. The lucky, comfortable person one minute can become a forgotten and injured person the next. The essential message of these two lessons is that we are all people, some luckier than others, but almost everyone is one adverse event away from a different life.

I have been a faculty member at several dental schools, teaching on the clinic floor and working as an associate dean. Through these experiences, I have learned an unwritten but common belief pervasive in many schools, one conveyed from opinionated faculty to their students: good dentists—quality dentists—do not serve Medicaid patients.

---

*This is a modified version of the article that appeared in the *American Journal of Public Health*. See: Batliner T. The dental professional. *Am J Public Health*. 2017;107(suppl 1):S12.

The message is conveyed through stories about "those people." They do not show up for their appointments; they come late and do not appreciate what you do for them; they make the other people in your waiting room uncomfortable—I can keep going, but the idea is apparent. Well, I could have been one of those people. The only difference between those people and me is luck. Most of us could have been one of those people.

It is time for those of us who serve Medicaid patients to speak up. We need more good dentists who care about people to join us. I do veneers on cash-paying patients, I restore implants for nice people working in high-tech jobs, and I help kids playing football in the suburbs get mouth guards, but I also serve Medicaid patients and treat them like anyone who has insurance. We are all people, and we all deserve respect and care. If you are a dentist, I believe you have a responsibility to serve those in need because, if not for luck, you could be on the other end of the phone at 3PM on a Friday.

23

Aetna and the National Dental Association: A Model Partnership for Racial and Ethnic Health Care Equity*

Hazel J. Harper, DDS, MPH, Mary L. Conicella, DMD, FAGD, Nicole C. Cranston, DDS, Janalyn C. Edmonds, PhD, RN, CNE, and Camesia O. Matthews, DDS

Although progress has been made, oral health is not universally recognized as a critical component of overall health. Coupled with the fact that the burden of disease has been shouldered by those who have been traditionally disenfranchised because of race, ethnicity, gender, age, and socioeconomic status, disparities in health continue to plague vulnerable populations. To address these disparities, Aetna created the Racial and Ethnic Health Care Equity Project and with long-term partner, the National Dental Association (NDA), developed programs to change perceptions about oral health and close the knowledge gaps between dental and nondental health professionals. This public–private partnership has evolved over the span of two decades and is changing the health landscape by moving the concept of interprofessional collaboration from visualization to actualization.

The NDA and the Aetna Foundation share a common mission: to improve racial and ethnic health equity. The Aetna Foundation began to address this issue and started working with national partners to reduce inequities in health outcomes through research, experimentation, and education. Aetna awarded funding to long-term partner, the NDA (the premier organization for African American oral health professionals), to create an initiative for interdisciplinary education that would bridge the gap between dental professionals and nondental health professionals. The vision was that, by working together, Aetna and the NDA could explore ways to develop more effective health teams to eliminate health disparities in communities of color and vulnerable populations.

*This is a modified version of the article that appeared in the *American Journal of Public Health*. See: Harper HJ, Conicella ML, Cranston NC, Edmonds JC, Matthews CO. The Aetna–NDA partnership for achieving racial and ethnic health equity. *Am J Public Health*. 2017;107(S1):S10–S11.

CURRENT EVIDENCE-BASED RESEARCH ON ORAL HEALTH AND DISEASE

Current research shows that oral health may have even more of an impact on overall health than previously thought. Periodontal disease has a significant impact, but inflammation may be more responsible for the association with specific conditions such as rheumatoid arthritis and prostatitis.[1] Clinical and research findings are increasingly unveiling links between oral health and such maladies as cancer, heart disease, and pancreatic disease.[2] These diseases have an impact on multiple organ systems throughout the body, and periodontal disease may play a major part.[3] Infection and inflammation associated with periodontitis have also been implicated in cardiovascular events and stroke, sleep disorders, pneumonia, and Alzheimer's disease.[4-6]

The significance of the oral–systemic link is not only because it *relates* to quality-of-health issues, but also because it has an *impact* on quality-of-life issues. Evidence-based research links oral health to systemic health in ways that can no longer justify separation of the health disciplines. Aetna's Racial and Ethnic Health Care Equity Project seeks to address health disparities and achieve health equity by supporting promising programs that promote coordinated, collaborative, patient-centered care. The Aetna–NDA partnership closes gaps in knowledge and creates better health teams through innovative interprofessional events.

THE AETNA–NATIONAL DENTAL ASSOCIATION PARTNERSHIP

The National Dental Association was formed in 1913. The NDA mission statement says, "The National Dental Association promotes oral health equity among people of color by harnessing the collective power of its members, advocating for the needs of and mentoring dental students of color, and raising the profile of the profession in our communities."[7] As both caregivers and citizens of the communities that they serve, NDA members seek to improve the health of the underserved, eliminate disparities, and promote health equity. The impact of the 20-year NDA–Aetna partnership (which began in 1996) has been far-reaching and continuously expanding. The shared vision and commitment to integrate medicine and dentistry to achieve better health has not only permeated throughout the NDA but has also been shared with and adopted by organizations outside the NDA. Now widely accepted, the concept is changing the health care landscape and continues to be strengthened by rapidly proliferating networks dedicated to patient-centered care and reducing disparities.

Since 2006, the Aetna–NDA partnership has addressed health equity and disparities in vulnerable communities. In 2008, the Aetna Foundation created a new funding focus area: racial and ethnic health care equity. The NDA approached Aetna with the vision of developing a national program to increase interprofessional collaborations and improve health outcomes in vulnerable populations. Initially, continuing education programs included primarily dentists and physicians and were hosted by the local NDA chapters. Early partnerships formed were with local chapters of the National Medical Association, the Association of Black Cardiologists, and health professional training institutions. Later, the NDA chapters formed partnerships and collaborations with other groups in their cities and states to improve health status in vulnerable populations, promote prevention, and increase awareness about the link between oral health and systemic health. Interprofessional programs have been conducted in 12 states (Alabama, California, Georgia, Kentucky, Louisiana, Maryland, New York, North Carolina, Ohio, Pennsylvania, South Carolina, and Texas) and the District of Columbia.

Over the years, the programs expanded to include not only local, but also national interprofessional symposia, and programs were also developed to address national and global health crises. In 2017, in response to public health crises, Aetna and the NDA sponsored two programs: (1) The NDA President's Symposium, "Combatting the Opioid Addiction Crisis: NEW Guidelines for Managing Pain and Prescribing Controlled Substances" (NDA Annual Convention; Dallas, Texas; July 2017) and (2) "The Impact of Social Determinants on Access to Care, Health and Healing" (Texas A & M University School of Dentistry Center of Excellence and Gulf State Dental Association; Dallas, Texas; November 2017). In 2018, the annual Women's Health Symposium Lecture was titled "Prenatal Dental Care and Birth Outcomes: The Consequences of Benign Neglect" (NDA Annual Convention; Orlando, Florida; July 2018).

The opioid addiction crisis symposium was developed to encourage dentists to consider nonopioid alternatives in managing their patients' pain before prescribing an opiate drug. The social determinants of health symposium increased awareness about the profound impact of external factors on health behavior and outcomes. The symposium on prenatal dental care and benign neglect provided a forum to discuss strategies and new techniques to care for expectant mothers, develop prenatal questionnaires, and create referral networks for dentists and obstetricians. It also raised awareness about negative birth outcomes associated with poor oral health. This is especially important when one considers recent findings from analyses of Aetna medical and dental claims data that found an association between intrauterine growth restriction (IUGR) and dental treatment related to infection and inflammation in a large national sample.[8] This association has potential implications for insurance design and for health care policy decisions on the national and state level. For example, a tentative policy recommendation would be that women of childbearing age should be encouraged to have their oral health examined to reduce the risk of IUGR by addressing any oral infection and inflammation well in advance of pregnancy.

INTERPROFESSIONAL COMMUNITY-BASED LEARNING

An innovative, hands-on oral health training program for nursing students was developed and piloted at the 2015 annual Greater New York Dental Meeting (GNYDM) at the Javits Convention Center in New York City. It has since become an annual feature of the GNYDM. It is titled "Inter-Professional Community-Based Learning for Health Professional Students—Oral Health and Nursing: A Team Approach to Population Health." The program is designed to encourage nurses to include oral health screening as a part of their routine health screenings. It spans four days and includes lectures; hands-on training for oral screening; an introduction to mobile dentistry on the Colgate Bright Smiles, Bright Futures van; fluoride varnish application; and nurse volunteer orientation for participation in the Greater New York Smiles children's program. The children's program reaches 1,500 third graders who are bussed to the Javits Center for three days of activities including dental screenings and referrals, interactive health education, oral health videos, and oral hygiene demonstrations. A massive network of volunteers participates in this event sponsored by Colgate, the DentaQuest Foundation, and a host of other dental companies. Collaborators include NDA HEALTH NOW (Health Equity, Access, Literacy, Technology, and Hope – National Outreach on Wheels) Advisory Committee members who support the unique program with resources, in-kind donations, speakers, trainers, and volunteers. Course training materials are donated by SUNSTAR, the Henry Schein Cares Foundation, Columbia Dentoform, and VOCO. The participating nursing students are from Columbia University and New York University

After the 2015 training, 96.9% of the respondents indicated that they are more likely to perform oral screenings, which would not have been the case without this training. At the end of the 2016 session, 100% of the pediatric nursing students answered in the affirmative that this training would help them promote oral health with their pediatric patients.

Finally, in 2017, Colgate Bright Smiles, Bright Futures brought a special guest to the Greater New York Smiles—baseball great C. C. Sabathia, who raised oral health awareness among the local elementary-school kids.

CONCLUSIONS

The strength of the Aetna–NDA partnership lies in its unwavering commitment to racial and ethnic health equity. This public–private partnership has evolved over the span of two decades to become a model for the nation. It is changing the health landscape by moving the concept of interprofessional collaboration from visualization to actualization and is an example of what can be achieved when groups combine their commitment and complementary talents for collective impact and social justice.

ACKNOWLEDGMENTS

Funding for the project came from the Aetna Foundation. In-kind donations for the New York nurses community-based programs were received from the Henry Schein Cares Foundation, Colgate, Sun-star, VOCO, Greater New York Dental Meeting, and Columbia Dentoforms. Funding for the Washington, DC, Healthier Nation program came from the Aetna Foundation, Colgate, the Henry Schein Cares Foundation, and The Pew Charitable Trusts.

REFERENCES

1. American Academy of Periodontology. Periodontal disease and systemic health. 2018. Available at: https://www.perio.org/consumer/gum-disease-and-other-diseases. Accessed August 23, 2018.

2. Jacob JA. Study links periodontal disease bacteria to pancreatic cancer risk. *JAMA.* 2016;315(24):2653–2654.

3. Rostami A, Sharifi M, Kalantari M, Ghandi Y. Oral health and coronary artery disease, a review article. *J Cardiothorac Med.* 2016;4(1):391–396.

4. Carra MC, Schmitt A, Thomas F, Danchin N, Pannier B, Bouchard P. Sleep disorders and oral health: a cross-sectional study. *Clin Oral Investig.* 2017;21(4):975–983.

5. Scannapieco FA, Harris KW. Oral health and pneumonia. In: Craig R, Kamer A, eds. *A Clinician's Guide to Systemic Effects of Periodontal Diseases.* Berlin, Germany: Springer; 2016:81–92.

6. Ide M, Harris M, Stevens A, et al. Periodontitis and cognitive decline in Alzheimer's disease. *PLoS ONE.* 2016;11(3):e0151081.

7. National Dental Association. About NDA. Available at: http://ndaonline.org/about-nda. Accessed November 7, 2018.

8. Albert D, Ananth C, Papapanou P, Ward A, Conicella ML, Andrews H. Utilizing national insurance data to examine the relationship between oral inflammation and infection and adverse pregnancy outcomes. Oral presentation at: American Public Health Association Annual Meeting and Expo; November 7, 2017; Atlanta, GA.

24

Integrating Preventive Oral Health Care Into Primary Care Nurse Practitioner Curriculum

Jan Odiaga DNP, CPNP-PC, Julianne Doucette, DNP, CPNP-PC, Ingrid Forsberg, DNP, FNP-BC, and Amy Manion, PhD, CPNP-PC

NEED FOR PARTNERSHIP BETWEEN PRIMARY CARE AND DENTAL HEALTH CARE PROVIDERS

In the United States, an estimated 21.5 million children lack access to basic dental care, which is greater than the unmet needs for medical care.[1,2] Currently, there are 45 million Americans who live in communities with a ratio of 1 dentist to 5,000 patients; therefore, 1 out of 16 children in the United States has never received oral health care.[2] Furthermore, disparities in preventive oral health care (POHC) exist and include racial and ethnic minorities, immigrant families, patients with lower socioeconomic status, and participants in Medicaid insurance. Children with dental caries have long-term health consequences associated with poor nutrition, chronic pain, loss of school days, and decreased self-esteem.[3] Unmet POHC needs can result in an increased economic burden to both families and the health care system. The Pew Center predicted that the annual spending on dental services would increase from $101.9 billion in 2009 to $161.4 billion in 2018, of which 35% will be spent on children.[4]

Qualis Health discussed the benefits of primary care providers partnering with dentists to reduce the consequences of oral diseases in "Oral Health: An Essential Component of Primary Care."[2] In addition, the Health Resources and Services Administration published a consensus report, "Integration of Oral Health and Primary Care Practice,"[5] which targeted nurse practitioners, nurse midwives, physicians, and physician assistants to become part of the solution. These reports reinforce the urgent need to incorporate POHC clinical competencies (oral health risk assessment, oral health examination, education on oral health promotion, fluoride varnish application, and dental referrals) into primary care education.[5]

RUSH COLLEGE OF NURSING PRIMARY CARE NURSING CURRICULUM

Rush College of Nursing is part of Rush University, located in urban Chicago, Illinois. Rush College of Nursing's mission is to educate a broadly diverse student body who will deliver exceptional health care, generate innovative knowledge, and provide transformative leadership to improve health outcomes for all populations. The vision is to lead health care transformation through innovative nursing education, practice, research, and scholarly inquiry. With the mission and vision in mind, the integration of POHC into Pediatric Primary Care Nurse Practitioner Program (PPCNP) began in 2013 and is ongoing. In 2017, the family nurse practitioner (FNP) program joined forces with the PPCNP and began the integration of POHC into its Doctor of Nursing Practice (DNP) programs.

Goal and Planning for Integration of Preventive Oral Health Care

The goal of the project was to develop a cost-effective integration of POHC into PPCNP education. The objectives of the intervention were to (1) provide a structured educational approach for PPCNP students to acquire knowledge of POHC, (2) provide opportunities for students to practice POHC clinical competencies, (3) evaluate student progress, and (4) develop a POHC educational model for other health education universities.

The populations affected by the integration of POHC into PPCNP education are (1) PPCNP nursing students, (2) other professionals in dental clinics where students participated in clinical practicum, and (3) patients.

Implementation of Preventive Oral Health Care Into the Curriculum

Integration was a four-step process:

- Step 1: Incorporating Smiles for Life: A National Oral Health Curriculum (SFL), a free online educational resource, into PPCNP clinical practicum courses.[6] The PPCNP students were required to complete courses 1 through 7, FNP students 1 through 8. To receive a Certificate of Completion and 1.0 contact hour of continuing education credit through New York University College of Nursing Center for Continuing Education in Nursing, students completed a post assessment with a mandatory passing score of at least 80%.
- Step 2: Incorporating a low-fidelity simulation experience for students to apply the knowledge gained from SFL and practice POHC competencies. A local dentist from the American Academy of Pediatrics presented Bright Smiles from Birth[7] and

supervised the clinical simulation. Students completed oral health risk assessments and oral examinations, applied fluoride varnish to each other, and were evaluated by the dentist.

- Step 3: Student participation in a four-hour interprofessional dental clinical practicum experience to observe and practice the POHC, including identification of early tooth decay, oral pathology, and when to refer to a dentist. Students submitted a clinical log of completed hours signed by the dentist.
- Step 4: Student documentation of the POHC clinical competencies in the Typhon Group's Nurse Practitioner Student Tracking System (Typhon Group LLC, Metairie, LA), which functions as a complete and secure electronic student tracking system including clinical skills logs and reports for faculty review.

Evaluation of the Results

Before integration, PPCNP students had limited knowledge or skills related to POHC. A total of 97 PPCNP students completed the four-step integration process. Demonstrating their clinical competence via the Typhon Tracking System, the PPCNP students documented performing oral examinations, identifying patients at risk, performing preventive oral health services, and appropriately referring patients to a dentist.

Three master's PPCNP students implemented a POHC program in their respective primary care clinics as a capstone project. One PPCNP DNP student initiated a POHC program at her clinical site within the US Navy. Because of the success of her project, the Navy is interested in adopting the program at multiple sites across the country. Two other DNP students completed DNP projects on integration of POHC, one in a rural primary care practice in Indiana and the other in a pediatric intensive care unit for children who were not intubated but were hospitalized long-term.

Student Typhon Tracking System documentation of POHC demonstrated limited opportunities to utilize the oral health risk assessment tool and application of fluoride varnish. The principal reason for the lack of documentation was attributable to few primary care clinics integrating POHC within the practice.

SUSTAINABILITY OF PREVENTIVE ORAL HEALTH CARE AS A PART OF PRIMARY CARE NURSE PRACTITIONER CURRICULA

Oral disease can have social and emotional consequences on children's ability to learn and succeed. Integration of POHC and associated clinical competencies into nurse practitioner primary care education will play a significant role in addressing oral health disparities and lack of access to POHC. In the past, large-scale, grant-funded POHC interprofessional projects at New York University and Washington University were extremely successful; but, without funding, most universities would not be able to replicate programs of this magnitude.[8] This project provides evidence that despite size or lack of funding, schools of nursing can integrate POHC and the associated clinical competencies into PPCNP education.

The straightforward four-step process of integration is easily reproducible, cost-effective, and sustainable. Faculty can easily track changes in the learners' behaviors and monitor translation of educational concepts into practice by utilizing the Typhon Tracking System. Translation into practice can have long-term positive effects on population health.

CONCLUSIONS

Dental caries in young children remains a serious public health crisis. The problem is exacerbated by lack of access to POHC and early dental referrals. Most children are exposed to medical care but not dental care at an early age. Nurse practitioners have a unique opportunity to see children on a frequent basis because of the required well-child physical examinations and immunizations. To address disparities and lack of access, educational innovation in expanding the oral health workforce is one of the most viable solutions.

ACKNOWLEDGMENTS

The initial pilot was partially funded by DentaQuest Foundation grant PO #UW507330, for the National Interprofessional Initiative on Oral Health for the provision of the Oral Health Nursing Education Project.

REFERENCES

1. The Pew Charitable Trusts. The state of children's dental health: making coverage matter. 2011. Available at: http://www.pewtrusts.org/en/research-and-analysis/reports/2011/05/23/the-state-of-childrens-dental-health-making-coverage-matter. Accessed October 23, 2016.

2. Qualis Health. Oral health: an essential component of primary care. 2015. Available at: http://www.safetynetmedicalhome.org/sites/default/files/White-Paper-Oral-Health-Primary-Care.pdf. Accessed October 23, 2016.

3. US Department of Health and Human Services, Health Resources and Services Administration. Oral health in America: a report of the Surgeon General. 2000. Available at: https://www.cdc.gov/oralhealth/publications/sgr2000_05.htm. Accessed October 23, 2016.

4. The Pew Center on the States. The cost of delay: state dental policies fail one in five children. 2010. Available at: http://www.pewtrusts.org/~/media/legacy/uploadedfiles/pcs_assets/2010/costofdelaywebpdf.pdf. Accessed October 23, 2016.

5. US Department of Health and Human Services, Health Resources and Services Administration. Integration of oral health and primary care practice. 2014. Available at: http://www.hrsa.gov/ publichealth/clinical/oralhealth/primarycare/integrationoforalhealth.pdf. Accessed October 23, 2016.

6. Clark MB, Douglass AB, Maier R, et al. Smiles for Life: a national oral health curriculum. 3rd ed. Society of Teachers of Family Medicine. 2010. Available at: http://www.smilesforlifeoralhealth.org/buildcontent.aspx. Accessed October 23, 2016.

7. American Academy of Pediatrics. Bright Smiles from Birth: an oral health educational program. 2010. Available at: http://www.brightsmilesfrombirth.org. October 23, 2016.

8. Haber J, Hartnett E, Allen K, et al. Putting the mouth back in the head: HEENT to HEENOT. *Am J Public Health*. 2015;105(3):437–441.

25

The Nurse Practitioner–Dentist Model: Improving Access to Primary Care for Dental Patients

Maria C. Dolce, PhD, RN, Jessica L. Parker, EdD, RDH, Lisa Simon, DMD,
R. Bruce Donoff, DMD, MD, and John Da Silva, DMD, MPH, ScM

DENTAL CARE SETTINGS AND ACCESS TO HEALTH CARE

Dental practices can serve as a gateway for patients to access primary care and preventive services. Access to care is a major concern in US health care reform. Despite historic gains in health insurance coverage under the Patient Protection and Affordable Care Act (ACA), approximately 29 million people aged younger than 65 years will not be insured in 2018.[1] This number is projected to increase to 35 million by 2022.[2] With the repeal of the ACA individual mandate provision, an additional 4 million people will remain without insurance coverage starting in 2019.[1] According to 2014 data from the Medical Expenditure Panel Survey, 20% of the total US population reported no usual source of health care.[3] Moreover, 27 million patients reported having a dental visit but not a general health care provider visit within the same year.[3]

Health care reform presents an opportunity to redefine the role of dental practices within the health care system.[4] Dental care settings are promising practice sites for increasing access to general health care.[5] In 2014, 60% of adults in the United States were living with one chronic health condition, and 42% were living with multiple chronic conditions.[6] This public health issue is exacerbated by the gap in access to general health care. Screening for undiagnosed chronic conditions has been found to be feasible in dental settings.[7] Furthermore, dental patients and providers believe that the dental visit is a good opportunity for early identification of chronic conditions such as diabetes.[7] Additional chairside chronic disease screening and increased referral from the dental setting could reduce health care costs and improve health for these and other patients who do not have a primary care provider.[8]

Access to primary care services, a central provision of the ACA, is a critical factor for prevention, detection, and treatment of chronic health conditions.[9] The ACA links this goal to the effective use of nurse practitioners (NPs) and optimization of health care delivery models.[10] Moreover, Medicare beneficiaries are eligible to receive an annual wellness visit as a free, preventive service under the ACA. In 2016, only 19.8% of Medicare Part B beneficiaries in the United States received an annual wellness visit.[11]

The integration of NP services within primary dental care settings is one strategy that may effectively increase access to primary care and preventive services for adults and older adults with diagnosed and undiagnosed chronic health conditions and increase utilization of annual wellness visits for Medicare beneficiaries. There is a sound rationale for this strategy. First, a proportion of dental patients do not regularly visit a physician.[5] Furthermore, dental care settings have a broad reach with 63% of US adults aged younger than 65 years reporting at least one annual dental visit.[12] Second, the prevalence of diagnosed, undiagnosed, and uncontrolled chronic health conditions is staggering.[13] Embedded within a dental practice, NPs can be utilized to provide preventive services, detect chronic health conditions, make timely patient referrals to general and specialty health care providers for diagnosis and treatment, and improve chronic disease management. Third, the provision of preventive and primary care services within a dental practice is within the scope of practice for NP, and these services may use existing medical coding, billing, and reimbursement infrastructures.[14]

In this chapter, we describe the NP-Dentist Model (NPD Model), an emerging patient-centered care model that seeks to improve access to primary care services for patients, improve population health through management of diagnosed and undiagnosed chronic health conditions, and prepare dentists and NPs to improve oral–systemic health.

THE NURSE PRACTITIONER–DENTIST MODEL

In 2015, Northeastern University, in partnership with Harvard School of Dental Medicine (HSDM), was awarded a three-year cooperative agreement by the US Department of Health and Human Services, Health Resources and Services Administration, to implement the NPD Model at the Harvard Dental Center (HDC) Teaching Practices. The study protocol was approved by HSDM institutional review board (protocol 17-0165). The HDC is a state-of-the-art dental facility located within HSDM in Boston, Massachusetts. The HDC Teaching Practices serve more than 5,000 dental patients each year, 17% of whom are beneficiaries of MassHealth, Massachusetts's Medicaid program. A needs assessment of adult (aged 18–64 years) and older adult (aged ≥ 65 years) dental patients indicated that 27% (n = 1,143) of adults and 21% (n = 180) of older adults did not have a usual source for medical care, 15% (n = 430) of adults and 49% (n = 420) of older adults had hypertension, and 4% (n = 126) of adults and 38% (n = 326) of older adults had type 2 diabetes.

Goals, Planning, and Development of the Model

Planning and development of the NPD Model took place over a six-month period, from July 2015 to January 2016. A multidisciplinary team comprising academic deans and program directors, an NP, a dentist, a clinical operations director, and a clinical applications director met frequently to generate ideas, establish a timeline, and set priorities. Common goals were identified between the partnering institutions, including meeting accreditation standards and advancing knowledge around interprofessional education and interprofessional collaborative practice.

To facilitate planning, surveys were conducted with HSDM faculty and students. A survey of third-year dental students highlighted what types of primary care services dental students believed would be beneficial to dental patients, targeted educational topics on the NP role and scope of practice, and identified potential barriers to implementation of the NPD Model. A survey of faculty and staff perceptions of teamwork indicated areas of improvement related to team function, leadership, and communication within the health care team. Findings were used to develop student education and faculty development activities. Quality measures, including clinical and educational measures, were developed and coordinated in a comprehensive program monitoring and evaluation plan.

Development of the NPD Model was guided by the Chronic Care Model, an integrated framework for improving chronic disease management and health outcomes.[15] The essential elements of the Chronic Care Model, including self-management support, delivery system design, clinical information systems, patient safety, and care coordination,[16] were addressed when planning the major activities and strategies for integrating NP and dental services in the HDC Teaching Practices. These activities and strategies consisted of (1) constructing and equipping a private examination room, (2) designing and testing clinical and operational workflow processes, (3) developing and implementing customized primary care elements into the electronic health record (EHR), and (4) developing practice-based experiences for dental and NP students.

Implementation of the Model

The integration of NP services began with the construction of a dedicated private examination room. The private examination room was specifically designed to be feasible in a typical private dental office and was furnished with both dental and medical equipment and supplies. The private room is equipped with a standard dental chair, eye-level height and weight scale, glycated hemoglobin (HbA1c) and glucose analyzer, stethoscope, otoscope, standard sphygmomanometer, point-of-care testing supplies, and personal protective equipment. A designated work station was located adjacent to the examination room and provided adequate space for administrative activities such as scheduling appointments, patient care coordination, and EHR documentation. The next major step was the redesign of key workflow processes, particularly patient intake, patient discharge, treatment planning, appointment scheduling, and referrals. A clinical microsystems approach was employed for designing and testing change ideas for improvement.[17]

An important determinant of successful implementation was the integration of primary care elements into axiUm (Exan, Las Vegas, NV), the HDC's electronic dental record, to allow documentation and clinical decision support. Medical components were derived from the Medicare annual wellness visit (AWV), which includes a health risk assessment and personalized prevention services.[18] Components of the Medicare AWV were included because of the focus on health risk assessment and health promotion, the higher rate of chronic illness in the older adult population, and the low rate of utilization for the examination.[19] We also integrated other components such as patient referrals, appointments, treatment planning, provider alerts, problem lists, educational resources, progress notes, medications, and patient education materials. New templates were embedded within a central location within the *forms* tab of the EHR (Figure 25-1) and included health risk assessment, chronic conditions, depression screening, fall risk, hearing, physical examination, and cognition. Data fields were programmed to facilitate data mining and reporting and to

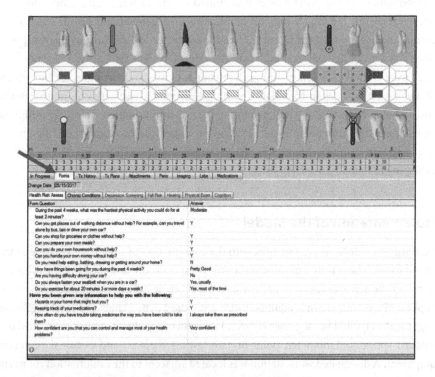

Source: Reprinted with permission from Harvard School of Dental Medicine.[20]

Figure 25-1. Electronic Health Record *Forms* Tab

generate alerts for providers. The NP utilized UpToDate (Wolters Kluwer, Waltham, MA), an evidence-based clinical decision support resource. An integrated medication inventory list was created so that all providers could access a patient's current medication list and view changes. A Health Insurance Portability and Accountability Act–compliant internal messaging system facilitated communication between the NP and dental providers.

Implementation of the NPD Model began in January 2016. A convenience sample of older adults (aged ≥ 65 years) seeking dental treatment at the HDC Teaching Practices were recruited to participate in the study. Older adults who self-reported having hypertension and/or type 2 diabetes were eligible to participate in the study. Individuals with renal failure and currently undergoing hemodialysis, with diminished cognitive functioning, or who were non–English-speaking, were not eligible to participate in the study. Potential study participants were screened by the NP on the same day as their dental appointment. Patients who met eligibility criteria and agreed to participate in the study were required to sign an informed consent form. Patients who declined participation in the study continued usual care with their dental provider.

Assessment and Interventions by the Nurse Practitioner

Patients were observed for a minimum of six months following the first study visit and were required to complete at least two study visits. Each study visit was conducted in the private examination room and lasted approximately 30 minutes, with the exception of the enrollment and final study, which lasted 60 minutes. The NP intervention consisted of the following activities:

- Review of family and medical history;
- Medication review;
- Review of systems;
- Review history of present illness;
- Blood pressure measurement;
- Height, weight, and body mass index (BMI) measurement;
- HbA1c measurement (diabetic patients only, taken every three months);
- Individualized care plan with self-confidence rating; and
- Patient education and skill building.

Before each study visit, the NP gathered clinical and patient experience data in the patient's chart and asked the patient to bring health monitoring information, such as blood pressure and blood glucose measurements. During each study visit, the NP asked the patients about goals to improve their health and helped develop action plans to build confidence in their ability to reach goals. The NP primarily focused on helping patients understand their central role in managing their conditions. A written care plan and visit summary was also prepared that included goals and action plans to ensure that the patients knew what to do when they left the office. Patient education and skill building focused on teaching patients how to understand the signs and symptoms of their hypertension and/or type 2 diabetes and training them in how to monitor clinical indicators such as blood pressure and glycemic control.[21]

Follow-up care was provided by the NP every 4 to 12 weeks. Frequency of care was based on individualized patient need, the patient's dental care treatment plan, and the ability to establish communication with the patient. Follow-up appointments were used to help patients meet goals established in the action plan and sustain healthy behaviors over time. The NP focused on incremental changes and regular contact with patients. Patients were also given contact information for community resources, such as community behavioral health centers. The NP engaged other members of the patient's health care provider team by sharing visit summaries with the patient's primary care provider and dental providers.

Evaluation of Patient Goals

The NP documented the patient's health goals and self-confidence in achieving goals by using the Action Plan form and Confidence Ruler provided in the Institute for Health Care Improvement's Partnering in Self-Management Support: A Toolkit for Clinicians.[22] These tools were developed by the New Health Partnerships initiative, a national program of the Robert Wood Johnson Foundation at the Institute for Healthcare Improvement to develop and test efficient approaches to empower patients and families to manage their chronic conditions.[23] The Action Plan is a tool that is administered by the NP to help patients set health goals, specify action planning steps, and anticipate barriers in reaching goals. The Confidence Ruler is a tool administered by the NP to help assess the patient's likelihood of success achieving the goals described in the action plan. The Confidence Ruler ask patients to rate their confidence on a scale of 0 to 10, with 0 being totally unconfident and 10 being extremely confident.

Relevant demographic, socioeconomic, and health information were captured in existing EHR forms. Pre- and postintervention blood pressure and HbA1c values were evaluated as the primary outcome measures. Pre- and postintervention values for body weight, BMI, self-confidence scores, advanced care planning status, and vaccination status were evaluated as secondary outcome measures. Data were collected from prospective review of patient health records. A pre–post design was used to evaluate the effectiveness of the intervention. Data were analyzed using descriptive statistics.

Results of the Study

From 2016 to 2018, the NP called 977 older adult patients scheduled for dental treatment to discuss potential inclusion in the study. Among these, 326 were unreachable and 322 met the exclusion criteria and were therefore excluded from the study. Among the remaining 329 potential study participants, 232 did not show for a screening visit or were not interested in participating in the study. Ninety-seven patients completed a screening visit with the NP to confirm study eligibility, and 49 agreed to participate in the study. Seven patients withdrew for reasons unrelated to the study and 11 patients dropped out of the study (did not complete more than one visit and/or stopped responding to requests to attend follow-up visits). Therefore, 31 patients completed the study. In addition, 205 students (105 dental students and 100 NP students) completed a practice-based experience in the NPD Model environment.

Table 25-1 presents the descriptive statistics of the 31 study participants who completed pre- and postintervention measures. The average age of the participants was 71.75 years. A majority of participants were male (n = 21; 68%), White (n = 27; 87%), and non-Hispanic (n = 21; 68%). Most of the participants (n = 21; 68%;) had hypertension

Table 25-1. Baseline Characteristics of Study Participants (N = 31)

Characteristic	Participants, No. (%)
Male	21 (68)
Female	10 (32)
Mean age (years)	71.75
Race	
White	27 (87)
African American	1 (3)
Unreported/refused to report race	2 (6)
More than one race	1 (3)
Ethnicity	
Non-Hispanic	21 (68)
Hispanic	6 (19)
Chose not to disclose	4 (13)
Sexual orientation	
Straight (not lesbian or gay)	26 (84)
Lesbian or gay	4 (13)
Choose not to disclose	1 (3)
Smoking status	
Nonsmokers	30 (97)
Smokers	1 (3)
Diagnoses	
Hypertension alone	21 (68)
Hypertension + type 2 DM	8 (26)
Type 2 DM alone	2 (6)

Note: DM = diabetes mellitus.

Table 25-2. Primary and Secondary Outcome Measures Comparison Between Preintervention and Postintervention

Outcome Measure	No.	Preintervention,[a] No. (%)	Postintervention,[b] No. (%)
HbA1c (< 8.0)	10	9 (91)	10 (100)
Systolic BP (< 140 mm Hg)	29	19 (65)	25 (86)
Diastolic BP (< 90 mm Hg)	29	26 (90)	29 (100)
Mean body weight, lbs	31	197	189
BMI, mean	31	31.7	30.6
Documentation of advance care planning	31	23 (73)	30 (97)
Report ever having a pneumococcal vaccination	31	27 (86)	30 (97)
Annual influenza vaccination	31	25 (81)	30 (97)
Mean self-confidence rating, scale of 1–10	31	7	9

Note: BMI = body mass index; BP = blood pressure; HbA1c = glycated haemoglobin.
[a]Number and percentage of participants who met the specific outcome or quality measure *before* the intervention.
[b]Number and percentage of participants who met the specific outcome or quality measure *after* the intervention.

only, 26% (n = 8) had both hypertension and type 2 diabetes, and 6% (n = 2) had type 2 diabetes only. Among the 31 patients who completed the study, 71% (n = 22) completed five or six study visits; 23% (n = 7) completed three or four study visits, and 6% (n = 2) completed the minimum two study visits. Patients were enrolled in the study an average of 8 months (range 6–13).

Table 25-2 presents a comparison between pre- and postintervention primary and secondary outcome measures. All (n =10) participants with diabetes achieved the targeted HbA1c measure (< 8.0). Among the hypertensive participants, 86% (n = 25) achieved the targeted systolic blood pressure (< 140 mm Hg) and 100% (n = 29) achieved the targeted diastolic blood pressure (< 90 mm Hg). The mean body weight of participants decreased by 4%, from 197 pounds to 189 pounds, and mean BMI decreased from 31.7 to 30.6. Improvements in documentation of advanced care planning, vaccinations, and self-confidence scores were also observed.

DISCUSSION OF THE RESULTS, ONGOING CHALLENGES, AND PLANS FOR THE FUTURE

This study provides preliminary evidence that the integration of an NP in a dental care setting has the potential to improve the care of older adults with hypertension and/or type 2 diabetes. This study demonstrated improvements in participants' HbA1c, blood pressure, body weight, BMI, self-confidence scores, advanced care planning status, and vaccination status. However, the small sample size limits our ability to determine the significance of results. Furthermore, a majority of participants had controlled blood pressure and HbA1c upon study enrollment.

Three ongoing challenges include engaging students in integrated practice, educating patients about the new model, and addressing medical billing in a dental environment. To ensure that students were aware of the model and its benefits for their patients, "student champions" have been selected across all years of training. These students take a leadership role in engaging their classmates, participating in the program's outcomes research, and providing feedback to the NPD team. We have also identified "student ambassadors" who are interested in providing peer teaching to NP students on basic oral health clinical competencies.

A communication strategy was developed to educate patients and increase interest and acceptance. Print materials were developed at a fifth-grade reading level; they featured a photograph of the NP and a description of services offered. Posters were placed in high-traffic locations such as the waiting area, and information cards were also made available at the check-in desk. The NP also makes daily calls to new patients who are scheduled for a new patient intake appointment.

A final challenge has been billing insurance companies for medical services. The team worked closely with the HDC administrative staff, many of whom were unfamiliar with medical billing, especially Medicare, given the very different reimbursement mechanisms present in dental insurance coverage. The HDC also needed to apply for a Clinical Laboratory Improvement Amendment Waiver through the Centers for Medicare and Medicaid Services so that the NP could perform point-of-care testing.

Increasing awareness of the relationship between oral health and overall health has led to increased interest in both the public and private sectors to improve communication and service integration between primary care and dental providers. In conclusion, our experience demonstrated the advantages of integrated, patient-centered care models and allowed us to test solutions for the challenges that emerging practice models will face. Continued program assessment will include monitoring patient and population health outcomes, nursing and dental student learning outcomes, and changes in patient and provider acceptability. The NPD model presents a feasible point of access to primary care while training future primary care and dental providers to work together as a team.

The next development phase of this emerging model will entail the testing of medical coding and billing processes for reimbursement through Medicare and third-party commercial insurers. We expect to demonstrate a sustainable financial model that can be replicated and scaled in a range of dental practice settings, including community health centers, private practices, and dental support organizations. We know that the prevalence of multiple chronic health conditions increases with age.[6] The NPD model will be expanded to serve the younger adult (aged 18–44 years) population and include tailored interventions for the prevention of chronic health conditions. In 2014, 36% of Americans in this age group reported no usual source of health care.[3] The HDC Teaching Practices will serve as a gateway to comprehensive primary care for younger adults without a usual source of health care.

CONCLUSIONS

The NPD model seeks to connect patients already seeking dental care with primary care services. This model serves two underserved groups: those who do not have a primary care provider and those with chronic illness who may benefit from closer or more frequent monitoring of their health conditions. In addition to meeting the needs of these patients, the NPD Model's placement within an academic dental practice and the involvement of NP students present the opportunity to train future primary care providers to better understand oral health, identify patients at risk of oral disease, and communicate more effectively with their dental colleagues.

ACKNOWLEDGMENTS

This project was funded by the US Department of Health and Human Services, Health Resources and Services Administration, through the Nurse Education, Practice, Quality, and Retention Program for Interprofessional Collaborative Practice (grant UD7HP28534).

REFERENCES

1. Congressional Budget Office. Repealing the individual health insurance mandate: an updated estimate. 2017. Available at: https://www.cbo.gov/system/files?file=115th-congress-2017-2018/reports/53300-individualmandate.pdf. Accessed July 19, 2018.

2. Congressional Budget Office. Federal subsidies for health insurance coverage for people under age 65: 2018 to 2028. 2018. Available at: https://www.cbo.gov/publication/53826. Accessed July 19, 2018.

3. Agency for Healthcare Research and Quality. Table 1: Usual source of health care and selected population characteristics, United States, 2014. Available at: https://meps.ahrq.gov/mepsweb/data_stats/quick_tables_search.jsp?component=1&subcomponent=0. Accessed November 8, 2018.

4. Agency for Healthcare Research and Quality. Medical Expenditure Panel Survey. Household component data. Generated interactively. 2014. Available at: https://meps.ahrq.gov/mepsweb/survey_comp/household.jsp. Accessed November 8, 2018.

5. Vujicic M. Health care reform brings new opportunities. *J Am Dent Assoc.* 2014;145(4): 381–382.

6. Strauss SM, Alfano MC, Shelley D, Fulmer T. Identifying unaddressed systemic health conditions at dental visits: patients who visited dental practices but not general health care providers in 2008. *Am J Public Health*. 2012;102(2):253–255.

7. Buttorff C, Ruder T, Bauman M. Multiple chronic conditions in the United States. RAND Corporation. 2017. Available at: https://www.rand.org/pubs/tools/TL221.html. Accessed July 19, 2018.

8. Rosedale M, Strauss S. Diabetes screening at the periodontal visit: patient and provider experiences with two screening approaches. *Int J Dent Hyg*. 2012;10(4):250–258.

9. Nasseh K, Greenberg B, Vujicic M, Glick M. The effect of chairside chronic disease screenings by oral health professionals on health care costs. *Am J Public Health*. 2014;104(4):744–750.

10. Patient Protection and Affordable Care Act, 42 USC § 18001 (2010).

11. Carthon JM, Barnes H, Sarik DA. Federal policies influence access to primary care and nurse practitioner workforce. *J Nurse Pract*. 2015;11(5):526–530.

12. Centers for Medicare and Medicaid Services. Beneficiaries utilizing free preventive services by state, 2016. 2016. Available at: https://downloads.cms.gov/files/Beneficiaries%20Utilizing%20Free%20Preventive%20Services%20by%20State%20YTD%202016.pdf. Accessed July 19, 2018.

13. Manski RJ, Cooper PF. Dental care use: does dental insurance truly make a difference in the US? *Community Dent Health*. 2007;24(4):205–212.

14. Ward BW, Schiller JS, Goodman RA. Multiple chronic conditions among US adults: a 2012 update. *Prev Chronic Dis*. 2014;11:E62.

15. Alfano MC. Connecting dental education to other health professions. *J Dent Educ*. 2012;76(1):46–50.

16. Coleman K, Austin BT, Brach C, Wagner EH. Evidence on the chronic care model in the new millennium. *Health Aff (Millwood)*. 2009;28(1):75–85.

17. Improving Chronic Illness Care. The Chronic Care Model: model elements. 2018. Available at: http://www.improvingchroniccare.org/index.php?p=Model_Elements&s=18. Accessed July 19, 2018.

18. Agency for Healthcare Research and Quality. Plan–Do–Study–Act (PDSA) Cycle. 2008. Available at: https://innovations.ahrq.gov/qualitytools/plan-do-study-act-pdsa-cycle. Accessed July 22, 2018.

19. Centers for Medicare and Medicaid Services, Medicare Learning Network. The ABCs of the annual wellness visit. 2014. Available at: https://www.cms.gov/Outreach-and-Education/Medicare-Learning-Network-MLN/MLNProducts/downloads/awv_chart_icn905706.pdf. Accessed October 23, 2018.

20. Harvard School of Dental Medicine. Electronic dental record. Boston, MA: Harvard School of Dental Medicine; 2016.

21. Dallman-Papke V, Scott K. The Medicare wellness exam: a population health innovation for the older adult. *Nurse Lead.* 2016;14(5):302–303.

22. Institute for Healthcare Improvement. Partnering in self-management support: a toolkit for clinicians. 2009. Available at: http://www.ihi.org. Accessed October 25, 2018.

23. Institute for Healthcare Improvement. New Health Partnerships Initiative. 2009. Available at: http://www.ihi.org/Engage/Initiatives/Completed/NewHealthPartnerships/Pages/default. aspx. Accessed November 7, 2018.

26

Expanding the Dental Workforce to Improve Access and Reduce Disparities in Oral Health[*]

Wendell B. Potter, BS

"Twelve-year-old Deamonte Driver died of a toothache Sunday."

Those were the first words of a 2007 *Washington Post*[1] story that identified by name a young victim of what former US Surgeon General David Satcher had called a "silent epidemic," seven years earlier.

After that unforgettable lead sentence, the reporter went on explain why this was such an unnecessary tragedy.

"A routine, $80 tooth extraction might have saved him," she wrote.

Driver's mother, however, did not have the money to pay for the extraction, and the family did not have dental insurance. They also had recently lost their Medicaid coverage. Even when they had it, finding a dentist who would accept Medicaid patients was a challenge.

What undoubtedly surprised many readers was that tooth decay is not only a painful annoyance but a serious infectious disease that, left untreated, can be fatal. And probably just as surprising to many was just how difficult getting timely and appropriate care can be for people of all ages who lack dental benefits—including most Medicare and Medicaid beneficiaries—or who live in areas where few dentists practice.

In his 2000 report,[2,3] Satcher wrote that the burden of dental and oral diseases affects members of racial and minority groups disproportionately. Nearly two decades later, that is still the case.[4]

Some progress has indeed been made. More children receive dental sealants to help prevent cavities now than in 2000, fewer adolescents have tooth decay, and more adults are retaining their natural teeth. But progress in other areas has been slow, especially among children in low-income families, as former US Surgeon General Vivek Murthy wrote in a 2016 report.[4] Here is just one statistic from that report: a fourth of preschool-aged children living in households below the federal poverty level have untreated tooth decay, compared with 1 in 10 living above the poverty level.[4]

[*]This is a modified version of the article that appeared in the *American Journal of Public Health*. See: Potter WB. Expanding the dental workforce to improve access and reduce disparities in oral health. *Am J Public Health*. 2017;107(suppl 1):S26–S27.

Among the reasons for the enduring disparities and lack of access are shortcomings that policymakers have not adequately addressed. Although members of Congress included dental care for children among the Affordable Care Act's essential health benefits, relatively few dentists accept new Medicaid patients—20% or fewer in some states. Medicaid reimbursement rates are considerably lower than are commercial reimbursement rates in most states, ranging in a recent year from 26.7% in Minnesota to 81.1% in Delaware.[5] And instead of narrowing, the difference between Medicaid reimbursement and commercial reimbursement actually widened in all but six states and the District of Columbia over a recent 10-year period.[5]

In the Medicare program, dental benefits remain very limited. Medicare Part A will pay for certain dental services provided during hospitalization, but routine visits and cleanings are not covered. The Affordable Care Act made preventive medical care a covered benefit but not preventive dental care.

It is little wonder, then, why an increasing number of both children and adults are seeking treatment in hospital emergency departments—where the cost is typically much higher than in a dentist's office—when a toothache becomes unbearable. According to an analysis by the American Dental Association (ADA), the number of dental emergency department visits doubled, from 1.1 million to 2.2 million, between 2000 and 2012. The ADA estimated that by 2012, emergency department dental visits cost the US health care system $1.6 billion annually, with an average cost of $749 per visit.[6]

There are other costs of America's continuing silent epidemic of dental disease. People with diseased and missing teeth are at a disadvantage when applying for employment. Pregnant women with untreated decay can pass disease on to their unborn children. Toothaches also contribute to children missing school and parents missing work.[7]

The ADA and state dental societies lobby lawmakers to increase Medicaid reimbursement, but few states have done so. What many lawmakers are showing more interest in are solutions that do not require government spending and that have the additional benefit of creating jobs.

Programs to improve access by strengthening the oral health workforce at little or no cost to taxpayers are underway in several states. They are to a certain extent the fulfillment of Murthy's recommendations to expand the capabilities of existing providers and to promote models that incorporate other clinicians.

The ADA, which maintains that there are enough dentists in the United States but acknowledges that many areas are underserved, launched a pilot project in 2006 to train community dental health coordinators. Community dental health coordinators, whose focus is education and prevention, are currently working in nine states.

Paul Glassman, director of the Pacific Center for Special Care at the University of the Pacific, has pioneered a dental telehealth project featuring a collapsible dental chair and other portable equipment that enable dental hygienists to examine patients in schools and other locations and transmit x-rays via a laptop computer to a dental office. The project is being piloted in several locations.

Several other states and tribal communities have broadened or are considering broadening the dental workforce to include midlevel providers, often called dental therapists, whose scope of practice is considerably broader than is that of the community dental health coordinators.

Although dental therapists practice in at least 50 countries (starting in New Zealand in the 1920s), they are relatively new to the United States. Alaska Native communities were the first to use them in this country. Dental disease had become so prevalent among Alaska Natives, most of whom live far from a dentist's office, that tribal leaders decided in 2004 to see if dental therapists—or dental health aide therapists, as they are called in Alaska—could make a difference.

More than 30 dental health aide therapists are now providing care to 45,000 people in 81 communities. As elsewhere, they work as part of a broader dental team and are supervised by dentists. Their scope of practice ranges from education and prevention to uncomplicated extractions and fillings. When a patient requires care beyond their scope of practice, they refer the patient to a dentist.

Dental therapists began practicing in Minnesota in 2009. The Minnesota Department of Health noted in a 2014 report that the state's dental therapists were providing quality care to predominantly low-income, uninsured, and underserved patients.[8]

Maine, Vermont, Washington, and Arizona are the most recent states to allow dental therapists to practice, and several other states may soon follow suit. In 2017, the Washington legislature approved a bill to allow the 29 Native American tribes in the state to use them.[9] The Swinomish Native American community did not wait for the state to act. Swinomish leaders exercised tribal sovereignty in early 2016 and recruited one of the Alaska-trained dental health aide therapists. His presence on the team enabled the Swinomish dental clinic to see 20% more patients last year than in 2015 and reduced wait times from three to four months to less than three to four weeks.

Legislation authorizing dental therapists to practice has received bipartisan support and usually has both Democrats and Republicans as sponsors. A growing number of dentists have become dental therapy champions, but the ADA and state dental societies have, for the most part, remained opposed. That appears to be changing. In New Mexico, the state dental association is working with advocates and lawmakers on a bill that would allow dental therapists to practice in that state.

Dental societies in other states should do the same. Strengthening and expanding the dental workforce, by broadening the capabilities of existing providers and encompassing new clinicians like dental therapists, can make a big difference in access—and in the lives of millions of people—at little cost to taxpayers.

REFERENCES

1. Otto M. For want of a dentist. 2007. Available at: http://www.washingtonpost.com/wp-dyn/content/article/2007/02/27/AR2007022702116.html. Accessed May 10, 2017.

2. Satcher D. *Oral Health in America: A Report of the Surgeon General.* Rockville, MD: US Department of Health and Human Services; 2000.

3. *Oral Health in America: A Report of the Surgeon General.* Rockville, MD: US Department of Health and Human Services; 2000.

4. Murthy VH. Oral health in America, 2000 to present: progress made, but challenges remain. *Public Health Rep.* 2016;131:224–225.

5. Nasseh K, Vujicic M, Yarbrough C. A Ten-Year, State-by-State Analysis of Medicaid Fee-for-Service Reimbursement Rates for Dental Care Services. Chicago, IL: American Dental Association; 2014.

6. Wall T, Vujicic M. *Emergency Use for Dental Conditions Continues to Increase.* Chicago, IL: American Dental Association; 2015.

7. Otto M. Teeth: The Story of Beauty, Inequality, and the Struggle for Oral Health in America. New York, NY: New Press; 2017.

8. Minnesota Department of Health; Minnesota Board of Dentistry. *Early Impacts of Dental Therapists in Minnesota.* Minneapolis, MN; 2014.

9. Myers A. Inslee signs bill to improve dental care for state tribes. 2017. Available at: http://www.seattletimes.com/seattle-news/inslee-signs-bill-to-improve-dental-care-for-state-tribes. Accessed May 10, 2017.

27

Educating Future Oral Health Professionals to Support Individuals and Communities Affected by Incarceration

Lisa Simon, DMD, Rachael Williams, AB, David Beckmann, MD, MPH, Marya Cohen, MD, MPH, and Matthew Tobey, MD, MPH

Since 1980, rates of incarceration in the United States have more than quadrupled; today, nearly 1 in 100 adults are incarcerated and 2 in 100 are on probation or parole.[1] US public health faces alarming challenges in this era of mass incarceration, with numerous downstream health and social consequences for affected individuals and their communities. Among these is poor oral health, which causes undue shame and suffering and even impacts the ability to seek employment upon re-entry into the community.[2,3]

STUDENT–FACULTY COLLABORATIVE CLINIC

Health professions education can help address these injustices. For more than three years, we have helped lead an interprofessional student–faculty collaborative clinic in an urban county jail, which has now facilitated experiences in correctional health for 25 dental students and more than 300 students across disciplines.[4] Across the country, more than one quarter of US dental schools provide rotations within correctional facilities to their students, but not all of these schools provide supportive education about mass incarceration and the criminal–legal system.[5] We believe this support and training is key to providing meaningful experiences in the correctional setting for dental students and to enhancing humanistic care for patients.

Exposure to the correctional setting and the oral health challenges faced by our patients can encourage both future dentists and other health professionals to help address the barriers to achieving oral health faced by justice-involved people (Table 27-1). First, dental students develop confidence while caring for individuals experiencing incarceration that extends beyond technical dental skills, such as the epidemiology, associated risks, and best practices in the care of such populations. Second, the clinic serves as an opportunity to train nondental providers—including future physicians, physician assistants, and nurse practitioners—in the importance of oral health and how to screen patients for dental needs. Lastly, the clinic trains students to partner with their patients to provide necessary services and advocacy that extend beyond clinical care.

Table 27-1. Potential Impact of Academic Institutional Participation on the Health Impact of Criminal Justice Involvement

Advancing Oral Health Equity With Learners in the Correctional Setting	
Educational Objective	Potential Impact
1. Empower future dentists to care for patients with a history of incarceration.	Improve access to care by increasing dentists working with underserved groups and in correctional facilities.
2. Train nondental providers to screen and counsel about oral health issues.	Improve referral networks and prevention of oral disease in the primary care setting.
3. Encourage advocacy and research for oral health equity.	Produce civic-minded health professionals who contextualize oral health within individual health, public health, and social justice.
Key Tenets for Sustainable Academic Dental–Correctional Facility Partnerships	
1. Active participation by supportive faculty in correctional-based student clinical experiences.	
2. Clear expectation setting for students about professional behavior, advocacy, and writing in the lay and academic press.	
3. Attention to logistical issues including facility access, background checks, and memoranda of understanding between partner institutions.	

Dentists exposed to vulnerable communities during training have a higher likelihood of caring for these communities during their career.[6] Students exposed to the correctional setting during training can come to understand the complex interaction of the social determinants of health with the health care experience of marginalized patients.[7] Given the high rate of dental need in incarcerated populations, dental trainees also have the opportunity to improve clinical outcomes for patients at high risk of poor oral health.[2]

In our clinic model, patients are selected from the triage list used by all dental providers in the jail's electronic health record. The patients are introduced to the dentist and students and are told that they can choose to be treated by the students or by the dentist alone. The patient, attending dentist, and students participate in a group discussion of the treatment plan that centers on the patient's wishes and goals, and all treatment is directly supervised by the attending dentist. Treatment includes the full range of services available at the jail, including restorative dentistry, periodontal treatment, and oral surgery; unfortunately, prosthodontic treatment is not available. Because of positive experiences with their student providers, multiple patients have specifically requested to return for follow-up when students are present.

Patients with dental pain who are unable to visit a dentist often seek care in emergency departments or primary care offices, and people with a history of incarceration are especially likely to lack dental access.[8,9] Our interdisciplinary correctional clinic gives nondental students exposure to the high dental needs of the incarcerated population, an overview of basic dental treatment, and even training in how to provide dental anesthesia and how to conduct an oral screening. All students come together for a preclinic education

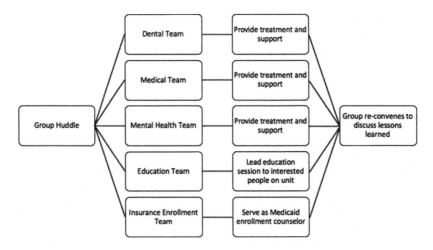

Source: Reprinted from Simon et al.[4]

Figure 27-1. Clinic Workflow

session, which may focus on oral health, substance use disorders, health policy, or another topic requested by the group. At the close of clinic, the group reconvenes and each team describes the services they provided that evening (Figure 27-1). Co-location with medical and psychiatric clinics allows a particular focus on how these disciplines intersect in ways that are often ignored in traditional medical training, such as the oral effects of systemic illness and the relationship between severe mental illness or substance use disorders and poor dentition.

RESULTS OF STUDENT–FACULTY COLLABORATIVE CLINIC EXPERIENCES

After one year of volunteering in our student–faculty collaborative clinic at a large urban jail, dental students indicated in a survey that they were significantly more comfortable caring for patients with a history of incarceration and indicated an increased agreement that they planned to work with vulnerable groups when practicing (before volunteering: 5.8 ± 2.2 [n = 10]; after volunteering: 8.1 ± 1.6 [n = 17]; $P = .005$ with unpaired student *t* test). Key to this clinical care is building trust with and ensuring as much agency as possible for our vulnerable patients.

Students have responded very positively to these interprofessional efforts. Students in primary care clinical roles requested consults from their dental colleagues after identifying dental pathology when examining a patient's mouth, and some requested to observe dental extractions and other procedures in the dental clinic. An oral health education module, originally developed by dental students, is now taught regularly by medical, nursing, and physician assistant students. After one year of volunteering in the clinic, students rated the importance of collaborating with oral health providers significantly higher (before volunteering: 7.8±2.3 [n = 48]; after volunteering: 8.7±1.7 [n = 66]; P = .02 with unpaired student t test).

CONCLUSIONS

To truly address the persistent oral health disparities in the United States, clinicians will also need to develop skills as advocates, researchers, and educators. Involvement in our correctional clinic can help develop these important competencies for health professions students. Dental students have the opportunity to train their colleagues in nursing and medicine in basic dental procedures such as oral examinations and anesthesia. At the request of their patients, students have developed and taught oral health and substance use disorder curricula, further honing their teaching skills and their partnership with their patients. The program also launched a team to enroll patients in Medicaid before release and piloted a care coordination effort to book dental and medical appointments for individuals when they return to the community. Dental students and their health professions colleagues have conducted research that has been shared in peer-reviewed journals and in national conferences.[5] Of the 12 alumni who have graduated from dental school after volunteering, 7 are currently working as general dentists or are enrolled in a general practice residency and are working at least part-time in a public setting.

Reflecting on her role, a long-time dental student volunteer wrote: "I'm constantly reminded of the importance of considering the patient as an individual human being with unique experiences and perspectives, while remembering that we are all linked by a common humanity." Academic–correctional partnerships present a hopeful future for dentistry and an opportunity for the next generation of health care providers to improve the oral health of all patients, and especially those affected by incarceration.

ACKNOWLEDGMENTS

The Crimson Care Collaborative is funded by the Stoeckle Center for Primary Care Innovation, Massachusetts General Hospital. Matthew Tobey's position in the clinic is supported by a charitable Crimson Care Expanded Support grant from the Gilead Foundation. Our most sincere gratitude goes to the Suffolk County Sheriff's Department and NaphCare for their continued partnership and support.

REFERENCES

1. Kaeble D, Glaze L. Correctional populations in the United States, 2015. Washington, DC: US Department of Justice, Office of Justice Programs, Bureau of Justice Statistics; 2016.

2. Treadwell HM, Formicola AJ. Improving the oral health of prisoners to improve overall health and well-being. *Am J Public Health.* 2005;95(10):1677–1678.

3. Brinkley-Rubinstein L, Adler N, Stewart J, et al. Incarceration as a catalyst for worsening health. *Health Justice.* 2013;1(1):3.

4. Simon L, Sue K, Williams R, Beckmann D, Tobey M, Cohen M. Dental student–delivered care at a student–faculty collaborative clinic in a correctional facility. *Am J Public Health.* 2017;107(suppl 1):S85–S87.

5. Candamo F, Tobey M, Simon L. Teaching dental students about incarceration and correctional dentistry: results from a national survey. *J Dent Educ.* 2018;82(3):299–305.

6. McQuistan MR, Kuthy RA, Heller KE, Qian F, Riniker KJ. Dentists' comfort in treating underserved populations after participating in community-based clinical experiences as a student. *J Dent Educ.* 2008;72(4):422–430.

7. Ferguson WJ, Cloud D, Spaulding AC, et al. A call to action: a blueprint for academic health sciences in the era of mass incarceration. *J Health Care Poor Underserved.* 2016;27(2A):5–17.

8. Cohen LA, Bonito AJ, Akin DR, et al. Toothache pain: a comparison of visits to physicians, emergency departments and dentists. *J Am Dent Assoc.* 2008;139(9):1205–1216.

9. Kulkarni SP, Baldwin S, Lightstone AS, Gelberg L, Diamant AL. Is incarceration a contributor to health disparities? Access to care of formerly incarcerated adults. *J Community Health.* 2010;35(3):268–274.

V. INTERVENING VARIABLES

28

An Oral Health Benefit in Medicare Part B: It's Time to Include Oral Health in Health Care

Krishna Aravamudhan, BDS, MS, David Preble, DDS, JD, CAE, Marko Vujicic, PhD, Cassandra Yarbrough, MPP, Kata Kertesz, JD, Wey-Wey Kwok, JD, Jeffrey Chaffin, DDS, MPH, MHA, MBA, Michael Monopoli, DMD, MPH, MS, Cheryl Fish-Parcham, MSW, Melissa Burroughs, BA, Patrick Willard, MA, Jennifer Goldberg, JD, LLM, Bianca Rogers, BS, Beth Truett, BS, MDiv, Judith A. Jones, DDS, DScD, MPH, Richard Manski, DDS, PhD, MBA, and Elisa M. Chávez, DDS

OVERVIEW OF MEDICARE COVERAGE AS RELATED TO DENTAL CARE

Medicare is the federal health insurance program created in 1965 for people aged 65 years and older, regardless of income, medical history, or health status. The program was later expanded to cover certain persons with disabilities who are aged younger than 65 years, as well as individuals who have end-stage renal disease or amyotrophic lateral sclerosis.[1] Today, Medicare plays a key role in providing health and financial security to 59 million older people and people with disabilities.[1] Yet, the oral health status of the Medicare population and its ability to afford and access oral health care are issues of serious concern that must be addressed.

Many people lose their dental insurance when they retire, and traditional Medicare does not include coverage for routine oral health care such as checkups, cleanings, and x-rays, or restorative procedures (fillings, crowns, bridges, and root canals), tooth extractions, and dentures. Although some Medicare beneficiaries may be able to obtain dental coverage through other sources such as private Medicare Advantage plans, employer-sponsored retiree health plans, or individually purchased dental plans, the scope of dental benefits varies widely across plans. Persons with low income may qualify for Medicaid in addition to Medicare, but whether Medicaid will provide oral health coverage at all and the scope of that coverage varies widely across the country, depending on individual state Medicaid policies.

Accordingly, an estimated 70% of seniors lack or have limited dental insurance and fewer than half access dental care each year.[2,3] The gap in coverage leads to high out-of-pocket expenses for those who do access dental care. For those on a fixed or reduced income who may not be able to afford dental care, it can lead to higher expenditures for medical and emergency care associated with untreated dental problems. About one in five older Americans has untreated tooth decay,[4,5] and more than 70% have periodontal disease.[6] Younger Medicare beneficiaries with disabilities also lack oral health coverage, and more than a third of these adults have untreated dental caries.[7] A significant percentage of this group, as well as the low-income Medicare population, have reported delaying or forgoing dental care because of cost.[7]

Oral health problems can adversely affect one's ability to maintain optimal nutrition, self-image, social interactions, and mental and physical health. Caries and gum disease may lead to chronic pain, tooth loss, and serious infections. It is also not uncommon for Medicare beneficiaries to have medical conditions and medications that worsen their oral health or oral health issues that exacerbate or complicate treatment of their other medical conditions.

Increasingly, studies are showing that oral health is closely correlated to overall health.[8] Adding comprehensive oral health coverage to Medicare would keep older adults and persons with disabilities healthier and reduce other health care costs. This chapter discusses the need and support for this policy change and proposes how a comprehensive oral health benefit could be integrated into Medicare Part B.

BARRIERS TO DENTAL CARE FOR MEDICARE RECIPIENTS

People who rely on Medicare face numerous barriers to maintaining their oral health, including lack of coverage and affordable care, as well as costly medical conditions that can have an impact on their oral health. While the importance of good oral health is generally accepted, dental care use among older adults diminishes with age for those with limited income or no dental insurance.[3,9] As income and dental insurance coverage are typically tied to employment, the ability to pay for dental services decreases with both age and retirement.[10] Similarly, people who leave work because of permanent disability lose dental coverage at a time that they also have lost income.

Medicare beneficiaries spend a significant portion of their income on health care. More than one third of beneficiaries in traditional Medicare spend at least 20% of their per-capita total income on out-of-pocket health care costs. Between 2013 and 2030, out-of-pocket health care costs are projected to increase from 41% to 50% of average per-capita Social Security income.[11] The spending burden is even greater for individuals in poor health, those aged 85 years and older, and those with modest income or who derive most of their income from Social Security. In fact, cost is the number-one reason that older adults cite for not having gone to a dentist in the past year.[3]

The majority of persons on Medicare are of modest means, and median per-capita income declines with age, which limits their ability to afford dental coverage and care.[11] The median incomes for White beneficiaries aged 65 years or older ($30,050) is significantly greater than for Black ($17,350) and Hispanic ($13,650) beneficiaries. Across all ages, median per-capita income was lower for beneficiaries aged younger than 65 years with permanent disabilities ($17,950) than among seniors. Between 2013 and 2030, median income and savings are projected to increase after adjusting for inflation, but much of that growth will be concentrated among a small subset of beneficiaries with relatively high incomes and assets.

Furthermore, Medicare beneficiaries also have limited savings. One out of four Medicare beneficiaries has savings less than $14,550, no savings, or is in debt. Half of Medicare beneficiaries have less than $75,000 in savings, including retirement accounts.[12] As with income, median per-capita savings vary greatly across demographic characteristics, with lower rates of savings among Black ($16,000), Hispanic ($12,250), disabled aged younger than 65 years ($33,300), and single ($25,750) beneficiaries. For people who have less than a high-school education, per-capita savings are only $11,450.[12]

While some seniors continue to have sufficient income to enjoy private dental benefits after turning 65, half of all Medicare beneficiaries live on annual incomes less than $26,200, and one quarter have incomes less than $15,250.[12] More than half of beneficiaries aged 85 years and older have incomes of less than $20,400. And 70% of all seniors have no dental coverage. Further complicating access to dental care is the belief by many retirees that oral health coverage is included within Medicare, and many of those that do report having dental insurance do not realize that their Medicare coverage does not include a dental benefit.[13] Numerous studies have documented that more than 50% of people aged 50 to 64 years do not know that Medicare does not include dental coverage.

A substantial segment of the Medicare population with fixed incomes and limited resources will need to spend more of their incomes on dental care if they choose to access care, while others may forgo this vital care except in emergency cases, while prioritizing other life necessities such as food and shelter.[11] Providing dental coverage to older Americans and people with disabilities would close previous gaps in dental use and expense between the uninsured and the insured[14,15] and ensure that America's seniors and people with disabilities have access to good oral health care [savings] throughout their lifetime.

RISK FACTORS AND ACCESS TO/DISPARITIES IN DENTAL CARE FOR OLDER ADULTS

Disparities in oral care for older adults are significant for those with few financial resources and limited oral health education, particularly if they are entering their senior years with a significant history of oral disease.[16] The prevalence increases for those who are homebound or institutionalized and is more pronounced among groups who have been traditionally underserved, such as Black, Asian, and Hispanic adults; persons with low incomes; and those without dental benefits.[17] Untreated decay and other oral diseases result in pain, chronic and acute infection, tooth fractures, and tooth loss, as well as compromised oral function and quality of life.[18]

To adequately address their oral health needs, older adults and persons with disabilities who receive health care through Medicare require a comprehensive oral health benefit. Given the importance of oral health as part of overall health, integrating a dental benefit into the Medicare structure is essential.[19] Medicare beneficiaries face increased risks to their oral health as direct and indirect consequences of systemic diseases, conditions, and medications common to older populations.[16] Oral pain and tooth loss can make it difficult to eat, leading to poor nutrition, weight loss or gain, and exacerbation of chronic conditions such as hypertension, diabetes, and hyperlipidemia—conditions that individuals are more likely to acquire later in life.[20] Furthermore, for older adults with weakened immune systems, oral infections can act as a source for ongoing infection.[17] Without the means to address oral health problems, many Medicare beneficiaries face adverse consequences to their overall health, oral health, quality of life, and financial stability.

There has been a paradigm shift in dentistry with increased focus on risk assessment, interprofessional collaboration, and minimally invasive treatment to maintain oral health, an approach that is especially critical for adults with multiple morbidities and frail older adults at the end of life.[14,15] Although the inclusion of oral health care as an integral part of health care is important, these models are not widespread. Lack of resources and an absence of coordinated care not only result in more extensive and expensive care but also prevent the collection of data that will further our knowledge about the relationship between general and oral health. Without the addition of a dental benefit to Medicare, many older adults will not have the resources to benefit from these changing models in health care that include oral health as part of comprehensive care. Access through Medicare Part B would provide a significant opportunity for more coordinated oral and primary health care.[16]

ADDING DENTAL COVERAGE TO MEDICARE PART B

As Medicare Part B is the part of the Medicare program that covers outpatient services, a comprehensive oral health benefit would be most effectively administered and delivered through Part B. Such a benefit would include medically necessary procedures, as well as preventive services—a set of services similar to those covered by Part B for other forms of medical care.

The Medicare Part B benefit would be amended to include dental services using the medically necessary and reasonable standard that applies to all Part B services: Part B would cover care that is medically necessary and reasonable to address the oral health condition. Preventive services such as cleanings, x-rays, screenings, and examinations would be defined and covered in a similar fashion to services already provided through Medicare wellness visits and preventive services.

An oral health benefit fully integrated into the Medicare Part B coverage would be subject to the same cost-sharing rules as other Part B components (i.e., the same deductible, co-insurance requirements, and protections). Additional costs would be funded as Part B is now, through general revenues and beneficiary premiums ($134 per month for beneficiaries paying the standard premium in 2018), using the current Medicare processes to determine premium amounts. Low-income individuals would receive the same level of financial assistance and protections regarding oral health services as they do for other Part B services. In addition, Medicare Advantage plans would be required to provide oral health coverage just as they cover all other Part B benefits.[21]

Medicare Part B Coverage and Costs

Medicare Part B covers physician services including surgery, consultations and visits, outpatient services, x-rays, laboratory work and other diagnostic tests, certain preventive benefits, durable medical equipment, and prosthetic devices. Part B benefits are subject to a deductible ($183 in 2018), and most Part B benefits are subject to co-insurance of 20%. No co-insurance or deductible is charged for an annual wellness visit or for preventive services that are rated "A" or "B" by the US Preventive Services Task Force.

Medicare is a defined benefit program. Coverage is grounded in the "medically reasonable and necessary" standard. Part B is funded by general revenues and beneficiary premiums. State Medicaid programs pay the Part B premiums, as well as cost-sharing for some low-income beneficiaries. Beneficiaries with incomes greater than $85,000 for individuals or $170,000 for married couples pay a higher, income-related monthly Part B premium, ranging from $187.50 to $428.60 per month in 2018.

In 2017, the majority of the 57 million people on Medicare were covered by traditional Medicare, with one third (33%) receiving their Medicare benefits through a private Medicare Advantage plan that may impose different premium and cost-sharing requirements. These plans must provide all items and services that are covered under Medicare Parts A and B, except for hospice.

Proposed Structure and Cost Analysis

As part of an ongoing investigation of alternatives to serve the dental care needs of a growing elder population, the American Dental Association (ADA) recently commissioned a study that analyzed the cost structure for various dental benefit designs within Medicare.* Pricing was based on 2016 self-insured market rates. This study estimated that a comprehensive benefit without dollar value caps would cost the federal government

---

*Inclusion of the results of the ADA studies on this issue is not intended as an endorsement of other statements included in this chapter.

$31.4 billion in 2016 dollars or $32.3 billion in 2018. This estimate assumes a general fund contribution of 75% of all costs, similar to the current Medicare Part B funding structure.

The estimated base premium increase for a Part B benefit is $14.50 per beneficiary per month. This cost estimate accounts for low-income beneficiary subsidies applied to premiums and cost-sharing and surcharges paid by high-income beneficiaries. A standard 20% co-insurance was applied across all services. In addition, this model assumes dental services are not subject to any additional deductible.

This study assumes a reimbursement rate at the median (50th percentile) fee (i.e., fees charged by at least 50% of dentists in the United States). Funding a benefit at appropriate levels to support participation is essential to ensure adequate access for Medicare beneficiaries. Apart from cost of services, overhead charges experienced by dental offices are significant. Unlike a typical physician's office, a dental practice that offers comprehensive services houses significant equipment, creating a relatively larger overhead. Unlike Part B, within Medicare Part A, hospitals are paid a facility fee to account for equipment costs for each service rendered in the hospital.

Furthermore, within dental fee-for-service reimbursement models, other unique costs such as dental laboratory material and supplies are included within the fee for each procedure. Practice viability is dependent upon a mix of patients who are eligible for various discounted rates versus full-fee-paying patients in a practice. Thus, practice overhead, along with total cost of the services relative to discounted fees, will be an important factor for dental practices considering whether to participate in Medicare.

Note that these estimates are based on the current coverage trends for working-age adults. For example, the cost of coverage for dental implants is not included within these estimates. Should dental coverage include services such as implants (necessary for some Medicare recipients), the utilization and cost of such services would need to be added to these estimates. Similarly, any current "pent-up" demand for dental services has not been modeled within these estimates. The ADA continues to consider many options to address care for elders.

Public Opinion and the Case for Inclusion of Dental Benefits in Medicare Part B

Surveys show that consumers widely support adding oral health coverage to Medicare. A recent survey of likely voters among the general public indicated that 86% support including dental coverage as part of Medicare.[22]

Regardless of income or education, a majority of older adults (52%) expect dental coverage in Medicare and do not realize that Medicare does not cover routine or preventive dental care.[23] To better understand older adults' views and attitudes on adding a dental benefit to Medicare, Oral Health America and the ADA's Health Policy Institute

(HPI), commissioned Wakefield Research to conduct a series of focus groups with adults aged 50 years or older. Findings showed that an increasing number of older adults[24] understand the link between oral health and overall health and virtually all (93%)—despite cost concerns—want dental coverage in Medicare.

Older adults prioritize two categories of care: checkups and pain treatment. One woman from Chicago, Illinois, explained, "I want to be pain-free. And that means getting my regular exam and cleaning, and then dealing with my crowns."

While research by Marketing for Change showed that 6 in 10 seniors had never thought about advocating a dental benefit in Medicare,[25] a local consumer pilot in Orlando, Florida, called Demand Medicare Dental provided an early indication of the power of grassroots organizing. When equipped with consumer-friendly advocacy tools, older adults are ready to take action including signing petitions and sending letters, postcards, and toothbrushes to their legislators demanding that Medicare include dental coverage.

Dental Provider View of Adding Dental Benefits to Medicare Part B

To better understand the views and attitudes of the dental provider community, the HPI, with input from the ADA Practice Institute, developed a survey to assess dentists' views and opinions on adding dental services to the Medicare program. Data were collected through an online survey administered to a random sample of licensed, professionally active US dentists between January 8 and 12, 2018, and responses were weighted to be nationally representative.

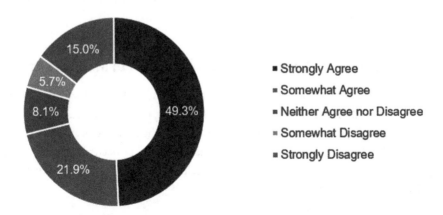

Figure 28-1. Overall, 71.2% of Dentists Agree That Medicare Should Include Comprehensive Dental Benefits

Overall, 71.2% of dentists agreed that Medicare should include comprehensive dental benefits (Figure 28-1).* Although provider reimbursement under such a benefit requires additional research, the majority of dentists indicated that they were willing to comply with typical Medicare practice requirements such as reporting diagnostic codes and using electronic health records.

Advantages of Adding Dental Coverage to Medicare Part B

Incorporating the oral health benefit into Part B has several advantages:

- It advances the goal of integrating oral health into total health care by incorporating the benefit administratively into the Medicare program that covers other health care providers. Administrative integration facilitates programmatic integration.
- It provides oral health coverage to everyone enrolled in Medicare, including those in Medicare Advantage plans, and ensures that public funding goes toward allowing the greatest number of beneficiaries access to a basic level of dental care and a healthy mouth. This is logical not only from a health equity standpoint but also because it would encourage provider participation.[16]
- Including an oral health benefit in Medicare Part B is simpler for beneficiaries and providers than setting up a separate benefit as was done for prescription drugs under Medicare. Beneficiaries would not have to navigate or enroll in a new, potentially confusing program. Oral health providers could interact with each other and the federal government in the same way that medical providers currently interact in the Part B system.
- There are established protections for both Medicare beneficiaries and providers. These include established Part B grievance and appeal procedures, existing precedent on medical necessity standards, and existing provider enrollment procedures, provider rate-setting processes, and payment protections for qualified Medicare beneficiaries. Including the Part B benefit avoids the need to create new systems and bureaucracies, saving significant time and costs.

Legislative Changes Needed to Add Dental Care to Medicare Part B

Currently, Medicare does not cover dental benefits because of the statutory exclusion in Section 1862(a)(12) of the Social Security Act. Removing this statutory exclusion is the most important legislative change to establish a comprehensive Medicare Part B oral health benefit.[16] However, additional statutory changes would be needed to ensure that a scope of services is established and that the oral health benefit is integrated into Medicare Part B as seamlessly as possible.

---

*For more information, contact the American Dental Association Health Policy Institute at hpi@ada.org.

Specifically, Congress would need to pass legislation to remove the exclusion of oral health benefits from the Medicare Program.[26] Furthermore, the legislation would need to establish dental coverage in Part B* and permit payment for services prescribed in the dental benefit.† Dental services would need to be defined in the Medicare statute, and various sections addressing provider payment would need to be amended to address oral health services.‡ Also, the Centers for Medicare and Medicaid Services would require the authority to promulgate any needed regulations to implement and administer oral health benefits as part of Medicare Part B.

CONCLUSIONS

Oral health is necessary for overall health. Older adults need timely and affordable access to dental care to age successfully. Oral health care is also essential for millions of those with permanent disabilities. A dental benefit in Medicare Part B will ensure that oral health care is integrated with, and elevated to, the same importance as the rest of health care. All older adults and people who are permanently disabled, regardless of socioeconomic status, need increased oral health literacy, along with access to oral health services and preventive care. Further research on the impact of oral health care coverage for Medicare Part B recipients would illuminate how this benefit would enhance overall health and better quality of life without excessive cost.

ACKNOWLEDGMENTS

Oral Health America would like to acknowledge the authors for their invaluable contributions to this chapter. This chapter was the result of a multidisciplinary collaboration with a shared commitment to improve the oral health and overall health of our nation's Medicare beneficiaries. Thank you to the representatives from the American Dental Association, Center for Medicare Advocacy, Families USA, Justice in Aging, and the Santa Fe Group.

REFERENCES

1. Kaiser Family Foundation. Centers for Medicare and Medicaid Services Medicare current beneficiary 2013 cost and use file. 2017. Available at: https://www.kff.org/medicare/issue-brief/an-overview-of-medicare. Accessed February 14, 2018.

---

*For example, this could be accomplished by amending section 42 USC § 1395k (section 1832 of the Social Security Act).
†Preventive services are addressed at 42 USC § 1395y(a)(1).
‡For example, dental could be included in the definition of Medical & Other Health Services at 42 USC § 1395x(s) or defined separately somewhere in 42 USC § 1395x (section 1861 of the Social Security Act).

2. Oral Health America. A state of decay, vol. II. 2013. Available at: https://oralhealthamerica. org/astateofdecay/archive. Accessed February 14, 2018.

3. Manski RJ, Rohde F. Dental services: use, expenses, source of payment, coverage and procedure type, 1996–2015: research findings. No. 38. Agency for Healthcare Research and Quality. 2017. Available at: https://meps.ahrq.gov/data_files/publications/rf38/rf38.shtml. Accessed April 23, 2018.

4. Dye BA, Thornton-Evans G, Li X, Iafolla TJ. Dental caries and tooth loss in adults in the United States, 2011–2012. NCHS data brief, no 197. National Center for Health Statistics. 2015. Available at: https://www.cdc.gov/nchs/data/databriefs/db197.pdf. Accessed April 23, 2018.

5. Vargas CM, Kramarow EA, Yellowitz JA. The oral health of older Americans. *Aging Trends.* No. 3. National Center for Health Statistics. 2001. Available at: http://www.cdc.gov/nchs/ data/ahcd/agingtrends/03oral.pdf. Accessed April 23, 2018.

6. Eke PI, Dye BA, Wei L, Thornton-Evans GO, Genco RJ. Prevalence of periodontitis in adults in the United States: 2009 and 2010. *J Dent Res.* 2012;91(10):914–920.

7. Kaiser Family Foundation. Oral health and Medicare beneficiaries: coverage, out-of-pocket spending, and unmet need. June 2012. Available at: https://kaiserfamilyfoundation.files. wordpress.com/2013/01/8325.pdf. Accessed February 14, 2018.

8. Jones JA, Monopoli M. Designing a new payment model for oral care in seniors. *Compend Contin Educ Dent.* 2017;38(9):616–624.

9. Manski RJ, Brown E. Dental use, expenses, private dental coverage, and changes, 1996 and 2004. MEPS Chartbook No. 17. Agency for Healthcare Research and Quality. 2007. Available at: http:// www.meps.ahrq.gov/mepsweb/data_files/publications/cb17/cb17.pdf. Accessed April 23, 2018.

10. Manski RJ, Moeller JR, Chen H, et al. Dental care coverage transitions. *Am J Manag Care.* 2009;15(10):729–735.

11. Cubanski J, Neuman T, Damico A, Smith K. Medicare beneficiaries' out-of-pocket health care spending as a share of income now and projections for the future. Kaiser Family Foundation. 2018. Available at: https://www.kff.org/report-section/medicare-beneficiaries-out-of-pocket-health-care-spending-as-a-share-of-income-now-and-projections-for-the-future-report. Accessed February 14, 2018.

12. Jacobson G, Griffin S, Neuman T, Smith K. Income and assets of Medicare beneficiaries, 2016–2035. Kaiser Family Foundation. 2017. Available at: https://www.kff.org/medicare/issue-brief/ income-and-assets-of-medicare-beneficiaries-2016-2035. Accessed February 14, 2018.

13. Moeller JR, Manski RJ, Mathiowetz N, Campbell N, Pepper JV. Response error in reporting dental coverage by older Americans in the Health and Retirement Study. *Inquiry.* 2014;51:1–10.

14. Manski RJ, Moeller JF, St Clair PA, Chen H, Schimmel J, Pepper JV. Dental use and expenditures for older uninsured Americans: the simulated impact of expanded coverage. *Health Serv Res.* 2015;50(1):117–135.

15. Manski RJ, Moeller JF, Chen H. Dental care coverage and use: modeling limitations and opportunities. *Am J Public Health*. 2014;104(2):e80–e87.

16. Griffin SO, Jones JA, Brunson D, et al. Burden of oral disease among older adults and implications for public health priorities. *Am J Public Health*. 2012;102(3):411–418.

17. Department of Health and Human Services. Oral health in America: a report of the Surgeon General. 2000. Available at: http://www.nidcr.nih.gov/DataStatistics/SurgeonGeneral/Documents/hck1ocv.@www.surgeon.fullrpt.pdf. Accessed November 15, 2017.

18. Hyde S, Dupuis V, Mariri BP, Dartevelle S. Prevention of tooth loss and dental pain for reducing the global burden of oral diseases. *Int Dent J*. 2017;67(suppl 2):19–25.

19. Slavkin HC; Santa Fe Group. A national imperative: oral health services in Medicare. *J Am Dent Assoc*. 2017;148(5):281–283.

20. Seligman HK, Laraia BA, Kushel MB. Food insecurity is associated with chronic disease among low-income NHANES participants. *J Nutr*. 2010;140(2):304–310.

21. US Centers for Medicare and Medicaid Services. Medicare costs at a glance. 2018. Available at: https://www.medicare.gov/your-medicare-costs/costs-at-a-glance/costs-at-glance.html. Accessed February 14, 2018.

22. Families USA. Public supports better insurance coverage for dental care, survey finds. December 14, 2017. Available at: http://familiesusa.org/blog/2017/12/public-supports-better-insurance-coverage-dental-care-survey-finds. Accessed February 12, 2018.

23. Oral Health America. Results of quick query omnibus survey conducted by Harris Poll, week of July 13, 2015 among Americans 50+. 2015. Available at: https://oralhealthamerica.org/wp-content/uploads/2015-Public-Opinion-Poll-Exec-Summary.pdf. Accessed February 12, 2018.

24. Oral Health America, American Dental Association Health Policy Institute. Results of instant-feedback qualitative sessions conducted by Wakefield Research on July 20–22, 2017, among Americans 50+. November 2017. Available at: https://oralhealthamerica.org/wp-content/uploads/MedicareToolkitOHA2018_InfographicWhatSeniorsWant.pdf. Accessed February 12, 2018.

25. Oral Health America. Demand Medicare dental pilot campaign report. September 2017. Available at: http://oralhealthamerica.org/files/OHA-DemandMedicareDental_PilotCampaignReport_September2017.pdf. Accessed February 12, 2018.

26. 42 USC § 1395y(a)(12) [section 1862(a)(12) of the Social Security Act].

29

Dental Homes for Older Americans*

Elisa M. Chávez, DDS, Jean Marie Calvo, DDS, MPH, and
Judith A. Jones, DDS, DScD, MPH

Good oral health is essential to overall health and well-being. Although the 2010 Affordable Care Act (ACA) improved access to oral health care for children and some Medicaid-eligible adults,[1] disparities remain in access to oral health care, especially for adults aged 65 years and older.[2] The majority of retired adults do not have coverage for dental care. A national 2016 survey showed that 57.5% of seniors with private insurance had visited a dental professional within the past 6 months, compared with 36.4% of those with Medicare alone and 25.9% eligible for both Medicare and Medicaid.[2]

Dental problems are exacerbated by comorbid medical, behavioral, and mental conditions, their treatments, and sometimes aging itself. Disparities in access to oral health care on the basis of income, insurance, race, and ethnicity result in higher costs to manage diseases and diminished quality of life for older adults.[3-5] Institutionalized and functionally or cognitively dependent older adults are disproportionately affected.[5] When people cannot afford basic dental services, society is called upon to pay for costly, complicated, or emergency procedures.[6,7] Older adults need dental homes (i.e., a long-term relationship with a dental provider to facilitate comprehensive oral health care) to receive appropriate, integrated prevention and dental care while they are well so that during the last stages of life the focus can be on maintenance and palliative care only.[8]

The World Health Organization (WHO) recognizes the value and efficiency of a life-course approach to improving oral health.[9] Improving population health and well-being depends on interventions aimed at individuals, families, communities, and health care systems within societal, behavioral, political, cultural, and economic contexts.[9] WHO suggests that "public health solutions for oral diseases are most effective when they are *integrated* with those for other chronic diseases and with national public health programmes."[10] Through the lens of WHO's Social Determinants of Health, this chapter focuses on what is needed to place and keep seniors in dental homes throughout their lives (Figure 29-1).

---

*This is a modified version of the article that appeared in the *American Journal of Public Health*. See Chávez EM, Calvo JM, Jones JA. Dental homes for older Americans: The Santa Fe Group call for removal of the dental exclusion in Medicare. *Am J Public Health*. 2017;107(suppl 1):S41–43.

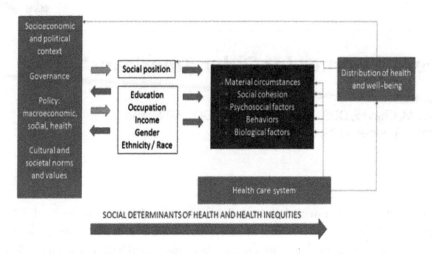

Source: Adapted from World Health Organization[11] and Solar and Irwin.[12]
Figure 29-1. Conceptual Framework: Social Determinants of Health

The oral health needs of America's older adults, gaps in access to care, and disparities in outcomes are examined. Actions for improving awareness and access are proposed. Potential medical cost savings data from the inclusion of dental care and the question of political feasibility are also considered. The goals and strategies outlined are aligned with the Institute for Healthcare Improvement's triple aim: lower costs, improved patient experience, and improved population health.[13,14]

CURRENT PUBLIC PROGRAM COVERAGE FOR ORAL HEALTH

While less than 2% of adults aged older than 65 years are medically uninsured, and most are publicly insured through Medicare, a reported 70% of those aged 65 to 74 years, 80% of those aged 75 to 84 years, and 84% of those aged 85 years and older lack dental insurance.[15,16] Thus, although most have resources to establish a medical home, where a regular primary care provider coordinates their medical care to achieve comprehensive, patient-centered care, fewer are guaranteed a dental home.

Medicare is a federal program that provides health benefits, with limited dental coverage for individuals aged 65 years and older.[17] Medicare Part A covers dental procedures that require inpatient hospitalization. Part B covers dental extractions in preparation for radiation therapy, inpatient oral examinations before kidney transplant, or in a rural/federally qualified health center before heart valve replacement.[17]

Medicaid is a state-managed health program available from birth.[17] Dually eligible Medicare–Medicaid enrollees *may* receive dental benefits. However, only 19 states provide adults extensive dental coverage, 16 limited, 13 emergency only, and three provide no coverage.[18] Sporadic dental benefits affect health and well-being and can strain other areas of the health care system.[6] Some older adults who are dually eligible participate in Programs of All-Inclusive Care for the Elderly (PACE). PACE enrollees have access to dental care on the basis of individual assessment of medical need, without additional fees or co-pays.[19] In addition to PACE, there has recently been growth in Medicare Advantage plans (i.e., private insurance alternatives to the government Medicare program). Some Medicare Advantage plans include dental benefits but benefits and costs vary among plans.[20]

SENIORS TODAY AND TOMORROW

Baby boomers began turning 65 in 2011, with 41.3 million persons aged 65 years and older in the United States. By 2030, one in five Americans (~72 million) will be aged 65 years and older.[21] The diversity of this generation is unlike any before. In 2017, an estimated 3% of adults aged 65 years and older lived in some form of institutional housing with the remainder living in the community. However, 9% of those aged 85 years and older resided in institutional settings.[22] The cohort aged 85 years and older is the fastest growing segment of the population and is expected to increase by 129% between 2016 and 2040 to 14.6 million people.[22] By 2060, approximately 32% of seniors will be foreign-born. The greatest growth among native-born older adults will be among Latinos, Blacks, and Asians, groups currently experiencing the greatest inequities in oral health.[21,23]

The median income of persons aged 65 years and older was $36,895 in 2014.[15] Ten percent were below the federal poverty level (FPL) and another 22.5% were between 100% of the 199% FPL; thus, a third (32.5%) of seniors fell below 200% of the FPL.[15] Importantly, a lower percentage of Whites (7.8%) fell below the FPL, compared with Asians (14.7%), Blacks (19.2%), and Hispanics (18.1%).[15]

With control for race and health behaviors, life expectancy of the poor can be 20 fewer years compared with nonpoor.[24] As income increases, so does quality of life (QOL).[25] Low educational levels are also associated with poorer psychological function, less optimal health behaviors, and poorer biological conditions.[26] Wu et al. found that, after control for education and access to care, disparities in edentulism (tooth loss) among racial groups were more evenly distributed, suggesting that they were largely a result of socioeconomic status.[27]

Similarly, insurance has been shown to be strongly tied to access. Manski et al. found that rates of dental coverage dropped steeply for persons aged 65 years and older. For adults aged 51 to 64 years, dental coverage was higher (64.65%) for those who were working compared with those who had retired (54.21%). This percentage dropped for working adults aged 65 to 74 years (40.08%) and dropped further still for those in this age group who were retired (36.30%). Working adults aged 75 years and older had even less coverage (23.37%), although those who were retired had slightly more coverage (26.47%), possibly due to Medicaid eligibility. Retired men aged 51 years and older were also more likely to have more coverage than retired women (38.68% and 32.27%, respectively). For those aged 65 to 74 years, Non-Hispanic Blacks had more insurance coverage than non-Hispanic Whites and Hispanics. Older adults with high incomes were more likely to have insurance than those with middle, low, or poor incomes, but poor older adults were more likely to have coverage than low-income adults, possibly because of Medicaid enrollment. Education, occupation, income, insurance, retirement, gender, ethnicity, and race all affect access to and outcomes of care for seniors in America.[16]

COMORBID MEDICAL CONDITIONS, LIMITED ACCESS, AND POOR ORAL HEALTH: A VICIOUS CIRCLE FOR OLDER ADULTS

Links between systemic inflammatory burden and chronic inflammation, such as what occurs from periodontal diseases, are well established.[28] There are many associations between poor oral health and systemic diseases: diminished chewing ability limits food choices and suboptimal nutrition poses a risk to general health and well-being[29,30]; periodontal disease and tooth loss have been associated with heart disease[31,32]; there is a bidirectional relationship between periodontal disease and diabetes[33,34]; and aspiration pneumonia in nursing home patients has been associated with poor oral hygiene.[35,36] Left untreated, chronic oral diseases diminish quality of life, foster social isolation, cause acute infections and conditions, and can result in hospitalization or death.[30,37]

Many age-related and prevalent systemic diseases and their treatments have clear and direct impacts on oral health[38] (e.g., heart disease, arthritis, cancer, diabetes, and polypharmacy). Poorly controlled diabetes increases the risk for periodontal diseases.[39,40] Cancer occurs as primary and metastatic disease in the oral cavity.[41,42] Bisphosphonates used to manage osteoporosis and some cancers increase risk of osteonecrosis of the jaw.[43] The temporomandibular joint is susceptible to arthritic destruction, altering food choices and nutriton.[44] Many medications reduce salivary flow increasing the risk of dental caries, soft-tissue trauma, altered taste, and difficulty swallowing. Older adults may not perceive diminished salivary flow resulting in delayed diagnoses, inadequate prevention, and poor oral outcomes.[5,45] Arthritis, depression, dementia, and history of stroke indirectly impact oral health. Arthritis and stroke limit dexterity to perform oral hygiene. People with depression, dementia, or stroke may be less able to care for themselves and experience changes in independence, living, economic, and social situations preventing them from receiving care.[5] People with depression may not address their own self-care; persons with dementia may not remember how or when to brush their teeth.[46] The consequences of cascading general and oral health problems mandate that aggressive prevention of oral diseases be part of a comprehensive care plan for patients living with chronic diseases or recovering from acute conditions (Figure 29-2).

Tooth loss, dental caries, periodontal diseases, and oral cancer incidence and mortality vary by age, race and ethnicity, education, and income. National Health Interview

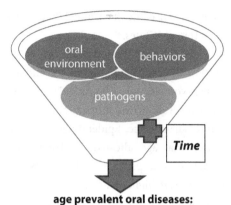

age prevalent oral diseases:
caries, periodontal and endodontic diseases, oral cancer and other oral pathology

exacerbated by:

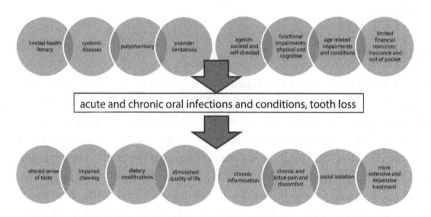

Source: Based on data from Griffen,[3] Pretty et al.[5] Neely et al.,[7] Finch and Crimmins,[28] Walls and Steele,[29] Nowjack-Raymer et al.,[30] Islam et al.,[34] Pace and McCullough,[35] Liantonio et al.,[36] US Department of Health and Human Services,[38] Mealey and Oates,[39] Noguti et al.,[41] Murillo et al.,[42] Ruggiero et al.,[43] Wiener et al.,[45] Ghezzi and Ship,[46] and Kiyak and Reichmuth.[47]

Figure 29-2. Cascade to Poor Oral Health and Its Sequelae

Survey data from 2014 show that complete tooth loss increases with age, affecting 16% of those aged 65 to 74 years, 25% of those aged 75 to 84 years, and 31% of those aged 85 years and older . Reports of complete edentulism in persons aged 65 years and older were higher among non-Hispanic Blacks (28.2%) and Hispanics (23.2%) than in Whites (19.6%).[15] National Health and Nutrition Examination Survey (NHANES) data from 1999 to 2004 showed that edentulism was higher in persons with poverty (< 100% FPL: 44%; 100%–199% FPL: 37%; ≥ 200% FPL: 17%).[48] The 2011–2012 data also showed that, among persons aged 65 years and older, untreated caries were highest among the poor (39.5%) and near poor (33%) versus nonpoor (12.2%) and untreated caries also varied by race and ethnicity[49]: 41% of non-Hispanic Black and 27% of Hispanic and Asian seniors had untreated caries versus 16% of Whites.[50]

NHANES 2009–2014 data showed "Periodontitis was highest in men, Mexican Americans, adults below 100% FPL, and current smokers" and more common in persons aged 65 years and older than younger age groups: 50.7% of persons aged 65 years and older had mild to moderate or severe periodontitis (9%).[51]

National Cancer Institute Surveillance, Epidemiology, and End Results (SEER) data from 2011 to 2015 showed that age-adjusted incidence rates per 100,000 of oral and pharyngeal cancers are highest in persons aged 65 years and older. While age- and gender-specific incidence rates were higher among White men (67.5 for those aged 65 to 69 years and 69.7 for those aged 70 to 74 years vs. 55.1 and 55.2 respectively for Black men), death rates were higher among Black men aged 65 to 69 years (19.5 for those aged 65 to 69 years, 23.7 for those aged 70 to 74 years olds vs. 14.0 and 15.6 respectively for White men).[52]

AGEISM AND ORAL HEALTH

Poor oral health is no more a consequence of normal aging than are systemic diseases such as diabetes and heart disease.[46] The World Health Organization defines oral health as "a state of being free from mouth and facial pain, oral and throat cancer, oral infection and sores, periodontal (gum) disease, tooth decay, tooth loss, and other diseases and disorders that limit an individual's capacity in biting, chewing, smiling, speaking, and psychosocial wellbeing."[10] Despite the presence of disease, infection, limited oral function, or significant risk factors for poor oral health, the impetus for seeking and justifying oral health care for seniors is often based solely on the presence of pain.[53] However, older adults often have atypical responses to diseases (e.g,. lack of pain, while some are unable to express pain because of cognitive impairment).[54] They may also experience financial strain as a result of trying to manage their medical conditions on fixed incomes, and dental care is often perceived as optional in the absence of pain, or oral health is anticipated to decline with aging. Older persons are challenged with economic issues and ageism, which condones less-than-optimal oral health for older Americans.[47,55]

IMPROVING ACCESS TO ORAL HEALTH FOR OLDER ADULTS

Four issues must be addressed to improve access to oral health care for older Americans:

1. The benefit of integrating oral health into the US health care system;
2. Determination of medical cost savings associated with dental treatment for persons with comorbid diseases;

3. Reversal of emerging trends of declining dental care access among older Americans and potential impact on workforce; and
4. Political feasibility of including a universal dental benefit in Medicare.

Oral Health and the Institute for Healthcare Improvement's "Triple Aim"

The ACA increased health care coverage and redirected US priorities toward innovation to increase health quality and effectiveness and reduce costs. The Centers for Medicare and Medicaid Innovation was created in 2010 and pilots innovations in health care, tests novel payment and delivery models, evaluates best practices, and engages stakeholders in developing new models of delivering health care.[17,56] Inclusion of a dental benefit in Medicare is consistent with the triple aim and would enable the dental care delivery system and patients to benefit from this innovation and integration with the rest of the health care system.

A first step toward stimulating research into the impact of maintaining oral health on aging and identifying opportunities for improving overall health outcomes and cost savings by improving oral health would be the development of an 80/20 goal for *Healthy People 2030* to promote a 10% increase in the percentage of persons aged 80 years and older with at least 20 teeth in reasonable chewing pairs to maintain function.[57] Establishment of additional target outcomes for oral health, and good oral health as a quality measure in chronic systemic disease management, will guide national focus and help to widely improve oral health and function.

A broad public health campaign is needed to raise oral health literacy and awareness about the value of oral health, the associations of poor oral health with systemic diseases, and the potential cost savings from the inclusion of oral health benefits to the health care system. A clearer understanding of oral health's inherent value is needed so that society is willing to incur some expense to create a benefit and for seniors to make use of the new resource.[54] The more seniors take advantage of the plans, the greater the impact and the better information we will have about the benefits of maintaining oral health and dental homes across the life span.

DENTAL CARE AND INSURANCE COST SAVINGS

Analyses of Insurance Claims by Insurance Providers and the American Dental Association Health Policy Institute

Three insurance providers (Cigna, United Concordia, and United Healthcare) and the American Dental Association Health Policy Institute retrospectively analyzed insurance claims data to examine the effects of the provision of dental care on the cost of treating US adult beneficiaries with stroke, congestive heart failure (CHF), and/or diabetes. Given the high prevalence of chronic diseases in the Medicare population, the potential cost savings of managing oral health are substantial.[58] Table 29-1 shows (1) the total costs to Medicare for treatment of stroke, CHF, and diabetes and the number of beneficiaries with those conditions; (2) for each insurance study the estimated annual cost savings per beneficiary when dental care was provided; and (3) the potential total annual savings to Medicare by dollars and percentages if provided for all beneficiaries with those conditions. To ensure that savings were not double-counted for beneficiaries with comorbid chronic diseases, we used the unique number of beneficiaries with a condition category of stroke, CHF, and diabetes as defined by the Center for Medicare and Medicaid Services.[59]

Data from Cigna estimated that routine dental treatment could result in medical cost savings of more than $19 billion for the US Medicare population with stroke, CHF, and diabetes annually.[60-62] The United Concordia study estimated $18.8 billion savings for persons with stroke, CHF, and diabetes,[63] and United Healthcare estimated $20 billion medical cost savings for those with CHF and diabetes.[64] The fourth study, by Nasseh et al., reviewed insurance claims data for patients newly diagnosed with diabetes, and quantified the medical cost savings of dental treatment to be $1,577 per beneficiary over two years or potentially $6.8 billion annually for the US Medicare population.[65] Interestingly, all four analyses found substantial medical cost savings when dental treatment was implemented.[61-65]

Limitations of the Studies

There were shortcomings in the insurance studies, particularly in the area of study design (retrospective, nonrandom allocation to groups). Furthermore, we do not know whether cost savings are a result of more compliant patients (that use dental services) who adhere to regular needed health care, and only one study was peer-reviewed. However, the United Healthcare study divided its study groups into persons who were medically compliant and not medically compliant. This study found that the medically noncompliant group demonstrated the greatest savings, but all groups demonstrated savings.[64] Additional research is needed to determine whether these insurance studies stand up to the scrutiny of peer review. Finally, none of these studies takes into account the overlap among diabetes, cardiovascular disease, and stroke. Demonstration programs using prospective study designs with random allocation of similar groups of persons (location, education, race and ethnicity, comorbidities) into test and comparison groups are needed to definitively test the hypothesis that providing dental care saves money in the Medicare population.[66]

TRENDS IN DENTAL CARE USE AND IMPACT ON WORKFORCE

American Dental Association reports show that US trends in adults accessing dental care have been level since 2010.[65] Dental care use among adults aged 65 years and older showed no changes from 2012 to 2013; however, dental care use among *poor* seniors fell

Table 29-1. Medicare Spending and Potential Savings for Stroke, Congestive Heart Failure (CHF), and Diabetes Based Upon Numbers of Beneficiaries and Insurance Data

	Stroke	CHF	Diabetes	Total
Estimates of total Medicare costs due to disease annually, 2014				
Medicare beneficiaries with diagnosis[59,60]	1,879,021	4,814,660	8,657,223	15,350,904
Unique Medicare beneficiaries within condition category	1,287,280	2,052,953	3,278,663	6,618,896
Average annual cost per beneficiary[59,60]	$45,840	$29,472	$18,108	$93,420
Total Medicare cost due to disease annually[59,60]	$59,008,915,200	$60,504,630,816	$59,370,029,604	$178,883,575,620
Four estimated insurance cost savings per beneficiary per year for select chronic diseases				
Cigna[61,62]	$10,142	$647	$1,418	$12,207
United Concordia[63]	$5,681	$1,090	$2,840	$9,611
United Healthcare[64]	N/A	$8,466	$923	N/A
American Dental Association[65]	N/A	N/A	$664	N/A
Potential annual savings to Medicare for stroke, CHF, and diabetes, by cited study				
Cigna[61,62]	$13,055,593,760	$1,328,260,591	$4,649,144,134	$19,032,998,485
United Concordia[63]	$7,313,037,680	$2,237,718,770	$9,311,402,920	$18,862,159,370
United Healthcare[64]	N/A	$17,380,300,098	$3,026,205,949	N/A
American Dental Association[65]	N/A	N/A	$2,177,032,232	N/A
Potential annual percentage of savings to Medicare for stroke, CHF, and diabetes, by cited study				
Cigna[61,62]	22%	2%	8%	
United Concordia[63]	12%	4%	16%	
United Healthcare[64]	N/A	29.50%	5.00%	
American Dental Association[65]	N/A	N/A	4%	

from 29.6% in 2010 to 24.0% in 2012 to 19.4% in 2013.[67] By contrast, seniors with private dental benefits increased dental utilization rates from 66.9% in 2012 to 68.6% in 2013.[67] Providing dental insurance to adults aged 65 years and older could help reverse the downward trends in US dental care use among poor and underserved seniors and reduce disparities in access between the poor (19.4% in 2013) and seniors with private dental insurance (68.6% in 2013).[67]

One concern regarding the expansion of Medicare to include dental benefits is the increased demand for dental services. Results from analyses of Medicaid dental expansion showed that dentists were able to increase the number of newly insured patients they saw without reducing the care they provided to other patients.[68] Increases in dental hygienist visits were 16% to 33% larger than increases in dentist visits following adult Medicaid dental expansion. Income increased by $15,096 to $20,365 per practice annually in those states. Thus, the supply of dental services was able to meet the demand for new dental services following the expansion of publicly funded dental insurance with a modest increase in wait time for patients (< 0.1 day).[68] However, as patients experience comorbidities, polypharmacy, and related oral pathology, practitioners must spend more time and resources to ensure that treatment is appropriate, timely, and safe.[5,46] This may be cost-prohibitive for providers if reimbursement rates cannot match the expenses incurred to provide appropriate care to a complex population with complex needs.

POLITICAL FEASIBILITY OF A MEDICARE DENTAL BENEFIT

Section 1862(a) of the Social Security Act (42 USC 1395y [a]), paragraph 12, states that dental coverage is excluded from Medicare

> where such expenses are for services in connection with the care, treatment, filling, removal, or replacement of teeth or structures directly supporting teeth, except that payment may be made under part A in the case of inpatient hospital services in connection with the provision of such dental services if the individual, because of his underlying medical condition and clinical status or because of the severity of the dental procedure, requires hospitalization in connection with the provision of such services.[69]

Federal legislation is needed to remove the exclusion, creating an opportunity for a dental benefit.

The inclusion of a Medicare dental benefit does not require new entities within the Center for Medicare and Medicaid Services for its administration. However, leaders in medicine, dentistry, geriatrics, insurance, and policy would need to work together to propose a benefit, determine the benefit's fiscal impact, build a constituency, and engender legislation to implement the benefit. Repurposing wasteful spending from the budget to fund a Medicare dental benefit would be more fiscally responsible than increasing the Medicare budget to support the benefit. Thus, testing whether or not there are costs savings from dental care may be a first step in the process. If true, inclusion of dental care in parallel with chronic disease treatment would present an opportunity to reduce Medicare spending while improving quality of care. Demonstration of such savings would require testing of benefit models and allowing components to evolve as more information on utilization and savings is gathered.

The inclusion of dental services for Medicare enrollees through Part B as an integral, rather than a supplemental program, is essential to improve access to dental homes for seniors. This would insure greater stability and longevity of access than currently available through Medicaid, access not guaranteed through the supplemental plans, and a reduction of the administrative burden of creating a stand-alone benefit. A universal benefit is a critical step toward increasing the public's perception about the value of oral health, raising the visibility and importance of oral health care to other health professionals, and encouraging timely and appropriate referrals for patients.

CONCLUSIONS

The mouth is essential for human health, function, and interaction. We use our mouths to eat, speak, and engage others. In the words of the late C. Everett Koop, MD, "You can't be healthy without good oral health."[38] We are faced with a generation of baby boomers with increased life expectancy, comorbid chronic health conditions, and evidence of a dynamic balance between oral and systemic health, yet only a limited percentage of older Americans will have the resources to maintain dental homes and good oral health to the end of life.[38,70] Can we say that we are successfully managing systemic disease or that people are aging successfully while oral health deteriorates? Oral diseases are preventable with routine care. Yet, for many older adults, a routine visit to their dental home must be abandoned because of disability or lack of knowledge, access, funds, and societal will. Are tooth loss, chronic inflammation, chronic and acute oral conditions, and lack of awareness acceptable? Oral health is integral to health to preserve dignity and function in old age. Federal legislation to remove the dental exclusion in Medicare would open the door for a dental benefit to be created and keep open the door to dental homes for millions of underserved older adults.

ACKNOWLEDGMENTS

The authors are grateful for the review and advice by The Santa Fe Group, especially Duskanka Kleinman, DDS, MScD, Claude Earl Fox III, MD, MPH, and Michael C. Alfano, DMD, PhD, who provided guidance and assistance in the development, organization, review, and editing of this chapter throughout the process. Elisa M. Chávez, DDS, is a Santa Fe Group Scholar and Judith A. Jones, DMD, DScD, MPH, is a member of The Santa Fe Group. We also thank Kendrick Smaellie for her superior editing and technical assistance.

REFERENCES

1. Vujicic M, Nasseh K. Gap in dental care utilization between Medicaid and privately insured children narrows, remains large for adults. Health Policy Institute Research Brief. American Dental Association. December 2015. Available at: http://www.ada.org/en/~/media/ADA/Science%20and%20Research/HPI/Files/HPIBrief_0915_1. Accessed November 27, 2018.

2. Blackwell DL, Villarroel MA. Tables of summary health statistics for US Adults: 2016 National Health Interview Survey. National Center for Health Statistics. 2018. Available at: https://ftp.cdc.gov/pub/Health_Statistics/NCHS/NHIS/SHS/2016_SHS_Table_A-6.pdf. Accessed November 27, 2018.

3. Griffin SO, Jones JA, Brunson D, et al. Burden of oral disease among older adults and implications for public health priorities. *Am J Public Health*. 2012;102(3):411–418.

4. Cohen LA, Manski RJ, Magder LS, et al. Dental visits to hospital emergency departments by adults receiving Medicaid: assessing their use. *J Am Dent Assoc*. 2002;133(6):715–724.

5. Pretty IA, Ellwood RP, Lo E, et al. The Seattle Care Pathway for securing oral health in older patients. *Gerodontology*. 2014;31(suppl 1):77–87.

6. Singhal A, Caplan DJ, Jones MP, et al. Eliminating Medicaid adult dental coverage in California led to increased dental emergency visits and associated costs. *Health Aff (Millwood)*. 2015;34(5):749–756.

7. Neely M, Jones JA, Rich S, et al. Effects of cuts in Medicaid on dental-related visits and costs at a safety-net hospital. *Am J Public Health*. 2014;104(6):e13–e16.

8. Jones JA, Brown EJ, Volicer L. Target outcomes for long-term oral health care in dementia: a Delphi approach. *J Public Health Dent*. 2000;60(4):330–334.

9. Marmot M, Friel S, Bell R, et al. Closing the gap in a generation: health equity through action on the social determinants of health. *Lancet*. 2008;372(9650):1661–1669.

10. World Health Organization Media Centre. Oral health fact sheet no. 318. 2012. Available at: https://www.mah.se/CAPP/Oral-Health-Promotion/WHO-Oral-Health-Fact-Sheet1. Accessed November 27, 2018.

11. World Health Organization, Commission on Social Determinants of Health. Closing the gap in a generation: health equity through action on the social determinants of health. Final Report of the Commission on Social Determinants of Health. Geneva, Switzerland: World Health Organization; 2008.

12. Solar O, Irwin A. A conceptual framework for action on the social determinants of health. Discussion paper for the Commission on Social Determinants of Health. Geneva, Switzerland: World Health Organization; 2007.

13. Institute for Healthcare Improvement. The IHI triple aim 2016. Available at: http://www.ihi. org/engage/initiatives/TripleAim/Pages/default.aspx. Accessed January 1, 2017.

14. Berwick DM, Nolan TW, Whittington J. The triple aim: care, health, and cost. *Health Aff (Millwood)*. 2008;27(3):759–769.

15. Federal Interagency Forum on Aging-Related Statistics. Older Americans 2016: key indicators of well-being. August 2016: 29, 94–95, 117. Available at: https://agingstats.gov/docs/LatestReport/ Older-Americans-2016-Key-Indicators-of-WellBeing.pdf. Accessed August 8, 2018.

16. Manski RJ, Moeller J, Schimmel J, et al. Dental care coverage and retirement. *J Public Health Dent*. 2010;70(1):1–12.

17. Klees B, Wolfe C, Curtis C. Brief summaries of Medicare and Medicaid: Title XVIII & Title XIX of the Social Security Act. Centers for Medicare and Medicaid Services, Department of Health and Human Services. 2017. Available at: https://www.cms.gov/Research-Statistics-Data-and-Systems/Statistics-Trends-and-Reports/MedicareProgramRatesStats/Downloads/ MedicareMedicaidSummaries2017.pdf. Accessed August 10, 2018.

18. Center for Health Care Strategies. Medicaid adult dental benefits: an overview. 2018. Available at: https://www.chcs.org/media/Adult-Oral-Health-Fact-Sheet_072718.pdf. Accessed August 9, 2018.

19. Center for Medicare and Medicaid Services. Program of All-Inclusive Care for the Elderly (PACE). 2016. Available at: https://www.cms.gov/Medicare/Health-Plans/PACE/Overview. html. Accessed November 27, 2018.

20. Center for Medicare and Medicaid Services. Health plans—general information. 2014. Available at: https://www.cms.gov/Medicare/Health-Plans/HealthPlansGenInfo/index.html. Accessed January 1, 2017.

21. Ortman JM, Velkoff VA, Hogan H. An aging nation: the older population in the United States. Current Population Reports, P25-1140 Washington DC: US Census Bureau; 2014.

22. Administration on Aging, Administration for Community Living. A profile of older Americans. US Department of Health and Human Services. 2017. Available at: https://www.acl.gov/ sites/default/files/Aging%20and%20Disability%20in%20America/2017OlderAmericansPro-file.pdf. Accessed August 8, 2018.

23. Colby SL, Ortman JM. Projections of the size and composition of the US population: 2014 to 2060. Washington, DC: US Census Bureau; 2015:25–1143.

24. Crimmins EM, Hayward MD, Saito Y. Differentials in active life expectancy in the older population of the United States. *J Gerontol B Psychol Sci Soc Sci*. 1996;51(3):S111–S120.

25. Huguet N, Kaplan MS, Feeny D. Socioeconomic status and health-related quality of life among elderly people: results from the Joint Canada/United States Survey of Health. *Soc Sci Med*. 2008;66(4):803–810.

26. Kubzansky LD, Berkman LF, Glass TA, et al. Is educational attainment associated with shared determinants of health in the elderly? Findings from the MacArthur Studies of Successful Aging. *Psychosom Med.* 1998;60(5):578–585.

27. Wu B, Hybels C, Liang J, et al. Social stratification and tooth loss among middle-aged and older Americans from 1988 to 2004. *Community Dent Oral Epidemiol.* 2014; 42(6):495–502.

28. Finch CE, Crimmins EM. Inflammatory exposure and historical changes in human life-spans. *Science.* 2004;305(5691):1736–1739.

29. Walls A, Steele J. The relationship between oral health and nutrition in older people. *Mech Ageing Dev.* 2004;125(12):853–857.

30. Nowjack-Raymer R, Sheiham A. Numbers of natural teeth, diet, and nutritional status in US adults. *J Dent Res.* 2007;86(12):1171–1175.

31. Vedin O, Hagström E, Budaj A, et al. Tooth loss is independently associated with poor outcomes in stable coronary heart disease. *Eur J Prev Cardiol;* 2016;23(8):839–846.

32. Humphrey LL, Fu R, Buckley DI, et al. Periodontal disease and coronary heart disease incidence: a systematic review and meta-analysis. *J Gen Intern Med.* 2008;23(12):2079–2086.

33. Iacopino AM. Periodontitis and diabetes interrelationships: role of inflammation. *Ann Periodontol.* 2001;6(1):125–137.

34. Islam SA, Seo M, Lee Y-S, et al. Association of periodontitis with insulin resistance, β-cell function, and impaired fasting glucose before onset of diabetes. *Endocr J.* 2015;62(11):981–989.

35. Pace CC, McCullough GH. The association between oral microorgansims and aspiration pneumonia in the institutionalized elderly: review and recommendations. *Dysphagia.* 2010;25(4):307–322.

36. Liantonio J, Salzman B, Snyderman D. Preventing aspiration pneumonia by addressing three key risk factors: dysphagia, poor oral hygiene, and medication use. *Ann Longterm Care.* 2014; 22(10):42–48.

37. Foltyn P. Ageing, dementia and oral health. *Aust Dent J.* 2015;60(suppl 1):86–94.

38. US Department of Health and Human Services. Oral health in America: a report of the Surgeon General. Rockville, MD: National Institute of Dental and Craniofacial Research, National Institutes of Health; 2000.

39. Mealey BL, Oates TW. Diabetes mellitus and periodontal diseases. *J Periodontol.* 2006; 77(8):1289–1303.

40. Kudiyirickal MG, Pappachan JM. Diabetes mellitus and oral health. *Endocrine.* 2015; 49(1):27–34.

41. Noguti J, Gomes de Moura C, de Jesus GP, et al. Metastasis from oral cancer: an overview. *Cancer Genomics Proteomics*. 2012;9(5):329–335.

42. Murillo J, Bagan JV, Hens E, et al. Tumors metastasizing to the oral cavity: a study of 16 cases. *J Oral Maxillofac Surg*. 2013;71(9):1545–1551.

43. Ruggiero SL, Dodson TB, Fantasia J, et al. American Association of Oral and Maxillofacial Surgeons position paper on medication-related osteonecrosis of the jaw—2014 update. *J Oral Maxillofac Surg*. 2014;72(10):1938–1956.

44. Hoffmann RG, Kotchen JM, Kotchen TA, et al. Temporomandibular disorders and associated clinical comorbidities. *Clin J Pain*. 2011;27(3):268–274.

45. Wiener RC, Wu B, Crout R, et al. Hyposalivation and xerostomia in dentate older adults. *J Am Dent Assoc*. 2010;141(3):279–284.

46. Ghezzi EM, Ship JA. Systemic diseases and their treatments in the elderly: impact on oral health. *J Public Health Dent*. 2000;60(4):289–296.

47. Kiyak HA, Reichmuth M. Barriers to and enablers of older adults' use of dental services. *J Dent Educ*. 2005;69(9):975–986.

48. National Institute of Dental and Craniofacial Research. Tooth loss in seniors (age 65 and over). 2016 Available at: http://nidcr.nih.gov/DataStatistics/FindDataByTopic/ToothLoss/ToothLossSeniors65andOlder.htm. Accessed January 1, 2017.

49. Table 66. Untreated dental caries, by selected characteristics: United States, selected years 1988–1994 through 2011–2012. Hyattsville, MD: National Center for Health Statistics: 2015.

50. Dye BA, Thornton-Evans G, Li X, et al. Dental caries and tooth loss in adults in the United States, 2011–2012. NCHS Data Brief. 2015;(197):197.

51. Eke PI, Thorton-Evans G, Liang W, Borgnakke WS, Dye BA, Genco R. Periodontitis in US adults. National Health and Nutrition Examination Survey 2009–2014. *J Am Dent Assoc*. 2018; 149(7):576–588.

52. National Cancer Institute. Surveillance, Epidemiology and End Results Program. Age-specific SEER incidence and death rates, US, 2011–2015. Available at: https://seer.cancer.gov/csr/1975_2015/browse_csr.php?sectionSEL=20&pageSEL=sect_20_table.08. Accessed November 27, 2018.

53. Slack-Smith L, Lange A, Paley G, et al. Oral health and access to dental care: a qualitative investigation among older people in the community. *Gerodontology*. 2010;27(2): 104–113.

54. Mitty E. Iatrogenesis, frailty, and geriatric syndromes. *Geriatr Nurs*. 2010;31(5):368–374.

55. Gilbert GH. "Ageism" in dental care delivery. *J Am Dent Assoc*. 1989;118(5):545–548.

56. Center for Medicare and Medicaid Services. Health Care Innovation Awards 2016. Available at: https://innovation.cms.gov/initiatives/Health-Care-Innovation-Awards. Accessed August 10, 2018.

57. Yamashina T, Kamijo H, Fukai K. The 8020 Campaign for oral health promotion in Japan: its history, effects, and future visions. In: *The Current Evidence of Dental Care and Oral Health for Achieving Healthy Longevity in an Aging Society.* Japanese Dental Association. 2015: 275–284.

58. Korda H, Erdem E. Prevalence and spending on diabetes for Medicare's fee-for-service population: US trends, 2010. *Chron Dis Int.* 2014;1:1–2.

59. Center for Medicare and Medicaid Services, Chronic Conditions Warehouse. CCW condition algorithms 2016. Available at: https://www.ccwdata.org/web/guest/condition-categories. Accessed August 10, 2018.

60. Marano A, Hahn M, Hall M, et al. Appropriate periodontal therapy associated with lower medical utlilization and costs. Paper presented at: International Association for Dental Research; March 20–23, 2013; Seattle, WA.

61. Jeffcoat M, Hall M, Hedlund C, et al. Periodontal treatment and medical costs in diabetes and cerebrovascular accident. Paper presented at: International Association for Dental Research Meeting; April 1–4, 2009; Miami, FL.

62. Jeffcoat M, Tanna NK, Hedlund C, et al. Does treatment of oral disease reduce the costs of medical care? *Medscape.* October 19, 2011. Available at: https://www.medscape.com/viewarticle/751609_1. Accessed August 10, 2018.

63. Jeffcoat MK, Jeffcoat RL, Gladowski PA, et al. Impact of periodontal therapy on general health: evidence from insurance data for five systemic conditions. *Am J Prev Med.* 2014; 47(2):166–174.

64. United Healthcare. Medical Dental Integration Study 2013. Available at: http://www.uhc.com/content/dam/uhcdotcom/en/Private%20Label%20Administrators/100-12683%20Bridge2Health_Study_Dental_Final.pdf. Accessed November 27, 2018.

65. Nasseh K, Vujicic M, Glick M. The relationship between periodontal interventions and healthcare costs and utilization. Evidence from an integrated dental, medical, and pharmacy commercial claims database. *Health Econ.* 2017;26:519–527.

66. Hawazin WE, Simon LS, Ticku S, Bain PA, Barrow J, Reidy CA. Does providing dental services reduce overall health care costs? A systematic review of the literature. *J Am Dent Assoc.* 2018;149(8):696–703.

67. Nasseh K, Vujicic M. Dental care utilization rate continues to increase among children, holds steady among working-age adults and the elderly. Health Policy Institute Research Brief. American Dental Association. October 2015. Available at: http://www.ada.org/~/media/ADA/Science%20and%20Research/HPI/Files/HPIBrief_1015_1.ashx. Accessed August 10, 2018.

68. Buchmueller T, Miller S, Vujicic M. How do providers respond to changes in public health insurance coverage? Evidence from adult Medicaid dental benefits. *Am Econ J Econ Policy.* 2016;8(4):70–102.

69. Center for Medicare and Medicaid Services. General exclusions from coverage. In: *2015 Medicare Benefit Policy Manual.* Available at: https://www.cms.gov/Regulations-and-Guidance/ Guidance/Manuals/downloads/bp102c16.pdf. Accessed August 10, 2018.

70. Slavkin HC; Santa Fe Group. A national imperative. *J Am Dent Assoc.* 2017;148(5):281–283.

Oral Health: Basic Tenets for a Healthy, Productive Life*

Louis W. Sullivan, MD

Our nation's history began with the appropriation of native lands, followed by the introduction of slavery, and then legally sanctioned discrimination against the sons and daughters of those slaves and others who reached our shores as immigrants. The socio-economic residue from these stark realities remains with us today. Individual and institutional racism continues in overt and covert ways in our society.

In my own life, overcoming obstacles to education and professional achievement has certainly grounded my perspective on how our nation can and must address the ongoing challenges for our country, for our health system, and for our society at large. The significant disparities in the health status of our poor and minority citizens, compared with the health of our majority White population, result in life expectancies for minorities and the poor that are as much as five to seven years shorter. The latter is a result of minorities having less access to health services, having fewer health professionals present in their communities, and often experiencing bias (conscious and unconscious) in their interactions with our health system.

The prerequisite for an optimal, fulfilling, and productive life for all our citizens is good health, which makes all of their other possibilities more achievable. And one of the most basic tenets for a healthy, productive life is good oral health: oral health is not only part of an individual's state of physical, mental, and social well-being, but also a key factor in maintaining such a state.

SIZE OF THE PROBLEM

Dental caries, or tooth decay, is the most common chronic disease in children and adults in the United States. And it is largely, if not entirely, preventable. Yet, millions of Americans—adults and children—lack access to preventive dental services and routine dental care. More than 70 million Americans obtain their water from community water systems with no access to fluoridation, although fluoridation is known to

*This is a modified version of the article that appeared in the *American Journal of Public Health*. See: Sullivan LW. Oral health: basic tenets for a healthy, productive life. *Am J Public Health*. 2017;107(suppl 1):S39–S40

significantly reduce tooth decay.[1] About 130 million Americans (43% of the population) have no dental coverage whatsoever.[2] Over the past 20 years, the number of Dental Health Professional Shortage Areas has grown six-fold—from 800 in 1993 to more than 4900 in 2014. These issues are exacerbated in minorities and the communities in which they live.

THE MANPOWER CHALLENGE

As our society continues to recognize and address the impact of racism on our individual behaviors and on our institutional and governmental actions, it is critical to the nation's health and economic vitality that the health workforce becomes more diverse, to better respond to the country's changing demographics.

Today, one in three Americans is a member of a racial/ethnic minority group, with African Americans, Hispanic Americans, and American Indians constituting more than 30% of the nation's population. However, these groups account for only 12.3% of physicians, 7% of dentists, 10% of pharmacists, and 11% of registered nurses. Minorities are also severely underrepresented among health profession faculties, deans, provosts, hospital administrators, and health policy experts. As we look toward the year of 2043, when the United States is projected to become a nation with no majority population, we should ask, "who will care for the racial/ethnic minority groups if today's children of color are not supported and encouraged to pursue a career in the health professions?"

Dentists, dental hygienists, and dental therapists for communities currently without regular dental care are needed to improve the oral health of Americans. Only 20% of the nation's 179,000 practicing dentists accept Medicaid.[3] And of those practitioners who do, fewer than 8500 devote a substantial part of their practice to serving the poor or rural residents.[3] By contrast, 62% of the members of the National Dental Association (whose members are predominantly African American) serve Medicaid patients (H. Harper, personal communication, September 2014). We must address the current insufficient reimbursement policies for dental care.

To improve our nation's oral health, we need more well–trained dental professionals to deliver care where it is lacking—in culturally appropriate ways, and in safe community settings. The coming decades will see more changes in our health delivery models (e.g., more team delivery of care and greater use of telemedicine). To improve the oral health of our communities, we need a more robust response to community health needs.

Oral health care must become an integral part of overall health care. For too long, our health system has treated the mouth separately. This is not an appropriate or sustainable model for improving population health. We must find ways to integrate oral health care patient centered comprehensive health care and wellness models at the community level. We need more oral health professionals in communities as part of health education teams.

ORAL HEALTH: A PRIORITY

The social determinants of health—socioeconomic conditions, safe housing, good nutrition, educational and job opportunities, access to transportation, and access to health care services (including oral health care)—all influence individual and community health. The issues are complex and the solutions hard to achieve. Changes can be difficult and fraught with lack of information, fear, and efforts to delay. However, changes resulting in a significant improvement in the lives and the futures of children and adults suffering from poor oral health are worth fighting for.

As our nation continues its quest for a more perfect union, for the elimination of racism and unequal opportunity, we can and must strengthen our commitment to improving the health of our citizens, including their oral health. Comprehensive access to oral health care and preventive services needs to be a priority for all. This affects the health and vitality of our nation. No child or adult in our nation should suffer—or die—because of a lack of affordable access to quality oral health care and preventive oral health services.[4]

These goals are important, they are worthy, and foremost, they are achievable.

REFERENCES

1. Wyckoff AS. Fluoride toothpaste should be used when child's first tooth erupts: AAP. *AAP News.* 2014;35(9):18. Available at: http://www.aappublications.org/content/35/9/18. Accessed December 8, 2016.

2. National Association of Dental Plans. Dental benefits improve access to dental care. Available at: http://www.nadp.org/docs/default-source/HCR-Documents/nadphcr-dentalbenefitsimprove-accesstocare-3-28-09.pdf. Accessed December 8, 2016.

3. Health Resources and Services Administration. Oral Health Workforce. Available at: http://www.hrsa.aquilentprojects.com/publichealth/clinical/oralhealth/workforce.html. Accessed December 8, 2016.

4. Sullivan LW. Grasping at the moon: enhancing access to careers in the health professions. *Health Aff (Millwood).* 2016;35(8):1532–1535.

31

Retaining Students to Develop a Diverse Oral Health Workforce: The Role of Need-Based Financial Aid

Denise Muesch Helm, RDH, EdD, and Robert A. Horn, PhD

In this chapter, we discuss the retrospective examination of the impact that Scholarships for Disadvantaged Students (SDS) has had on the diversity of the oral health workforce. A dental hygiene program at a midsize university in the southwestern United States has received SDS for the past 14 years. One hundred thirty-six dental hygiene students have received funds to support half the cost of their education.

The central question concerns the impact of SDS on oral health workforce diversity. The second question discusses the success of dental hygiene students who received SDS funds. The research described in this chapter focuses on how financial aid, in the form of need-based scholarships, can mitigate the shortage of diverse oral health care providers.

ORAL HEALTH DISPARITIES AND CURRENT WORKFORCE DIVERSITY

Despite attempts to eliminate gaps in oral health care, health disparities persist in this country. It is anticipated that this inequity will only worsen as our population increases in diversity. Oral health affects an individual's overall health and quality of life. Millions of adults and children in the United States do not receive dental care on an annual basis. In 2015, 36% of the adults aged 18 to 65 years did not visit a dentist.[1] Access to care is a multifactorial issue; however, one issue is the lack of diverse oral health care providers.[2] In addition, proven barriers to health knowledge and oral health care are language and individual health beliefs.

Oral health disparities, like health disparities, closely align with gender, race or ethnicity, education, income, disability, or geographic location.[3] Worse oral health and less access to oral health care continues in individuals from poor, non-White families; non-Hispanic Blacks/African Americans; Hispanics; and American Indians/Alaska Natives. The poorest oral health of all racial and ethnic groups in the United States is seen in American Indians/Alaska Natives.[1,2] Racial and ethnic minorities are less likely to seek health care, and, when they do, they are less likely to ask questions of their health care provider.[4]

More specifically, poor and culturally diverse groups visit the dentist less frequently and have more untreated dental caries than middle- and upper-income groups and Whites. Thirty-eight percent of Hispanics had untreated dental caries during 2011 to 2012.[1] In addition, untreated dental caries were found in 38% of those individuals with incomes 100% below the federal poverty level.[1] The only groups in which dental caries has increased from 1999 to 2012 are those aged 65 years or older who are Hispanic (from 38% to 48%) or Black/African American (from 37% to 41%). At the same time, caries decreased slightly in Whites (15%, 16%) in a matching age group.[1]

Increasing the number of diverse providers that serve the underserved is one approach that may address the gross inequity that poor access to health care presents.[2,5-7] Patients are more comfortable with health care providers who share their cultural beliefs, language, and traditions and are more likely to seek additional information from them. Minority physicians are more likely to treat underserved populations than are White physicians.[8-10] Likewise, underrepresented minority dentists are more likely than their White peers to practice in racial and ethnic minority communities.[11] Because racially and ethnically diverse health care professionals are significantly more likely than their White peers to serve underserved communities, graduating more diverse individuals is essential.

In spite of their willingness to practice in underserved areas, there exists a shortage of health care providers of color.[5-7] To address the inequity of health care, *Healthy People 2020* was established, outlining specific goals, objectives, and outcomes that target general and oral health.[12] One goal of *Healthy People 2020* is to "Prevent and control oral and craniofacial diseases, conditions, and injuries, and improve access to preventive services and dental care."[12]

Inasmuch as one of the goals of Health Resources and Services Administration (HRSA) and *Healthy People 2020* is to increase the health care workforce diversity, we have examined the current US population and oral health workforce. Currently, the vast majority of dental hygienists, dentists, and dental assistants are non-Hispanic White, which does not reflect the US population, as shown in Table 31-1. As is true with most health professions, Whites make up the greatest number.[13] In terms of gender diversity, a large majority of dental hygienists and dental assistants are female, and the majority of dentists are male; again, these demographics do not reflect the US population, which is shown in Table 31-2.

FINANCIAL AID FOR RETENTION AND GRADUATION OF ORAL HEALTH CARE PRACTITIONERS

Success of a diverse oral health student body will result in workforce diversity that is essential to achieving the goals of improving oral health and quality of life, and eliminating health disparities.[15] Recruiting and retaining diverse students by utilizing resources

Table 31-1. Race/Ethnicity of Oral Health Providers in the United States, 2015

Race/Ethnicity	Profession			
	DH, %	DA, %	Dentists, %	US, %
White (non-Hispanic)	92	81	81	77
Black/African American (non-Hispanic)	3	9	3	13
Asian	4	7	15	6
American Indian/Alaska Native	.4	1	.1	1
Native Hawaiian and other Pacific Islander	NR	.1	NR	.2
More than one race	2	2	2	3
Hispanic or Latino	6	23	6	18

Source: Based on data from US Department of Health and Human Services.[13]
Note: DA = dental assistant; DH = dental hygienist; NR = not reported; US = US citizens.

over which there is control is the responsibility of institutions of higher education.[7] Retention and college completion are especially important when one considers the increasing cost of obtaining a degree. There are several factors that contribute to the academic success of students in allied health professions such as reading and writing skills,[16] background mathematics courses, success in college biology,[17] integration into campus life,[18] mentorship,[19] and financial aid.[2,20]

Financial aid is one of many tools educational programs can use to enhance the success of students from low-income and diverse backgrounds.[2] Retention is correlated with whether or not a student completes a Free Application for Federal Student Aid (FAFSA). The likelihood that a student will be retained is 72% greater for those who complete a FAFSA than for those who do not.[21] By contrast, students not eligible for Pell Grants because of income are about twice as likely to graduate as those who were eligible.[22] Financial aid, especially in the form of grants, can mitigate the influence that a student's income has on graduation.[20]

Need-based financial aid amounts relative to the cost of tuition and fees predict how likely a low- to middle-income student is to graduate within six years.[23] (Six years is considered the typical time to graduate with a bachelor's degree.) Even small grants each semester have been found to positively influence college retention.[24] A $1,000-per-semester scholarship can result in 60% of the recipients graduating in six years. However, it seems that, in this case, size matters. The more generous the aid package, the more likely a student is to be retained from year to year.[25] The greater the aid package, the more likely a student is to graduate. Reducing the net cost of tuition seems to be key. Furthermore, financial aid awards have a greater impact on specific groups of students. In Indiana, the persistence in school for Hispanic students was influenced by state grants, primarily need-based, more so than any other racial/ethnic group.[26] Findings like these have caused experts to make recommendations for financial aid that covers at least half the cost of tuition and fees and 20% to 30% of the total price of attendance.[23]

Table 31-2. Gender of Oral Health Providers Compared With US Population, 2015

Profession	Percentage of US Workforce	
	Female	Male
Dental hygienists	97	3
Dental assistants	95	5
Dentists	25	75
US citizens	50	50

Source: Based on data from US Department of Health and Human Services,[13] US Census Bureau.[14]

HISTORY OF FEDERAL NEED-BASED AID

Promoting and supporting higher education had been integral in this country since its inception. Financial provisions for higher education in the United States started through the Seminary Land Grants and the land grants of the Morrill Act of 1862 with the establishment of the Federal Bureau of Education and the Morrill Act of 1890. In 1965, President Lyndon Johnson signed the Higher Education Act, a bill that was to provide financial support for students who were academically prepared for college. The Higher Education Act established a federal role in providing need-based grants, work–study opportunities, and loans to students. Since 1965, the Higher Education Act has created opportunity for millions of qualified students. Revisions to the Higher Education Act include the addition of Title IV, which created the student aid programs and the TRIO programs and the Basic Education Opportunity Grant, now the Pell Grant.

In recent years, financial aid has shifted toward more merit-based aid and less need-based aid, but overall federal grants and scholarships have increased. The College Board[27] reports that federal student aid increased: in 2002–2003, 68% of the students received financial aid and in 2012–2013, 71% received aid. In 2012–2013, $238.5 billion in financial aid including grants, federal work–study, federal loans, and federal tax credits and deductions were distributed to undergraduate and graduate students.[27] In 2007–2008, 60% of White, 80% of Black, 85% of Hispanic, 68% of Native Hawaiian or Pacific Islander, 76% of American Indian/Alaska Native, and 67% of students who are two or more races received financial aid.[28]

The average Pell Grant in 2012–2013 was only $3,650, and 63% of the aid awarded was in the form of federal loans,[27] resulting in debt upon graduation. Of the graduates who completed a bachelor's degree in 2011–2012, 60% had an average debt of $26,500.[27] The average student loan debt was between $15,000 and $17,000 from 1993 to 2004. In a study by the Brookings Institution, it was estimated that Blacks graduate with $23,400 in debt, 32% more than their White counterparts' debt of $16,000.[29] Health professions students have higher cost for their education because of additional fees charged by programs to offset the cost of expensive laboratory and classroom equipment and supplies. Large debt upon graduation causes health professionals to seek practice locations with the greatest income potential—not serving the underserved.[30]

To reduce student debt, HRSA offers scholarship and loan programs to support colleges and universities that train health care professionals to practice in health professions shortage areas. The goals of HRSA are to promote diversity within the health professions and to meet critical workforce shortages. HRSA's mission is to "improve health and achieve health equity through access to quality services, a skilled health workforce, and innovative programs."[31] One way that HRSA achieves its mission is by offering SDS funds to accredited US health professions schools.

SCHOLARSHIPS FOR DISADVANTAGED STUDENTS AT A MIDSIZED SOUTHWESTERN UNIVERSITY

In 2002, a faculty member at a midsized southwestern university applied to HRSA for and received SDS that funded baccalaureate dental hygiene students for the 2002–2003 academic year. The dental hygiene program was awarded $38,342. Recipients were selected by a department scholarship committee; the reporting process was completed by the grantee while the awards were managed by the university office of financial aid. After the initial grant, the awardee has submitted annual applications to HRSA resulting in funding dental hygiene students' scholarship from 2002 to 2016. In 2011, HRSA revised its award process to fund for four years, instead of one year at a time. During this same year, the student selection and award process was moved to the office of financial aid.

To be eligible to receive SDS, students must demonstrate that they are from either an educationally/environmentally disadvantaged background or have a current financial need. HRSA defines disadvantaged as the following:

> Educationally/environmentally disadvantaged means an individual comes from an environment that has inhibited the individual from obtaining the knowledge, skills, and abilities required to enroll in and graduate from a health professions school, or from a program providing education or training in an allied health profession. Economically disadvantaged means an individual comes from a family with an annual income below a level based on low-income thresholds, according to family size, established by the U.S. Census Bureau, adjusted annually for changes in Consumer Price Index, and adjusted by the Secretary of the U.S. Department of Health and Human Services (HHS), for use in all health professions. The Secretary updates these income levels in the *Federal Register* annually.[32]

Furthermore, the students must be enrolled full time in the accredited health professions program and be US citizens.

Methods Used in the Analysis of Scholarships for Disadvantaged Students

Study Sample of Scholarships for Disadvantaged Students Recipients

The study sample consisted of 136 SDS recipients and 62 nonrecipients. Of the 136 SDS recipients, 131 (96.3%) were female, 4 (2.9%) were male, and 1 (0.8%) did not identify gender. Of the 62 SDS nonrecipients, 56 (89%) were female and 6 (11%) were male.

Race and ethnicity data were collected on the application for the SDS. They were used in the analysis because, as previously stated, oral health providers of color are more likely than their White counterparts to practice in underserved and diverse communities. Students self-identified on their application as Hispanic or non-Hispanic as well as American Indian/Native American, Native Hawaiian or other Pacific Islander, Black/African American, White, or more than one race. These classifications were selected because they are used by HRSA. Just over one third (n = 51; 37.5%) identified as Hispanic/Latino. Recipients' race/ethnicity. Almost half of the sample (n = 60; 44%) were aged between 24 and 30 years, with 42 (30.9%) aged between 17 and 23 years, 16 (11.8%) aged between 31 and 40 years, 2 (1.5%) aged 51 years or older, and 16 (11.8%) not identifying their age range, with no one aged between 41 and 50 years. These data were not available for the nonrecipients.

Dental hygiene students completed an application with appended documentation to determine eligibility for SDS. Our analysis included dental hygiene students who received SDS since 2002. Financial need was determined for each student using HRSA guidelines based on the Department of Education financial need guidelines. These guidelines consider a student's cost of attendance and expected family contribution.

For a student to be considered to be from a disadvantaged background, the student must demonstrate meeting at least one qualifying factor. For example, the student may be from a health professions shortage area, have lived in a rural community, or attended an underperforming high school. HRSA uses components of two federal definitions of rural, one of which is produced by the US Census Bureau and the other by the Office of Management and Budget. Rural eligibility is determined by using the Rural Health Grants Eligibility Analyzer found at https://datawarehouse.hrsa.gov/tools/analyzers/geo/Rural.aspx. Underperforming schools are determined by state report cards and the percentage of free and reduced lunches.

For the individuals who identified as Hispanic/Latino, 11 (21.6%) had one qualifier, 25 (49%) had two, 12 (23.5%) had three, and three (5.9%) had four eligibility qualifiers for the SDS. By comparison, for the individuals who did not identify as Hispanic/Latino, 20 (23.5%) had one qualifier, 38 (44.7%) had two, 25 (29.4%) had three, and two (2.4%) had four eligibility qualifiers for the SDS.

Procedure and Analysis

To determine the breakdown of gender and race/ethnicity of the SDS recipients, data were imported into SPSS version 20 (IBM, Somers, NY) from the data spreadsheet. The 136 dental hygiene SDS recipients were first identified as having reported as Hispanic/Latino. A crosstabs analysis was conducted to sort the participants by race and gender.

Results of the Analysis

As noted earlier, all of the SDS recipients graduated on time from the dental hygiene program. By contrast, of the students in the cohorts that were not offered SDS, six (10%) did not complete the program because they either dropped out or were dismissed. Of the six students who dropped out, four (67%) were from an educationally or economically disadvantaged background. Of these, five (83%) were female and one (17%) was male. The majority of the SDS recipients were female (n = 131; 96.3%), which is consistent with the percentages in the US workforce. More than half (n = 69; 51%) of SDS recipients were culturally/ethnically diverse, which is notably higher than the diversity of the workforce.

Discussion of the Results

To our knowledge, this is the first study to investigate the role of need-based financial aid on oral health workforce diversity. By drawing on data from recipients of SDS over a 14-year period, we found that a greater number of diverse dental hygienists who received funding graduated during the 14-year period compared with those currently practicing. These results are consistent with previous studies that indicate that financial aid has a positive impact on graduating students of color. Our results add to the literature in that these graduates contribute to the diversity of oral health professions, specifically dental hygienists.

Although scholarships enhance students' ability to graduate, schools must continue to actively engage in ways to recruit those who are diverse and will practice in underserved areas. Diverse students must first be enrolled full-time in a health professions program to be eligible to receive SDS. Schools can draw on their ability to consistently award scholarships as a recruitment tool inasmuch as low-income students prefer institutions that are able to reduce their net cost of education.

We found that SDS successfully supported students of racial/ethnic diversity but, because only a few recipients were male (n = 4; 2.9%), the funding had little impact on changing the gender balance in practicing dental hygienists. Dental hygiene programs should actively seek to recruit more male students, and dental schools should recruit more female students.

While financial aid is one way to improve workforce diversity, it is important to couple these efforts with other programs that promote academic retention for students of color. Because the student retention issue is a multifactorial problem, mentorship, a culturally competent faculty, and academic support in the sciences and English are pieces to the success puzzle that must be utilized alongside financial support.

When we examine these results, we must ask if it is possible that students who received SDS would have been successful without financial support. Typically, only highly academically successful students gain entrance to health professions programs with competitive application processes. One can assume that these students would have been successful without the SDS. However, without large debt upon graduation, health professionals are more inclined to practice in medically underserved areas.

IMPLICATIONS FOR PUBLIC HEALTH

This work has implications for public health because dental caries is the most common preventable disease in children, five times more common than asthma. Early intervention reduces dental caries, especially in children, and the lifelong dental treatment associated with the disease. The negative impact of dental caries can continue throughout life resulting in expensive health care in later years. An estimated 51 million school hours are lost each year because of oral disease in children.[33] In 2014, dental care expenditure in the United States reached $113.5 billion[34] not including emergency department visits, school days lost, the cost of systemic diseases exacerbated by poor oral health, or worse health outcomes from common oral infections. Increasing the diversity of oral health providers can reduce the burden that oral diseases present.

CONCLUSIONS

The importance of oral health equity has come to the forefront in recent years. To address this epidemic, dental hygienists are taking on a greater role in public and community health settings. In many states, the scope of practice for dental hygienists is expanding to better serve those in need. Dental hygienists are now able to provide oral health care in school-based settings, hospitals, and federally qualified health centers with less supervision. It is important to support and graduate those who are more inclined to serve in underserved populations to combat the most common disease in children.

ACKNOWLEDGMENTS

This project was supported by the Health Resources and Services Administration (HRSA) of the US Department of Health and Human Services (HHS) Scholarships for Disadvantaged Students, under award numbers T08HP25236, T08HP22378, T0AHP18390,

T08HP13146, T08HP09476, T08HP07214, T08HP04951, total award amount of $1,703,122.00, 0% financed with nongovernmental funds. This information or content and conclusions are those of the authors and should not be construed as the official position or policy of, nor should any endorsements be inferred by HRSA, HHS, or the US government.

REFERENCES

1. US Department of Health and Human Services, Centers for Disease Control and Prevention, National Center for Health Statistics. Oral and dental health. Available at: https://www.cdc.gov/nchs/fastats/dental.htm. Accessed July 22, 2018.

2. Smedley B, Butler A, Bristow L; Committee on Institutional and Policy-Level Strategies for Increasing the Diversity of the US Health Care Workforce. *In the Nation's Compelling Interest: Ensuring Diversity in the Health Care Workforce.* Washington, DC: Institute of Medicine; 2004.

3. Winter PA, Butters JM. An investigation of dental student practice preferences. *J Dent Educ.* 1998;62(8):565–572.

4. Blaxter M. Health services as a defence against the consequences of poverty in industrialised societies. *Soc Sci Med.* 1983;17(16):1139–1148.

5. Sullivan LW. Missing persons: minorities in the health professions, a report of the Sullivan commission on diversity in the healthcare workforce. Available at: http://health-equity.lib.umd.edu/40. Accessed December 14, 2018.

6. National Institutes of Health, National Institute of Dental and Craniofacial Research. Oral health in America: a report of the Surgeon General. Rockville, MD: US Department of Health and Human Services; 2000.

7. Mitchell DA, Lassiter SL. Addressing health care disparities and increasing workforce diversity: the next step for the dental, medical, and public health professions. *Am J Public Health.* 2006;96(12):2093–2097.

8. Komaromy M, Grumbach K, Drake M, et al. The role of Black and Hispanic physicians in providing health care for underserved populations. *N Engl J Med.* 1996;334(20):1305–1310.

9. Moy E, Bartman A. Physician race and care of minority and medically indigent patients. *JAMA.* 1995;273(19):1515–1520.

10. Cantor JC, Miles EL, Baker LC, et al. Physician service to the underserved: implications for affirmative action in medical education. *Inquiry.* 1996;33(2):167–181.

11. Solomon ES, Williams CR, Sinkford JC. Practice location characteristics of Black dentists in Texas. *J Dent Educ.* 2001;65(6):571–574.

12. US Department of Health and Human Services, Centers for Disease Control and Prevention, Office of Disease Prevention and Health Promotion. Healthy People 2020. Available at: https://www.healthypeople.gov/2020/about/History-and-Development-of-Healthy-People. Accessed October 18, 2016.

13. US Department of Health and Human Services, Health Resources and Services Administration. Sex, race, and ethnic diversity of US health occupations (2010–2012). January 2015. Available at: https://bhw.hrsa.gov/sites/default/files/bhw/nchwa/diversityushealthoccupations_2012.pdf. Accessed December 14, 2018.

14. US Census Bureau. Quick facts. Population estimates, 2017. Available at: https://www.census.gov/quickfacts/fact/table/US#viewtop. Accessed July 22, 2018.

15. Noonan AS, Evans CA. The need for diversity in the health professions. *J Dent Educ.* 2003; 67:(9)1030–1033.

16. Moore R. The importance of a good start. In: Duranczyk IM, Higbee JL, Lundell DB, eds. *Best Practices for Access and Retention in Higher Education*. Minneapolis, MN: Center for Research on Developmental Education and Urban Literacy, General College, University of Minnesota; 2004:115–123.

17. Black P, Heep H. Predictors of the successful completion of a biology college course with a laboratory component. *Educ Pract Innovation.* 2014;1(4):94–102.

18. Tinto V. *Leaving College: Rethinking the Causes and Cures of Student Attrition.* 2nd ed. Chicago, IL: University of Chicago Press; 1993.

19. Kreuter MW, Griffith DJ, Thompson, et al. Lessons learned from a decade of focused recruitment and training to develop minority public health professionals. *Am J Public Health.* 2011;101(suppl 1):S188–S195.

20. Condon VN, Morgan CJ, Miller EW. A program to enhance recruitment and retention of disadvantaged and ethnically diverse baccalaureate nursing students. *J Transcult Nurs.* 2013;24(4):397–407.

21. Novak H, McKinney L. The consequences of leaving money on the table: examining persistence among students who do not file a FAFSA. *J Student Financial Aid.* 2011;41(3):5–23.

22. DiAmico AM. Trends in Pell Grant receipt and the characteristics of Pell Grant recipients: selected years, 1999–2000 to 2011–12. National Center for Educational Statistics. 2015. Available at: https://nces.ed.gov/pubsearch/pubsinfo.asp?pubid=2015601. Accessed August 10, 2016.

23. Price DV, Davis RJ. Price institutional grants and baccalaureate degree attainment. Washington, DC: National Association of Student Financial Aid Administrators; 2006.

24. Thomas B, LeBlanc A, MacGregor C. Promoting student success in community college and beyond: the opening doors demonstration. New York, NY: MDRC; 2005.

25. Singell JD. Come and stay a while: does financial aid effect retention conditioned on enrollment at a large public university? *Econ Educ Rev.* 2004;23:459–471.

26. Gross JPK, Torres V, Zerquera D. Financial aid and attainment among students in a state with changing demographics. *Res Higher Educ.* 2013;54:383–406.

27. College Board. Trends in student aid. Trends in higher education. Available at: https://trends.collegeboard.org/student-aid. Accessed August 10, 2016.

28. National Center for Educational Statistics, Institute of Educational Sciences. Status and trends in the education of racial minorities 2007–2008. Available at: http://nces.ed.gov/pubs2013/2013037.pdf. Accessed August 10, 2016.

29. Scott-Clayton J, Thursday JL. Black–White disparity in student loan debt more than triples after graduation. *Evidence Speaks Reports.* 2006;(2)3:1–9.

30. Heller D. Debts and decisions: student loans and their relationship to graduate school and career choice. *Lumina Foundation for Education. A New Agenda Series.* 2001;3(4):2–50.

31. US Department of Health and Human Services, Health Resources and Services Administration. Strategic plan FY 2016–2018. Available at: https://www.hrsa.gov/about/strategic-plan/index.html. Accessed July 22, 2018.

32. US Department of Health and Human Services, Health Resources and Services Administration. Student financial aid guidelines; Health workforce programs: Scholarships for Disadvantaged Students. 2016. Available at: https://bhw.hrsa.gov/loansscholarships/schoolbasedloans/sds. Accessed July 22, 2018.

33. Gift HC, Reisine ST, Larach DC. The social impact of dental problems and visits. *Am J Public Health.* 1992;82(12):1663–1668.

34. Wall T, Vujicic M. US dental spending continues to be flat. Chicago, IL: American Dental Association, Health Policy Institute; 2015.

32

Attitudes Toward Emerging Workforce Models Among Underrepresented Minority Dentists: Implications For Improving the Oral Health of the Public

Elizabeth Mertz, Phd, MA, Cynthia Wides, MA, Matthew Jura, MSPH, Aubri Kottek, MPH, Christopher Toretsky, MPH, and Paul Gates, DDS, MBA

WORKFORCE DIVERSITY IN DENTAL HEALTH CARE

Among dentists in the United States, Black, Hispanic/Latino, and American Indian/ Alaska Native (AI/AN) dentists are considered underrepresented minority (URM) dentists.[1] Recent data show both the extensive gap in parity between URM dentists and their share of the general US population as well as the disproportionate share of dental care that URM dentists provide for underserved minority populations in the United States.[1-4] While URM dentists are critical to improving oral health equity in the United States, the daunting shortage of URM providers limits their ability to address minority community needs. The negative impact on access to care and public health from this lack of diversity has been well established in multiple high-level reports over several decades.[5-9] Yet efforts to improve racial/ethnic workforce diversity are falling short, and the gap in parity continues to grow.[4]

Workforce diversity is not limited to the race/ethnicity of the dentist. Diversity among the dental team members is an important component to expanding access and improving quality of care. One way in which diversity among other dental team members is being addressed is through state-level efforts to expand scopes of practice for dental hygienists and assistants and the deployment of two new workforce models: dental therapists (DTs) and community dental health workers (CDHWs). These efforts are intended to enhance care provision in underserved and minority communities and are viewed as potentially improving the cultural, racial, and ethnic diversity of the oral health workforce by attracting individuals who might not otherwise seek a career in dentistry.[10,11]

DTs vary in preparation and scope across the United States and the world; however, they generally share the ability to perform restorative procedures on patients without direct supervision by a dentist.[12] This skill can free dentists to provide more complex care, but it can also be perceived as a competitive threat to dentists' scope of practice. CDHWs are entry-level providers similar to community health workers, who also vary in preparation and scope, but who share a focus on health education, care coordination, and linking patients to dentists. One variant of this, the community dental health coordinator, was introduced and pilot tested by the American Dental Association (ADA).[13] The exact model varies by state, and, in some instances, expansion of the dental hygiene workforce overlaps with these efforts, and, in other states, extended-function dental assisting shares some of the new model's tasks or attributes.[14]

Research on emerging workforce models has focused on the important issues of care quality, political hurdles, patients' experiences, and practice economics, with empirical findings supporting the safety and efficacy of new models.[10,15–20] Research on attitudes toward new models is often conducted in the states where workforce development is already under consideration. In Minnesota in 2012, 59% of dentists surveyed were skeptical that DTs would expand access to care and were opposed to DTs practicing in their state.[21] Among dental faculty at the University of Minnesota, where one training program was instituted in 2009, disagreement was found in the belief that these models might work, but there was little resistance to their own role as educators of DTs.[22] Among dental school deans nationally, the attitude toward emerging workforce models was overwhelmingly positive, and the dental education community has generally evolved to view support of educational adaptation to new competencies or program requirements as necessary.[23]

One factor that has been shown to influence perceptions is prior experience with expanded-function hygiene or assisting staff, which now exist in the majority of states.[24] However, even in these states, research shows that allied providers are not often working to the top of their scope of practice because of lack of delegation from dentists.[24] For example, among dentists surveyed in Minnesota, it was also found that many did not delegate the responsibilities to allied staff that they legally could.[21] This may be in part attributable to the model of dental education whereby dentists are rarely trained in team models with the full complement of dental clinical staff.

Previous research on attitudes toward new workforce models has generally focused on measuring perceptions of both the need for new providers and the potential barriers or facilitators to implementation but has not examined what factors might drive an individual provider's opinions. As well, none of the research previously conducted has focused primarily on those dentists who provide a disproportionate share of care to underserved and minority patients. URM dentists are more likely to work in high-minority-population communities and with public-pay patients compared with non-URM dentists.[4] This may result in conflicting opinions by this group on the new model—on one hand, these providers can benefit from adding new providers to their team, but they also may perceive an economic threat in a substitute labor force created explicitly to expand access to underserved patients. The study discussed in this chapter provides an additional lens on the factors related to acceptance of change on the dental care team by examining predictors of URM dentists' attitudes toward new workforce models.

METHODS USED IN THIS RESEARCH

Source of the Data

In 2012 and 2013, a national sample survey was conducted to assess URM dentists in the United States. The study was conducted under institutional review board approval from the University of California, San Francisco. The sample was selected from the 2012 ADA Masterfile on the basis of geographic location of the dentists and identification in the Masterfile as a member of a URM group. The survey received 1,489 eligible, unique responses—a 34% response rate. These responses were weighted to be nationally representative, yielding the population of 12,481 URM dentists. The full survey methodology, including details on the response rate and evaluation of the response quality, has been previously published.[25] This analysis included only respondents who identified themselves as being Hispanic/Latino, Black, or AI/AN, and who were practicing clinical dentistry (weighted n = 11,408).

Statistical Analysis of the Research

Independent variables of theoretical relevance to the model were examined from the survey based on factors that would likely influence one's opinion on new models at the individual and group levels. At the *individual level,* standard control variables such as age, gender, and race were included. Factors that might influence perceived need for or competition with these new models were selected, including the dentists' practice setting, educational debt at graduation, income, and patient characteristics. Finally, personal experiences with racial, language, gender, sexual orientation, disability, or religious discrimination as a dentist or dental student was included (range of 0 to 32+ times) as a factor that might influence sympathy with perceived "outsider" status.

At the *group level,* we examined whether the dentist was US-born and/or US-trained as the global presence of these workforce models might influence dentists' opinions. We also examined if URM dentists reported working collaboratively with other dental and medical providers (coded 0–9 based on count of collaborations). Finally, we examined geographic location and membership in both minority dental professional associations and the ADA. We tested each variable for correlation against both the dependent variables and against each other.

We constructed the *primary outcome variables* from survey responses to the following statements on a five-point Likert scale (strongly disagree, disagree, neutral, agree, strongly agree):

1. A well-trained, licensed mid-level provider such as a dental therapist should be developed as part of the dental team.
2. A well-trained dental community health worker should be developed as part of the dental team.

Responses were combined into a binary variable coded "1" if support was indicated (strongly agree or agree = 1) or coded "0" if any other answer was indicated (strongly disagree, disagree, or neutral = 0). A second binary variable was created to indicate opposition, in which the variable was coded "1" for opposition (strongly disagree or disagree = 1) and "0" for any other answer (strongly agree, agree, or neutral = 0). This produced four dependent variables: (1) support of DTs, (2) support of CDHWs, (3) opposition to DTs, and (4) opposition to CDHWs.

We ran iterative logistic models for each dependent variable to estimate predictors of providers' attitudes in support of and opposition to the new dental team members. To validate the magnitude of the estimates, we created additional models with the neutral statements coded as "1" and all others as "0" to estimate the impact of the neutral opinions on the outcomes (results not shown).

Results of the Research

Characteristics of clinically active survey respondents by race/ethnicity are shown in Table 32-1. Each URM dentist group is distinct and varies in geographic distribution, country of origin, gender, association membership, and practice characteristics. Among URM dentists, 22.4% expressed support for DTs, 45.7% expressed opposition, and 31.9% indicated neither support nor opposition. An inverse distribution existed for the CDHWs, with 42.8% expressing support and 22.5% expressing opposition, while 34.7% indicated neither support nor opposition. Among the three URM groups, Black dentists were most likely to support both models, and all groups indicated greater support for CDHWs than for DTs.

Approximately 70% of URM dentists worked in a state that allows expanded-function allied staff, and, among these, just over half reported that they personally work with this type of staff (Table 32-2). Black dentists were more likely to employ allied providers if it was legal in their state. Among all URM dentists, those who worked with extended-function staff reported higher support (26.0% vs. 18.9% support for DTs and 47.3% vs. 39.6% support for CDHWs) than those who do not work with these staff.

The URM dentist workforce also reported the frequency and type of discrimination they have experienced in dental education and practice (Table 32-3). Black dentists reported having had a higher frequency of discrimination experiences in dentistry than

Table 32-1. Demographic Profile of Clinically Active Underrepresented Minority (URM) Dentists and Indicated Support for New Workforce Models, US National Sample Survey of URM Dentists, 2012

	URM Total	Hispanic/Latino	Black	American Indian/ Alaska Native
Independent variables				
Sample weighted, no.	11,408	5,342	5,641	425
Age, y, mean	49	48	50	46
Gender, no. (%)				
Male	6,784 (59.5)	3,322 (62.2)	3,162 (56.1)	300 (70.6)
Female	4,624 (40.5)	2,020 (37.8)	2,479 (43.9)	125 (29.4)
Census division, no. (%)				
East North Central	1,183 (10.4)	413 (7.7)	731 (13.0)	39 (9.1)
East South Central	662 (5.8)	69 (1.3)	586 (10.4)	7 (1.7)
Mid-Atlantic	1,258 (11.0)	607 (11.4)	651 (11.5)	0 (0.0)
Mountain	609 (5.3)	402 (7.5)	165 (2.9)	42 (9.9)
New England	283 (2.5)	154 (2.9)	126 (2.2)	4 (0.9)
Pacific	1,820 (16.0)	1,340 (25.1)	378 (6.7)	102 (23.9)
South Atlantic	3,794 (33.3)	1,470 (27.5)	2,242 (39.7)	83 (19.4)
West North Central	295 (2.6)	137 (2.6)	136 (2.4)	22 (5.1)
West South Central (Ref)	1,504 (13.2)	751 (14.1)	626 (11.1)	127 (29.9)
US-born, total count, no.	11,335	5,318	5,592	425
Yes, no. (%)	7,696 (67.9)	2,612 (49.1)	4,666 (83.4)	417 (98.1)
No, no. (%)	3,640 (32.1)	2,706 (50.9)	926 (16.6)	8 (1.9)
ADA member, no. (%)				
Yes	6,147 (53.9)	3,231 (60.5)	2,618 (46.4)	297 (69.8)
No	5,261 (46.1)	2,111 (39.5)	3,022 (53.6)	128 (30.2)
Work collaboratively, total count, no.	10,649	5,006	5,239	404
Mean no. of collaborating providers	2.3	2.2	2.4	2.5
Primarily serves underserved patients at one practice location, no.	10,443	4,896	5,143	404
Yes, no. (%)	5,598 (53.6)	2,410 (49.2)	2,982 (58.0)	205 (50.8)
No, no. (%)	4,845 (46.4)	2,486 (50.8)	2,160 (42.0)	199 (49.2)
Had no education loans, no.	11,408	5,342	5,641	425
Yes, no. (%)	2,482 (21.8)	1,371 (25.7)	994 (17.6)	117 (27.6)
No, no. (%)	8,926 (78.2)	3,971 (74.3)	4,646 (82.4)	308 (72.4)

(Continued)

Table 32-1. (Continued)

	URM Total	Hispanic/Latino	Black	American Indian/ Alaska Native
Ever attended a CODA-accredited dental school, no.	11,408	5,342	5,641	425
Yes, no. (%)	10,304 (90.3)	4,384 (82.1)	5,504 (97.6)	415 (97.6)
No, no. (%)	1,104 (9.7)	958 (17.9)	136 (2.4)	10 (2.4)
Accepts public insurance, no. (%)				
Yes	6,461 (64.0)	2,798 (58.3)	3,463 (70.1)	200 (55.8)
No	3,636 (36.0)	1,998 (41.7)	1,480 (29.9)	158 (44.2)
Quartile of patient panel covered by public insurance, no.	8,342	3,733	4,338	271
0%–24%, no. (%)	4,530 (54.3)	2,175 (58.3)	2,191 (50.5)	164 (60.5)
25%–49%, no. (%)	1,421 (17.0)	534 (14.3)	830 (19.1)	57 (21.1)
50%–74%, no. (%)	1,351 (16.2)	530 (14.2)	792 (18.3)	30 (11.0)
75%–100%, no. (%)	1,040 (12.5)	494 (13.2)	526 (12.1)	20 (7.5)
Dependent variables (n = 10,660)				
Support no. (%)				
Dental therapist	2,370 (22.4)	851 (17.4)	1,427 (27.0)	92 (23.3)
Community dental health worker	4,532 (42.8)	1,731 (35.3)	2,654 (50.1)	147 (37.5)
Opposition, no. (%)				
Dental therapist	4,838 (45.7)	2,375 (48.5)	2,251 (42.5)	212 (53.8)
Community dental health worker	2,383 (22.5)	1,261 (25.7)	985 (18.6)	137 (35.0)

Note: CODA = Commission on Dental Accreditation.

their URM counterparts. Black dentists also reported the highest rates of racial discrimination. Hispanic/Latino dentists reported the highest rate of language discrimination. Half of AI/AN dentists reported no discrimination experiences. Among all URM dentists, more than a quarter reported having experienced gender discrimination.

Predictive Models of Support and Opposition

Dental Therapists

The strongest significant predictors of *support* of the DT model were primarily treating underserved patients in at least one of the respondent's practice locations (odds ratio [OR] = 1.747; 95% confidence interval [CI] = 1.095, 2.787) and the amount of

Table 32-2. Clinically Active Underrepresented Minority (URM) Dentists' Prior Experience With Expanded-Function Staff, US National Sample Survey of URM Dentists, 2012

	Total URM, No. (%)	Hispanic/Latino, No. (%)	Black, No. (%)	American Indian/ Alaska Native, No. (%)
Not legal in my state	2,422 (30.3)	1,098 (29.1)	1,225 (31.3)	99 (30.1)
Legal but my practice does not employ	2,693 (33.6)	1,399 (37.1)	1,184 (30.3)	110 (33.5)
Legal and my practice does employ	2,888 (36.1)	1,270 (33.7)	1,499 (38.4)	120 (36.4)
Total	8,004 (100)	3,767 (100)	3,908 (100)	329 (100)

discrimination the respondent reported having experienced as a dentist or dental student (OR = 1.030; 95% CI = 1.004, 1.057; Table 32-4). Alternately, individuals in the Mountain Division (OR = 0.419; 95% CI = 0.183, 0.961), members of the ADA (OR = 0.467; 95% CI = 0.310, 0.704), and those with a higher percentage of public insurance patients (OR = 0.766; 95% CI = 0.620, 0.946) had lower odds of supporting DTs. Demographic variables were not predictive of support of DTs.

The strongest predictors of *opposition* to the DT model included being located in the Census divisions of either West North Central (OR = 4.030; 95% CI = 2.069, 7.850) or Mountain (OR = 2.235; 95% CI = 1.212, 4.124), membership in the ADA (OR = 2.111; 95% CI = 1.563, 2.850), and being US-born (OR = 1.633; 95% CI = 1.150, 2.318). Conversely, individuals who collaborated with more types of health providers were significantly less likely to oppose the DT model (OR = 0.899; 95% CI = 0.833, 0.970). Age was slightly significant, with older dentists having lower odds of opposing DTs (OR = 0.983; 95% CI = 0.970, 0.997).

Community Dental Health Workers

The strongest significant predictors of *support* of the CDHW model were primarily treating underserved patients in at least one of the respondent's practice locations (OR = 1.852; 95% CI = 1.365, 2.513) and a higher level of collaboration with other health providers (OR = 1.132; 95% CI = 1.049, 1.222; Table 32-5). Age was also slightly significant with older dentists being more supportive of CDHWs (OR = 1.014; 95% CI = 1.000, 1.029). Dentists who are Hispanic/Latino (OR = 0.515; 95% CI = 0.373, 0.710) or AI/AN (OR = 0.576; 95% CI = 0.333, 0.998) were significantly less likely to support the CDHW model than Black dentists. Unlike the DT model, no significant regional variation was found.

When we reversed the model to examine predictors of *opposition* to the CDHW model, the strongest factors included being AI/AN (OR = 2.141; 95% CI = 1.159, 3.954), Hispanic/Latino (OR = 1.531; 95% CI = 1.035, 2.265), or a member of the ADA (OR = 1.507;

Table 32-3. Types of Discrimination Ever Experienced by Clinically Active Underrepresented Minority (URM) Dentists, US National Sample Survey of URM Dentists, 2012

	Total	Hispanic/Latino	Black	American Indian/ Alaska Native
No.	10,658	4,934	5,338	386
Mean no. of discrimination experiences in dental education or practice (range 0–32)	7.5	5.4	9.7	4.9
Types of discrimination, no. (%)				
Race	6,704 (62.9)	2,275 (46.1)	4,344 (81.4)	85 (22.0)
Gender	2,866 (26.9)	1,059 (21.5)	1,696 (31.8)	111 (28.6)
Language	989 (9.3)	769 (15.6)	213 (4.0)	7 (1.7)
Sexual orientation	115 (1.1)	44 (0.9)	63 (1.2)	7 (1.8)
Disability	35 (0.3)	23 (0.5)	11 (0.2)	0 (0.0)
Religion	204 (1.9)	126 (2.6)	61 (1.1)	17 (4.3)
Other	600 (5.6)	214 (4.3)	373 (7.0)	13 (3.4)
Never	2,941 (27.6)	2,018 (40.9)	727 (13.6)	196 (50.8)

Note: Percentages do not add to 100 as multiple choices were allowed.

95% CI = 1.043, 2.176). Those who collaborated with more types of health providers (OR = 0.911; 95% CI = 0.833, 0.996) and accepted any public insurance (OR = 0.637; 95% CI = 0.447, 0.909) were significantly less likely to oppose the CDHW model. Neither age nor gender predicted opposition to CDHWs.

Discussion of the Results and Analysis of the Findings

Our findings support the hypothesis that URM dentists' opinions on emerging workforce models are shaped by both life experiences and factors related to shared group identity as dentists. URM dentists are more likely than other dentists to work in high-minority-population communities and with public-payer patients.[4] Their practices (and their patients) may benefit from the addition of new providers to their team as these communities are often classified as underserved. Both the DT and the CDHW models are designed to increase access to care in collaboration with a dentist, with DTs performing simple dental restoration procedures and CDHWs focusing on patient education. We found that indeed those dentists who self-reported primarily treating underserved populations supported the new models. Acute workforce shortages are more likely in

Table 32-4. Predictors of Attitudes Toward Dental Therapists Among Underrepresented Minority (URM) Dentists, US National Sample Survey of URM Dentists, 2012

Independent Variables	Support for Dental Therapist, OR (95% CI)	Opposition to Dental Therapist, OR (95% CI)
Age (continuous)	1.000 (0.980, 1.021)	**0.983 (0.970, 0.997)**
Gender (0 = male; 1 = female)	0.926 (0.583, 1.472)	1.125 (0.817, 1.548)
Race (Ref: Black)		
Hispanic	0.710 (0.449, 1.121)	1.250 (0.890, 1.757)
American Indian/Alaska Native	1.247 (0.571, 2.722)	1.150 (0.669, 1.975)
Census Region (Ref: West South Central)		
East North Central	0.729 (0.331, 1.607)	1.582 (0.885, 2,828)
East South Central	1.208 (0.422, 3.464)	0.966 (0.400, 2.333)
Mid-Atlantic	1.043 (0.469, 2.318)	1.430 (0.756, 2.704)
Mountain	**0.419 (0.183, 0.961)**	**2.235 (1.212, 4.124)**
New England	0.722 (0.274, 1.905)	1.284 (0.639, 2.580)
Pacific	0.654 (0.318, 1.343)	1.072 (0.630, 1.825)
South Atlantic	0.718 (0.318, 1.343)	1.147 (0.691, 1.903)
West North Central (Contains MN)	0.581 (0.233, 1.453)	**4.030 (2.069, 7.850)**
Born in the United States (0 = no; 1 = yes)	- -	**1.633 (1.150, 2.318)**
Member of the ADA (0 = no; 1 = yes)	**0.467 (0.310, 0.704)**	**2.111 (1.563, 2.850)**
Currently has no dental school loans (0 = no; 1 = yes)	1.660 (0.995, 2.769)	- -
Practice serves primarily underserved (0 = no; 1 = yes)	**1.747 (1.095, 2.787)**	- -
Collaboration index (0–7 types of providers)	- -	**0.899 (0.833, 0.970)**
Accepts public insurance (0 = no; 1 = yes)		0.760 (0.558, 1.036)
Quartiles of patients on public insurance (1 = 0%–24%; 2 = 25%–49%; 3 = 50%–74%; 4 = 75%–100%)	**0.766 (0.620, 0.946)**	- -
Degree of discrimination experienced in dental career (Range 0 times to 32+ times)	**1.030 (1.004, 1.057)**	- -
	Un/Weighted Obs = 923/7,649 F(17, 906) = 2.63 Prob > F = 0.0003	Un/Weighted Obs = 1,166/9,646 F(16, 1136) = 5.12 Prob > F = 0.0000

Note: ADA = American Dental Association; CI = confidence interval; CODA = Commission on Dental Accreditation; OR = odds ratio. Bold values are statistically significant.

high-need areas, and, therefore, these new models may be valued as providing high-skill services at lower costs. URM dentists who reported treating publicly insured patients were less likely to oppose CDHWs; however, those treating larger shares of publicly insured patients were also less likely to support DTs. This seemingly mixed result may indicate that URM dentists treating a high volume of publicly insured patients are not

Table 32-5. Predictors of Attitudes Toward Community Dental Health Workers Among Underrepresented Minority (URM) Dentists, US National Sample Survey of URM Dentists, 2012

Independent Variables	Support for Community Dental Health Worker, OR (95% CI)	Opposition to Community Dental Health Worker, OR (95% CI)
Age (continuous)	**1.014 (1.000, 1.029)**	0.997 (0.981, 1.013)
Gender (0 = male; 1 = female)	1.000 (0.724, 1.383)	1.098 (0.746, 1.615)
Race (Ref: Black)		
Hispanic	**0.515 (0.373, 0.710)**	**1.531 (1.035, 2.265)**
American Indian/Alaska Native	**0.576 (0.333, 0.998)**	**2.141 (1.159, 3.954)**
Census Region (Ref: West South Central)		
East North Central	1.048 (0.563, 1.949)	1.165 (0.584, 2.322)
East South Central	0.772 (0.314, 1.895)	1.234 (0.474, 3.214)
Mid-Atlantic	0.804 (0.425, 1.522)	0.806 (0.379, 1.715)
Mountain	0.840 (0.456, 1.545)	1.362 (0.709, 2.618)
New England	1.297 (0.637, 2.644)	0.575 (0.229, 1.446)
Pacific	1.342 (0.778, 2.316)	1.022 (0.560, 1.865)
South Atlantic	0.833 (0.497, 1.396)	0.758 (0.421, 1.365)
West North Central (contains MN)	0.928 (0.482, 1.786)	1.286 (0.613, 2.698)
Born in the United States (0 = no; 1 = yes)	- -	- -
Attended a CODA school (0 = no; 1 = yes)	- -	1.914 (0.976, 3.755)
Member of the ADA (0 = no; 1 = yes)	0.798 (0.590, 1.079)	**1.507 (1.043, 2.176)**
Practice serves primarily underserved (0 = no; 1 = yes)	**1.852 (1.365, 2.513)**	- -
Collaboration index (0–7 types of providers)	**1.132 (1.049, 1.222)**	**0.911 (0.833, 0.996)**
Accepts public insurance (0 = no; 1 = yes)	- -	**0.637 (0.447, 0.909)**
Degree of discrimination experienced in dental career (Range 0 times to 32+ times)	- -	0.991 (0.969, 1.014)
	Un/Weighted Obs = 1,182/9,776 F(15, 1152) = 4.41 Prob > F = 0.0000	Un/Weighted Obs = 1,150/9,476 F(17, 1109) = 3.26 Prob > F = 0.0000

Note: ADA = American Dental Association; CI = confidence interval; CODA = Commission on Dental Accreditation; OR = odds ratio. Bold values are statistically significant.

opposed to CDHWs (the practice extender), but are opposed to DTs (the dentist substitute). Other variables that would indicate economic concerns (income, overall debt, practice cost, specialty practice status) did not correlate with attitudes and were not included in the model.

We were unable to statistically model previous exposure to extended-function staff (see Table 32-2) as a factor as the question only asked about current exposure, not any exposure. However, we found other indicators of exposure to different models of care that influenced opinions on DTs and CDHWs. For example, collaboration with multiple types of health providers, shown to be more common for dentists in public health and safety-net settings, predicted lower opposition to both DTs and CDHWs and predicted support for CDHWs.[1-3] In addition, foreign-born URM dentists were less likely to oppose the DT model, possibly because of either positive exposure to those models in the international context or because foreign-born dentists may not have the same level of inculcation to the dental professional identity in the United States, possibly indicating some level of marginalization of this group of professionals. We also found geographic variation in attitudes toward DTs, with stronger opposition from the Mountain and West North Central Divisions (which contains the only state, Minnesota, where DTs were legally able to practice at the time of data collection), but geography did not predict attitudes toward CDHWs, which are more broadly spread across the country.

Finally, the results stemming from group-identity factors can best be understood in the context of sociological literature around professionals' power and identity. Professionals identify themselves with the larger group and defend their boundaries against perceived threat to their social and economic power.[26] Accordingly, membership in the ADA was one of the strongest predictors of negative attitudes toward both emerging workforce models. Organized dentistry, in particular the ADA, has been adamantly opposed to any perceived encroachment on dentists' scope of practice and has been very active at the state and national levels in lobbying against the DT model.[27] However, ADA membership also predicts opposition to CDWHs, the very model backed and supported by the ADA as an alternative to DTs. It is unclear whether the official ADA policy positions reflect the previously held opinions of its membership or whether the ADA drives its membership's opinions on this issue. The finding that ADA membership is so strongly a predictor of opposition to DTs and CDHWs is an indicator of both the power of the professional group identity holding all else constant and that nuances of the ADA's official stances on emerging workforce models are not reflected in the opinions of this segment (URMs) of their membership.

A different and overlapping group identity for minority dentists is their own racial or ethnic identity. Culturally, the three racial/ethnic groups we examined are very distinct and focus their work in different communities and parts of the country.[1-3] Historically, URM dentists formed their own associations as a place to create an agenda that might otherwise be unwelcome or muted in the larger field, which t   ᴵⁱn degree can be seen as a reflection of that group's shared social identity. dentists responding to our survey indicated their membership in minorit ciations, we know that, among Black dentists, 36% reported memb

National Dental Association (NDA); among Hispanic/Latino dentists, 15% reported membership in the Hispanic Dental Association (HDA); and, among AI/AN dentists, 14% reported membership in the Society of American Indian Dentists (SAID). At the time of this survey, the NDA, HDA, and SAID were not formally supportive (via policy statements or resolutions) of DTs or CDHWs. Yet we found that minority association membership was not predictive of attitudes independently of or in conjunction with ADA membership.

Among URM dentists, Hispanic/Latino and AI/AN dentists were more likely than Black dentists to oppose CDHWs. The reason for this racial group difference in opinions, holding all else constant, is unclear. At the time of our survey in 2012, the NDA, HDA, and SAID had not produced a formal position statement on new dental providers; however, in 2014 (less than one year after our survey closed) the NDA publicly voiced support for studying emerging workforce models and has furthered that support in a 2016 policy statement.[28,29] As of July 2018, the SAID and the HDA had no formal positions on emerging workforce models. The greater support for these models expressed among Black dentists at the time of the study prefaced the subsequent formal policy support, indicating that, at least among this group of dentists, the support may be growing over time. With DTs in particular being deployed in American Indian communities (including Alaska, Washington, Oregon, and Arizona), future work may examine how the AI/AN dentist community opinions change in either direction over time.

Shared identity and group association develops early for professions through the preparation and desire to become a dentist. While formal association membership is one way to express group identity, it may also reflect values instilled in the process of professionalization. Protection of professional borders from scope-of-practice encroachments is a well-established phenomenon and, therefore, is not a surprising finding.[26]

An important result of our study is that the degree of discrimination experienced by URM dentists correlated with support for DTs. If the dental profession is exerting generalized peer pressure to reject new models, that pressure may be less effective on already marginalized groups, in this case as measured by discrimination experiences. Unfortunately, we found that URM dentists reported a wide variety of types and frequency of discriminatory experiences in their dental education and career, indicating that there may be a substantial number of individuals who do not feel fully welcomed into the professional fold. Likewise, individuals employing the new workforce roles of DTs or CDHWs have also experienced hostility from the dental field broadly writ as their qualifications and legitimacy are continually challenged.

At the time of data collection in 2012, these workforce models were fairly new: the Alaska DT program was seven years old, Minnesota DTs had just entered practice a year before, and the ADA's CDHW program launched six years before.[12,30] Dental workforce odels will likely continue to expand given the number of states where they are under ¹eration along with the continued funding from advocates of these new models, pressures from the rapidly evolving environment of health care, and the trend toward consolidation into larger systems of care.[31,32] In fact, as of July 2018, DTs have been legally authorized in four states (Minnesota, Maine, Vermont, and Arizona), while three more (Alaska, Washington, and Oregon) have DTs working in tribal organizations and through pilot programs, and a number of other states are actively exploring authorizing DTs and campaigning heavily. For CDHWs, the ADA's community dental health coordinators are currently working in 26 states and the programs to train them have graduated 275 students with another 120 enrolled in programs.[33]

With growing national interest in these models since the time of data collection in 2012, and, importantly, more exposure to working with new providers, it is likely that dentists' perceptions are changing. Understanding what factors drive acceptance or rejection can help those seeking to increase the pace of adoption and implementation of new models. Previous research on dentist attitudes toward new workforce models has been limited by their focus on individuals in states or institutions where the new models were being deployed already, indicating a high likelihood that providers' opinions were shaped in the local context of a highly politicized issue. This study adds to our knowledge by examining attitudes toward new workforce models among dentists who have not necessarily been exposed to these models personally and, specifically, among URM dentists, whose perspectives have not been previously included despite being key stakeholders in addressing oral health equity. Finally, this study provides actionable evidence in support of greater inter- and intraprofessional education for the dental education community seeking to prepare the highly functional dental teams of the future.

CONCLUSIONS

Personal and professional identity drives provider attitudes toward innovations in the dental team. In addition to vital clinical skills, dental education provides important training related to interpersonal skills, empathy, critical thinking, and professional ethics. Greater intraprofessional and interprofessional training can enhance teamwork skills and increase the likelihood that dentists will take part in dental teams with other clinicians who work at the top of their scope of practice. Despite a mounting body of evidence to the contrary, some forces in organized dentistry continue to message that new care models are a threat to professional identity and standards rather than a complement, enhancing practice economics and care delivery. Efforts to enhance diversity and inclusion in dental education and practice should continue to focus on valuing the racial/ethnic and socioeconomic diversity of our workforce and expand to valuing the diversity in team member type and skills toward common goals of high-quality, patient-centered care and health equity. Finally, developing ethics in the professional dental workforce includes not just patient care but also providers who are capable of critical thinking around health care policy and engagement in creating a shared future delivery system that can flexibly and efficiently address the oral health needs of the nation.

ACKNOWLEDGMENTS

We acknowledge support from the following: W.K. Kellogg Foundation, Bronx–Lebanon Hospital Center & Dental Department, The Dentaquest Foundation, National Institute for Dental and Craniofacial Research Award P30DE020752, University of California San Francisco Department of Preventive and Restorative Dental Sciences, HealthPlex, and Henry Schein.

REFERENCES

1. Mertz E, Calvo J, Wides C, Gates P. The Black dentist workforce in the United States. *J Public Health Dent.* 2017;77(2):136–147.

2. Mertz E, Wides C, Calvo J, Gates P. The Hispanic/Latino dentist workforce in the United States. *J Public Health Dent.* 2017;77(2):163–173.

3. Mertz E, Wides C, Gates P. The American Indian and Alaska Native dentist workforce in the United States. *J Public Health Dent.* 2017;77(2):125–135.

4. Mertz E, Wides C, Kottek A, Calvo J, Gates P. Underrepresented minority dentists: quantifying their numbers and characterizing the communities they serve. *Health Aff (Millwood).* 2016;35(12):2190–2199.

5. Health Resources and Services Administration. The rationale for diversity in the health professions: a review of the evidence. Rockville, MD: US Department of Health and Human Services; 2006.

6. Institute of Medicine. *In the Nation's Compelling Interest: Ensuring Diversity in the Health-Care Workforce.* Washington, DC: National Academies Press; 2004.

7. Institute of Medicine. *Improving Access to Oral Health Care for Vulnerable and Underserved Populations.* Washington, DC: National Academies Press; 2011.

8. Sullivan L. Missing persons: minorities in the health professions, a report of the Sullivan commission on diversity in the health care workforce. The Sullivan Commission. 2004. Available at: http://health-equity.lib.umd.edu/40/1/Sullivan_Final_Report_000.pdf. Accessed October 30, 2018.

9. Oral health in America: a report of the Surgeon General. Rockville, MD: US Department of Health and Human Services; 2000.

10. Wetterhall S, Burrus B, Shugars D, Bader J. Cultural context in the effort to improve oral health among Alaska Native people: the dental health aide therapist model. *Am J Public Health.* 2011;101(10):1836–1840.

11. Williard M. The Alaska Native tribal health system dental health aide therapist as a dentist-centric model. *J Am Coll Dent.* 2012;79(1):24–28.

12. Nash DA, Friedman JW, Mathu-Muju K. *A Review of the Global Literature on Dental Therapists.* Battlecreek, MI: W.K. Kellogg Foundation; 2012.

13. American Dental Association. Community dental health coordinator: empowering communities through education and prevention. *Action for Dental Health.* Chicago, IL: American Dental Association; 2016.

14. Baker B, Langelier M, Moore J, Daman S. The dental assistant workforce in the United States. School of Public Health, State University of New York, Albany. 2015. Available at: http://www.oralhealthworkforce.org/wp-content/uploads/2015/11/Dental_Assistant_Workforce_2015.pdf. Accessed August 20, 2018.

15. Bader JD, Lee JY, Shugars DA, Burrus BB, Wetterhall S. Clinical technical performance of dental therapists in Alaska. *J Am Dent Assoc.* 2011;142(3):322–326.

16. Friedman JW. The international dental therapist: history and current status. *J Calif Dent Assoc.* 2011;39(1):23–29.

17. Beazoglou TJ, Bailit HL, DeVitto J, McGowan T, Myne-Joslin V. Impact of dental therapists on productivity and finances: II. Federally qualified health centers. *J Dent Educ.* 2012;76(8):1068–1076.

18. Beazoglou TJ, Lazar VF, Guay AH, Heffley DR, Bailit HL. Dental therapists in general dental practices: an economic evaluation. *J Dent Educ.* 2012;76(8):1082–1091.

19. Phillips E, Shaefer HL. Dental therapists: evidence of technical competence. *J Dent Res.* 2013;92(7 suppl):11S–15S.

20. Gwozdek AE, Tetrick R, Shaefer HL. The origins of Minnesota's mid-level dental practitioner: alignment of problem, political and policy streams. *J Dent Hyg.* 2014;88(5):292–301.

21. Blue CM, Rockwood T, Riggs S. Minnesota dentists attitudes toward the dental therapist workforce model. *Healthc (Amst).* 2015;3(2):108–113.

22. Lopez N, Blue CM, Self KD. Dental school faculty perceptions of and attitudes toward the new dental therapy model. *J Dent Educ.* 2012;76(4):383–394.

23. Aksu MN, Phillips E, Shaefer HL. US dental school deans' attitudes about mid-level providers. *J Dent Educ.* 2013;77(11):1469–1476.

24. Blue CM, Funkhouser DE, Riggs S, et al. Utilization of nondentist providers and attitudes toward new provider models: findings from the National Dental Practice-Based Research Network. *J Public Health Dent.* 2013;73(3):237–244.

25. Mertz E, Wides C, Cooke A, Gates P. Tracking workforce diversity in dentistry: importance, methods and challenges. *J Public Health Dent.* 2016;76(1):38–46.

26. Abbott AD. *The system of professions: An essay on the division of expert labor.* Chicago, IL: University of Chicago Press; 1988.

27. Kitchener M, Mertz E. Professional projects and institutional change in healthcare: the case of American dentistry. *Soc Sci Med.* 2012;74(3):372–380.

28. National Dental Association position statement: Access to care and emerging workforce models. Greenbelt, MD: National Dental Association; 2014.

29. National Dental Association position statement: Access to care: patients, providers and workforce. Greenbelt, MD: National Dental Association; 2016.

30. American Dental Association. Solutions: about CDHCs. 2018. Available at: https://www.ada.org/en/public-programs/action-for-dental-health/community-dental-health-coordinators. Accessed August 21, 2018.

31. Koppelman J. States expand the use of dental therapy. Pew Charitable Trusts Dental Campaign. 2016. Available at: http://www.pewtrusts.org/en/research-and-analysis/analysis/2016/09/28/states-expand-the-use-of-dental-therapy. Accessed September 29, 2016.

32. Vujicic M, Israelson H, Antoon J, Kiesling R, Paumier T, Zust M. A profession in transition. *J Am Dent Assoc.* 2014;145(2):118–121.

33. American Dental Association. Community dental health coordinators: provide solutions now. 2018. Available at: https://www.ada.org/~/media/ADA/Public%20Programs/Files/ADA_CDHC_Infographic.pdf?la=en. Accessed August 21, 2018.

33

Community Water Fluoridation: A Health-Equitable Prevention Strategy

Raymond Gist, DDS, MPH

It has become second-nature to me, as a former president of the American Dental Association, to be continually aware of certain issues within the national public health arena. This chapter offers the facts about community water fluoridation from a health-equity perspective.

I have been a general dentist in Flint, Michigan, for more than 45 years, and it has been my privilege to be heavily involved in community activities. I have been on the board of directors of Genesee Health Plan, with a dedication to help the underprivileged residents in Genesee County; the board of the Alumni Association of the University of Michigan, with a goal of recruiting and mentoring underprivileged students; the Flint Rotary, with a goal of giving aid globally; and now the Delta Dental Board of Michigan, where the Healthy Kids Dental program sets a national example of equitable dental access for all children.

In 1945, Grand Rapids became the first city in history to fluoridate its water supply, and the benefits were dramatic. The rate of tooth decay among Grand Rapids children, born after fluoride was added to the water supply, decreased as much as 60%.[1] Fluoridation spread across the United States as other communities asked to have this effective public health measure made available to their residents. By 1965, when Genesee County became fluoridated, approximately half the US population on public water supplies was enjoying the decay-preventive benefit of fluoridated water.

Today, more than 91% of Michigan residents are served by a public water supply; nationally, nearly 75% of the population on public water supplies receives fluoridated water.[2] In addition to scientific research, more than 70 years of practical experience has consistently demonstrated that an optimal level of fluoride in community water is safe and effective in preventing tooth decay in both children and adults. Despite the many issues Flint has been addressing in regards to its water supply, the community support for water fluoridation has never wavered. In fact, today, Flint receives its water from Detroit, Michigan, which has enjoyed the benefits of fluoridated water since August 1967.

Fluoridation is cost-effective and cost-saving. When compared with the cost of other prevention programs, water fluoridation is the most cost-effective means of preventing tooth decay for both children and adults in the United States. The cost of a lifetime of water fluoridation for one person is less than the cost of one filling.[3] It reaches all members of a community where they live, learn, work, and play and requires no additional action on the part of the recipient except for the daily routine of drinking water.

Recognizing the benefits of community water fluoridation, the United States has set a national goal of 80% of the US population on public water supplies to receive fluoridated water by the year 2020.[4] The health professionals throughout the country can attest to the differences they see in the dental health of residents who are served by fluoridated water and those who are not.

Water fluoridation has been endorsed by not only the American Dental Association, but also the National Dental Association,[5] Hispanic Dental Association,[6] American Academy of Pediatrics,[7] the American Medical Association,[8] the American Public Health Association,[9] the Association of State and Territorial Dental Directors,[10] and the World Health Organization.[11-13] In addition, more than 100 national and international organizations have recognized the public health benefits of fluoridation for preventing tooth decay.

Yet there are voices in this country who have claimed that because African Americans suffer disproportionately from kidney disease and diabetes, fluoridated water must be the cause. These voices have appealed to civil rights leaders to join their cause to discontinue community water fluoridation throughout America.[14]

The best available scientific evidence indicates that individuals with chronic kidney disease or diabetes can consume optimally fluoridated water without negative health consequences.[15-17] In fact, good oral health, provided in part by fluoridation, can assist individuals with these conditions to have fewer overall health issues.

Community water fluoridation is not a "Tuskegee experiment." As the vast majority of public health experts agree, it is the single most effective and influential public health measure of the 20th century to prevent tooth decay. It is not, and has not been, targeted to harm the health of the African American community. I want to stress that there is a great deal of misinformation regarding water fluoridation being circulated, especially on the Internet and through social media. No charge against the benefits and safety of fluoridation has ever been substantiated by generally accepted scientific evidence.

In fact, fluoridation is a socially equitable means of preventing tooth decay. Water fluoridation reaches everyone in a community regardless of age, race, education, income level, or access to routine dental care. Studies have shown that populations from a lower socioeconomic status within a fluoridated community have less tooth decay compared with their peers in nonfluoridated communities.[18-21] In the first-ever Surgeon General's

Report on Oral Health issued in May 2000, US Surgeon General David Satcher noted that community water fluoridation is safe and effective in preventing dental decay in both children and adults.[22] In 2001, Satcher issued a statement on fluoridation in which he noted, "community water fluoridation continues to be the most cost-effective, practical and safe means for reducing and controlling the occurrence of dental decay in a community . . . water fluoridation is a powerful strategy in efforts to eliminate health disparities among populations."[23]

Some of us remember the days before fluoridation was implemented, when it was almost an expectation that patients would lose all of their teeth by the time they were in their 30s. But children growing up today are far less likely than their grandparents were to experience the rampant tooth decay that caused this type of loss, in part because of the implementation of community water fluoridation. Discontinuing fluoridation would jeopardize that positive trend.

We also know that brushing with a fluoride toothpaste, flossing, eating a healthy diet, and regular cleanings and examinations are all critical to good dental health. But, despite a number of initiatives by the dental profession designed to raise awareness about the consequences of untreated tooth decay and mouth disease and to improve the safety net for those who are most vulnerable, we realize that surmounting barriers to proper care is challenging for many citizens. Access to fluoridated water from the tap in their own homes will help to prevent tooth decay while we search for strategies to end the disparities that exist in dental and health care.

REFERENCES

1. Arnold FA Jr, Likins RC, Russell AL, Scott DB. Fifteenth year of the Grand Rapids fluoridation study. *J Am Dent Assoc.* 1962;65(6):780–785.

2. Centers for Disease Control and Prevention. Community water fluoridation. Fluoridation statistics. 2014. Available at: https://www.cdc.gov/fluoridation/statistics/2014stats.htm. Accessed October 31, 2018.

3. Fluoridation facts. Question 68. Chicago, IL: American Dental Association; 2018.

4. US Department of Health and Human Services, Office of Disease Prevention and Health Promotion. Healthy People 2020. Topics and objectives. Oral health objectives. Available at: https://www.healthypeople.gov/2020/topics-objectives/topic/oral-health/objectives. Accessed October 31, 2018.

5. National Dental Association. Position on water fluoridation. 2012. Available at: http://www.ndaonline.org/position-on-water-fluoridation. 2012. Accessed October 31, 2018.

6. Hispanic Dental Association. Advocacy: HDA working for you. Community water fluoridation. Hispanic Dental Association endorses community fluoridation. Available at: http://hdassoc.org/about-us/advocacy. Accessed October 31, 2018.

7. American Academy of Pediatrics Section on Oral Health. Maintaining and improving the oral health of young children. *Pediatrics.* 2014;134(6):1224–1229.

8. American Medical Association. Water fluoridation H-440.972. American Medical Association Policy Finder. Available at: https://www.ama-assn.org/about-us/policyfinder. Accessed October 31, 2018.

9. American Public Health Association. Policy 20087. Community water fluoridation in the United States. 2008. Available at: https://www.apha.org/policies-and-advocacy/public-health-policy-statements. Accessed October 31, 2018.

10. Association of State and Territorial Dental Directors. Community water fluoridation policy statement. June 2015. Available at: https://www.astdd.org/a-z-topics. Accessed October 31, 2018.

11. Petersen PE, Lennon MA. Effective use of fluorides for the prevention of dental caries in the 21st century: the WHO approach. *Community Dent Oral Epidemiol.* 2004;32(5):319–321.

12. Petersen PE. World Health Organization global policy for improvement of oral health— World Health Assembly 2007. *Int Dent J.* 2008;58(3):115–121.

13. Petersen PE, Ogawa H. Prevention of dental caries through the use of fluoride—the WHO approach. *Community Dent Health.* 2016;33(2):66–68.

14. Fluoride Action Network. Environmental justice. 2017. Available at: http://fluoridealert.org/wp-content/uploads/FAN-Environmental-Justice-Brochure-Final.pdf. Accessed December 14, 2018.

15. Ludlow M, Luxton G, Mathew T. Effects of fluoridation of community water supplies for people with chronic kidney disease. *Nephrol Dial Transplant.* 2007;22(10):2763–2767.

16. Kidney Health Australia. 2011 Review of Kidney Health Australia fluoride position statement. 2011. Available at: http://kidney.org.au/cms_uploads/docs/2011-review-of-fluoride-position-statement.pdf. Accessed October 31, 2018.

17. National Kidney Foundation. Fluoride intake in chronic kidney disease. April 15, 2008. Available at: https://www.kidney.org/atoz/content/fluoride. Accessed October 31, 2018.

18. Cho HJ, Lee HS, Paik DI, Bae KH. Association of dental caries with socioeconomic status in relation to different water fluoridation levels. *Community Dent Oral Epidemiol.* 2014;42(6): 536–542.

19. McGrady MG, Ellwood RP, Maguire A, Goodwin M, Boothman N, Pretty IA. The association between social deprivation and the prevalence and severity of dental caries and fluorosis in populations with and without water fluoridation. *BMC Public Health.* 2012;12: 1122–1139.

20. Jones CM, Worthington H. Water fluoridation, poverty and tooth decay in 12-year-old children. *J Dent.* 2000;28(6):389–393.

21. Jones CM, Worthington H. The relationship between water fluoridation and socioeconomic deprivation on tooth decay in 5-year-old children. *Br Dent J.* 1999;186(8):397–400.

22. US Department of Health and Human Services. Oral health in America: a report of the Surgeon General. National Institute of Dental and Craniofacial Research, National Institutes of Health. 2000. Available at: https://profiles.nlm.nih.gov/ps/retrieve/ResourceMetadata/ NNBBJT. Accessed October 31, 2018.

23. US Department of Health and Human Services, Public Health Service, Surgeon General David Satcher. Statement on community water fluoridation. Office of the Surgeon General. 2001. Available at: https://www.cdc.gov/fluoridation/guidelines/surgeonsgeneral-statements. html. Accessed October 31, 2018.

34

Racial/Ethnic Minority Older Adults' Perspectives on Proposed Medicaid Reforms' Effects on Dental Care Access*

Mary E. Northridge, PhD, MPH, Ivette Estrada, MA, MPhil,
Eric W. Schrimshaw, PhD, Ariel P. Greenblatt, DMD, MPH,
Sara S. Metcalf, PhD, and Carol Kunzel, PhD

Because of increased life expectancy and improvements in oral health over the past 60 years in the United States, older adults are retaining greater numbers of their natural dentition.[1] Nonetheless, oral health disparities exist in the aging population regarding untreated dental caries (cavities) and edentulism (complete tooth loss) related to income, gender, race/ethnicity, and education.[2]

We devised a conceptual model titled, "ecological model of social determinants of oral health for older adults" for thinking about mechanisms whereby social determinants at various scales influence oral health and related health outcomes, toward promoting healthy aging.[3] In this frame-work, oral health in older adults is owing to the lifelong accumulation of advantageous and disadvantageous experiences at multiple scales, from the microscale of the mouth to the societal scale that involves inequalities in the distribution of material wealth and educational attainment and ideologies such as ageism and racism. Note that this model is compatible with the life course perspective, because both view oral disease as cumulative.[4,5]

It has also been argued that disparities in public policy regarding oral health for older adults nationally and on a state-by-state basis may compound social inequities.[2] Nearly 70% of older US persons currently have no form of dental insurance.[6] At the federal level, the Medicare program, which covers elderly adults and nonelderly adults with disabilities, provides no dental benefits for preventive or routine care.[7] At the state level, 42% of states provide no dental benefit or only emergency coverage through adult Medicaid.[8]

At present, market-based solutions that are part of Medicaid expansion plans may be appealing from a cost perspective but may have untoward consequences for vulnerable populations, including racial/ethnic minority older adults. For instance, the main

---

*This is a modified version of the article that appeared in the *American Journal of Public Health*. See: Northridge ME, Estrada I, Schrimshaw EW, Greenblatt AP, Metcalf SS, Kunzel C. Racial/ethnic minority older adults' perspectives on proposed Medicaid reforms' effects on dental care access. *Am J Public Health*. 2017;107(suppl 1):S65–S70.

elements of the Kentucky Health plan—with the stated intention of preparing people with expansion Medicaid coverage to become active consumers of health care—are (1) monthly premiums that increase over time; (2) a volunteer or work requirement; (3) the elimination of benefits, including vision and dental and nonemergency medical transportation; and (4) an incentivized "My Rewards" account in which credits would be accumulated for approved behaviors deemed appropriate, such as community service or work, and debited for behaviors deemed inappropriate, such as nonurgent emergency department use.[9] Of course, these elements are also part of other Medicaid reform plans submitted by the governors of states such as Arizona, Arkansas, Tennessee, and Indiana and are not new or innovative in and of themselves.[9]

A recent critique of the Medicaid reform plan proposed by the governor of Kentucky, Matt Bevin, underscored the need for evidence to guide policy.[9] In an ecological model derived from a systematic review of the complex factors that influence disparities in access to and quality of services, the endpoints of interest included clinical outcomes, avoidable hospital admissions, equity of services, and costs, along with patient experiences of care.[10] A simplified schematic of this framework that focuses on level 4 (policy and community), its associated intervention targets (neighborhood and community resources), and the health care processes (principally, interactions between patients and support networks and their health care providers) leading to outcomes (notably patient experiences of care) is provided in Figure 34-1.

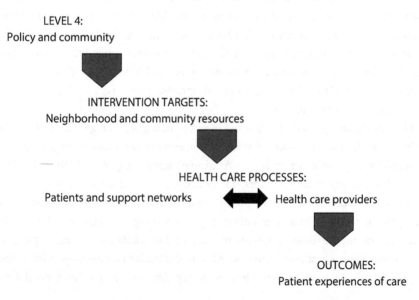

LEVEL 4:
Policy and community

INTERVENTION TARGETS:
Neighborhood and community resources

HEALTH CARE PROCESSES:
Patients and support networks ⬌ Health care providers

OUTCOMES:
Patient experiences of care

Source: Based on the conceptual model called "factors that influence disparities in access to care and quality of health care services, by level," from Purnell et al.[2]

Figure 34-1. Policy and Community Level Factors That Result in Patient Experiences of Care

We addressed the patient perspective on proposed Medicaid reforms, particularly that of racial/ethnic minority older adults, who are the focus of ongoing social science research to promote oral health equity (Northridge ME, Shedlin MG, Schrimshaw EW et al., unpublished data).[11]

The question that guided our qualitative analysis was this: How might the elements of proposed Medicaid reform plans be experienced by racial/ethnic minority older adults and what are the implications for their ability to access dental care through Medicaid?

METHODS

As part of an ongoing study funded by the US National Institutes of Health to understand factors that serve as barriers to oral health and health care among racial/ethnic minority older adults, we conducted 24 focus groups with 194 African American, Dominican, and Puerto Rican participants aged 50 years and older living in northern Manhattan, New York, New York. We approached and screened older adults for possible participation in the study at senior centers located throughout northern Manhattan. Details of the recruitment and screening procedures are available elsewhere (Northridge ME, Shedlin MG, Schrimshaw EW et al., unpublished data).

Following standard focus group techniques,[12] we conducted separate groups on the basis of important characteristics that may influence either the issues discussed or the ability of the members to build rapport, notably, gender, race/ethnicity, and history of dental care. Groups consisted of an average of 8 participants (SD = 2.4) and lasted an average of 1.3 hours (SD = 13 minutes). We audio-recorded and transcribed for analysis all group discussions.

Trained moderators conducted focus groups using a series of semistructured questions about the factors that serve as facilitators or barriers to obtaining dental care. Among the topics explored in each group were factors affecting the affordability of care and whether there was an understanding of what services Medicaid covers.

We transcribed group discussions conducted in Spanish in Spanish and then translated the transcription into English. To ensure accurate transcription and translation, the assistant moderator (IE), who was present for all focus group discussions, compared the resulting transcripts with the original audio-recordings. We analyzed the transcripts using thematic content analysis.[13]

The research team members began the analysis by familiarizing themselves with the data, which involved independently reading and rereading the focus group transcripts to immerse themselves in the data and become intimately familiar with its content. The subsequent phase involved generating succinct labels (codes) to identify important features of the data that might be relevant to the research question. Next, the team met to discuss the topics identified and to construct a list of 20 topic codes. Although many (15) of these topics were directly explored with questions in the interview guide, we collapsed some of the original guide topics and identified unanticipated codes and included them in our analysis. We achieved consensus among all research team members.

One of the codes identified was "financial and insurance." This code included Medicaid, Medicare, insurance, cost issues, policies regarding what dental procedures are and are not covered, and changes owing to retirement. To identify the text in which participants discussed Medicaid reform proposals, we read all transcripts to identify sections of text in which groups discussed Medicaid, and we took detailed notes on the specific comments participants made about their views of the Medicaid program. Participants reported difficulties in using Medicaid and confusion over what dental services were covered. We have reported the most commonly reported views. We selected quotations that best represented the perceptions that the majority of participants described regarding the implications of 4 proposed Medicaid reforms on the lives of Medicaid recipients and their ability to access care through the program: (1) monthly premiums, (2) a volunteer or work requirement, (3) eliminating covered services, and (4) behavioral incentives.

RESULTS

The sociodemographic characteristics of the focus group participants by race/ethnicity and for the total sample are presented in Table 34-1. Approximately half (53.6%) of the participants were women, and nearly half (48.5%) spoke primarily Spanish at home. We have presented representative focus group quotations that relate to each of these 4 proposed reforms.

Reform 1: Monthly Premiums

First, regarding the suitability of monthly payments that increase over time, many of the older adult participants reported problems with affording care at current copayment levels.

Group 1 (African American women with dental care).

Moderator (M): Great, so in terms of the affordability, what [have] been other people's experiences?

Participant 1 (P1): Like she said the expense. Seniors or whatever, the way they have the insurance now, you got the copayments. A lot of them don't accept Medicaid. And, seniors [have] basically Medicare now. Then certain work that you're getting done, your insurance.

P2: It's not covered.

P1: ... may not cover it or a lot of it's still coming out of your pocket. Very expensive.

Table 34-1. Sociodemographic Characteristics of Older Adult Focus Groups Participants by Race/Ethnicity and Total Sample: New York, NY, 2013–2015

Characteristic	African American	Dominican	Puerto Rican	Total
Participants, no.	72	69	53	194
Focus groups, no.	8	8	8	24
Age, y				
Mean ± SD	68.3 ± 10.2	71.6 ± 9.6	68.5 ± 10.0	69.5 ± 10.0
Range	50-92	50-90	50-91	50-92
Age group, y, % (no.)				
50-54	11.1 (8)	4.3 (3)	13.2 (7)	9.3 (18)
55-59	6.9 (5)	1.4 (1)	7.5 (4)	5.2 (10)
60-64	15.3 (11)	20.3 (14)	17.0 (9)	17.5 (34)
65-69	20.8 (15)	15.9 (11)	11.3 (6)	16.5 (32)
70-74	23.6 (17)	15.9 (11)	20.8 (11)	20.1 (39)
75-79	8.3 (6)	21.7 (15)	18.9 (10)	16.0 (31)
80-84	5.6 (4)	11.6 (8)	7.5 (4)	8.2 (16)
85-89	4.2 (3)	5.8 (4)	0.0 (0)	3.6 (7)
> 90	4.2 (3)	2.9 (2)	3.8 (2)	3.6 (7)
Gender, % (no.)				
Male	44.4 (32)	49.3 (34)	45.3 (24)	46.4 (90)
Female	55.6 (40)	50.7 (35)	54.7 (29)	53.6 (104)
Time of last dental visit, % (no.)				
Within past year	54.2 (39)	59.4 (41)	47.2 (25)	54.1 (105)
1-3 y ago	26.4 (19)	29.0 (20)	26.4 (14)	27.3 (53)
> 3 y ago	19.4 (14)	11.6 (8)	26.4 (14)	18.6 (36)
Primary language, % (no.)				
English	100.0 (72)	0.0 (0)	18.9 (10)	42.3 (82)
Spanish	0.0 (0)	98.6 (68)	49.1 (26)	48.5 (94)
Both	0.0 (0)	1.4 (1)	32.1 (17)	9.3 (18)
Neighborhood of residence, % (no.)				
Inwood	4.2 (3)	13.0 (9)	1.9 (1)	6.7 (13)
Washington Heights	13.9 (10)	58.0 (40)	5.7 (3)	27.3 (53)
East Harlem	15.3 (11)	5.8 (4)	79.2 (42)	29.4 (57)
Central Harlem	30.6 (22)	4.3 (3)	5.7 (3)	14.4 (28)
West Harlem	20.8 (15)	8.7 (6)	3.8 (2)	11.9 (23)
Other	15.2 (11)	10.1 (7)	3.8 (2)	10.3 (20)

Note: The racial/ethnic groups did not differ significantly on any of the listed sociodemographic characteristics, with the exceptions of primary language and neighborhood of residence in accordance with the sampling strategy.

Group 13 (African American men without dental care).

P1: Copayments. That's one of the [reasons] why I don't go to the doctor too much. I'm telling you: I haven't been to the doctor in a while. I'm 80 years old.
P2: That's the reason why.
P3: I haven't been to the doctor in almost 2 years now.
P4: Damn.

Group 1 (African American women with dental care). There was uncertainty regarding what is covered under Medicaid.

M: So, in terms of yourselves and other seniors in the senior center, is there a good understanding, do you think, of what Medicaid pays…
P1: No.
M: …for what Medicare pays for, what other—and what services are paid for, what that'll do?
P2: No.
P3: No.
P4: … Most people are not aware of their rights in terms of copayments, the different [types of coverage].

Group 17 (African American men with dental care).

M: Does Medicare cover anything for dental?
P1: No. No.
P2: No. No. But see: when you retire…. OK, so before you retire, you know like. You are indirectly to the union. But they'll put you … in Healthfirst[14] [provides no-cost do you and low-cost health insurance plans] …. And then that—they take that out of your Medicaid. So you pay for it out of that. So now you're covered on that end. Like see, now, I got Healthfirst. Right? So now Healthfirst is paying for my glasses. And they'll pay for my teeth. My teeth and all that. You know? But they get their money from my social security.

Group 5 (Dominican men with dental care; translated from Spanish). In addition to stated confusion over what plans cover what services, participants also expressed the desire for government to lend a helping hand.

P1: One point that is outside of what we are discussing is, for example, if the government here, for example, helps people; we get help with food coupons. It helps us with programs designed to help us. If it weren't for that, we would live in worse conditions than the ones that we are in. We couldn't live like that. It's hard. The situation is not easy.

P2: Look, [names moderator].

P3: It's not easy.

P4: Those are the insurance plans I have.

P2: I changed plans—from Medicaid to Medicare, no?

P5: Tell her about that.

P2: And I was doing better because there was a dentist at the medical center who went to fix my little mouth there. To all of us, where I lived. But, what happens? When I changed insurance, trying to find someone who would deign [to] fix my mouth, I changed from Obama[care], from Medicaid to Medicare, to get my mouth fixed and they have refused to fix it for me. And I am going to quit from that insurance and see if someone accepts me so I can get my mouth fixed. My mouth has deteriorated completely.

Reform 2: Volunteer or Work Requirement

Second, regarding a volunteer or work requirement, many of the participants reported complicated health and social issues that would interfere with fulfilling this obligation.

Group 24 (Puerto Rican men with dental care translated from Spanish).

P1: … First my plan dropped. They changed me to a crazy plan just because they don't take Medicaid … They sent me to a dentist far away. I'm in disability, I can't walk too much … find me a place close to my house and refer me. "Look this is close to your house. Check." So, you choose your best option. But the plan force[s] you to take what they have available only. I do not agree with only choosing what the plan has available.

Group 8 (African American men without dental care).

P1: … But I'm not concerned about myself now. I'm [gonna] talk to you about my wife. I'm worried about her.

P2: There you go!

P1: While she had to go through so much changes. And she, she's a diabetic and she's had cancer and her teeth, they [were] decaying and they told her—now she had enough to have Medicaid. Why she had Medicaid? 'Cause she had to pay some money and she had to go to the counseling program so—I don't know if you've ever heard of it, Sloan Kettering. That's one of the bigger counselors, doctors and hospitals. . .

P3: Like in New York, by NYU.

P1: Yeah, and so she goes there. Sometime[s] we go every day. Last month we went every day, in a row …. She was doing alright for about 20 years. Went in remission and it came back now if, she go again. It's started. It's in her ribs now. It came back. It's in her inner rib or something like that. And plus, she's a diabetic. So we have to go through all that travel—I'm not worried about myself. I'm just trying to say that she had this Medicaid— it used to be every 4 years. Now, they changed it to 8 years. So what she [has] to do for 8 years? And she's losing a lot of weight because—her teeth, she had teeth need to be extracted, and she [needs] teeth to be put in. Went to Columbia. They extracted teeth, but that's all they do.

P4: Well, people don't realize that your mouth take. . .

P1: You understand? That's a big part of your life.

P5: Part of your health.

P6: Oh yeah!

Reform 3: Eliminating Covered Services

Third, the loss of benefits, including dental coverage for adults, would undermine the ability of older adults to access preventive care.

Group 13 (African American men without dental care).

P1: 'Cause for me, since my father passed—been 8 months, 9 months. It seems like, 'cause I was taking care of him. He was 87. It seems like since he passed, all of the sudden I notice all of these things that need to be done before my body goes. I don't know if they were there before and I was so focused on him that I wasn't paying attention or it's just, you know, the natural progression of age but I mean as far as dentists and doctors, I need to get my Medicaid back, just go like up there and, you know, get checked in the office.

Group 9 (African American women with dental care). There is empathetic agreement among racial/ethnic minority older adult participants that providers ought to accept the coverage that community members are entitled to so that they can access needed health services.

P1: You got to be able to take Medicaid ... you gotta be able to take all of that. Don't come and say, "We don't do this." Well, f*** you. You need to be out. You don't need to come to a neighborhood if you are not going to be able to service the people who are here.

P2: That's right.

[Note that several women are echoing and following this speaker as she explains.]

P3: Why refuse us when you are here in our community?

P1: Just make sure that they come in knowing that you are not going to make a million dollars here for your practice.

P2: Right.

P1: 'Cause we don't have it like that.

P4: All these dentists, they should take so many people.

Reform 4: Behavioral Incentives

Fourth, an incentivized My Reward account that rewards older adults (e.g., for work or community service) and penalizes older adults (e.g., for nonurgent emergency department use) would no doubt prove even more confusing and stigmatizing for older adults than Medicaid coverage already is at present.

Group 20 (Puerto Rican men with dental care; in English).

P1: … My problem was Medicaid to pay for my dentures. I fought Medicaid. It took me 8 years to get my dentures because every time. First it started with 4 years, so I had to wait 4 years because they did some bad dentures. Now I gotta live with 4 years of dentures sitting in a cup looking at me. So I wait 4 years. I go to a dentist. They changed they law!

Group 20 (Puerto Rican men with dental care; in English).

P1: I got a letter from a doctor because it was 8 years and no dentures. I lost a lot of weight.

P2: Yeah!

P3: I had a, a doctor wrote me a letter that I was lacking vitamins in my body. I can't chew meat because I tried once and I almost choked. So I had to be careful with what I was eating. Now I'm eating. And they made a letter for me and I gave it to Medicaid. I made a copy—kept me a copy and I sent it to Medicaid. I waited and waited. Because of not having dentures, it cost me a deficiency. A vitamin deficiency. That's the only way I got an approval to go ahead and get the dentures then. Other than that …

P3: That still don't make no sense.

Group 23 (African American men with dental care).

P1: Now listen, listen to you and listen to me. You paying and they are happy. I'm welfare recipient, and you are paying. They are going to treat you better than they treat me, and we both live in the same building and you live next door to me. 'Cause you are paying cash, they are going to give you a more special service, than I'm going to pay with Medicaid they are going to treat me different. Maybe I have the same problem. They might say well we can save your teeth to you 'cause you are paying cash, and to me oh we are going to take your teeth out cause you are using Medicaid. See that is the problem.

The Patient Perspective

Our qualitative findings add a valued perspective that complements the quantitative evidence reported in the literature to date. For instance, Neely et al. found that dental-related emergency department visits increased 2% the first and 14% the second year after Medicaid cuts in Massachusetts.[15] Further, percentage increases were highest among older adults, minorities, and persons receiving charity care, Medicaid, and Medicare.[15] Hence, it appears likely that certain elements of the Kentucky First and of similar Medicaid expansion plans would be in direct opposition; for example, eliminating adult dental benefits would increase emergency department use and associated costs, thus further exacerbating the health and welfare of already disadvantaged and disabled older adults.

Instead Medicaid needs to be responsive to the experiences of older adults who seek care through the program. In the words of study participants, provision of respectful and comprehensive health care ought to be the guiding principle.

Group 8 (African American men without dental care).

P1: You have to be cordial. You have to show that you are really concerned about their health. So, listen. We adapt very well to people who show us respect.
P2: Right.
P1: Seniors like respect because we've paid our dues. We really have. We've suffered some real indignities and now that we've gotten older, they got worse. [Group laughs.]
P1: I mean they really have! We shouldn't have to have discussions about senior health. This should have been a foregone conclusion years ago. All that's been happening is that stuff has been taken away from us. It's made it more difficult for us to live like decent human beings.

Group 15 (Dominican men with dental care translated from Spanish). Racial/ethnic older adults need information on oral health and health care delivered in the formats that are accessible to them and their peers.

P1: I think that in this community, we need a lot more information. Many times we are orphaned of information. Those of us who have information are those of us who go to the centers, are paying attention to what is happening. But there are a lot of people who don't even know what is happening in their community. We need a lot of communication at the level of the [senior] centers, public offices, the libraries. We need information via radio.
P2: At the drug store!

P1: On television. The Hispanic community needs television. In other words, more information. Because it's through more information that you do consciousness building. More conscientious people [access] more easily those services [than] those who don't know that those things exist.

Group 5 (Dominican men with dental care translated from Spanish). Focus group participants underscored the need for affordable services.

P1: I say, if a clinic is there or there, I'd choose any of them but they have to treat me for free and it belongs to the government.
P2: Yup.
P1: But that doesn't exist.
P3: Or at least a clinic that charges low fees so one can pay.
P1: A minimum fee.
P3: Something that's not free, but that is reasonable.
P1: According to your income.
P2: It's not possible another way. It's too expensive.

Group 3 (African American women without dental care). Mobile services, such as those currently available through select dental schools, were also endorsed.

M: What kinds of things would you do to try to get seniors to go who aren't already going?
P1: They have the children's dental truck. They have it for children. Vans. So why don't they have one for grown-ups?
P2: That's a good idea.
P3: People would just go, take a morning and do all the screening and then once a month they'll do it or something every other week. Because it's easy. They don't have to travel anyplace ..... They offered screening, or everything, even if they're just a screening, okay. And then I refer you back to your own dentist or back to a regular dentist.

Group 24 (Puerto Rican men with dental care translated from Spanish). Dental home visits were another idea.

P1: I would get nurses or dentists, you know, go check the teeth out and in your apartment, you know.
M: Home visits?
P1: Visits to your apartment to check all the elderly people. So they don't have to come. Give me all the number of all the elderly people and all the kids. You go to the families; you check all the families. People are scared. If there was one person or a women

who says let's check your teeth, they open their mouth to check them and do not take anything out.... In Puerto Rico they have buses that go for the elderly people to fix their teeth and everything.

DISCUSSION

A critical step toward reducing racial/ethnic inequities in oral health and health care for older adults is to fund Medicaid well enough to deliver the standard of care for everyone, not just the privately insured.[5] Clearly just the provision of public dental insurance is not sufficient to eliminate disparities in the receipt of oral health care.[16]

Previously suggested public health priorities for reducing disparities in oral health and health care for older adults include better integrating oral health into medical care, implementing community programs to promote healthy behaviors and improve access to preventive services, developing a comprehensive strategy to address the oral health needs of the homebound and long-term care residents, and assessing the feasibility of ensuring a safety net that covers preventive and basic restorative services to eliminate pain and infection.[17]

To these we would add incorporating the views of older adults into public health programs and policies. Scientific approaches exist, including collaborative, interdisciplinary systems science inquiry, that provide opportunities to meaningfully integrate the experiences of both patients and providers in efforts to promote oral health equity.[18] Finally, instead of cutting Medicare, Medicaid, and other critical health care programs serving our nation's most vulnerable populations, policy makers ought to improve public health and modernize our largest insurance programs by expanding coverage and benefits, including comprehensive dental care.[8]

ACKNOWLEDGMENTS

This study was supported by the National Institute for Dental and Craniofacial Research and the Office of Behavioral and Social Sciences Research, National Institutes of Health for the project titled Integrating Social and Systems Science Approaches to Promote Oral Health Equity (grant R01-DE023072).

REFERENCES

1. Douglass CW, Jiménez MC. Our current geriatric population: demographic and oral health care utilization. *Dent Clin North Am.* 2014;58(4):717–728.

2. Friedman PK, Kaufman LB, Karpas SL. Oral health disparity in older adults: dental decay and tooth loss. *Dent Clin North Am.* 2014;58(4):757–770.

3. Northridge ME, Ue FV, Borrell LN, et al. Tooth loss and dental caries in community-dwelling older adults in northern Manhattan. *Gerodontology.* 2012;29(2):e464–e473.

4. Northridge ME, Lamster IB. A life course approach to preventing and treating oral disease. *Soz Praventivmed.* 2004;49(5):299–300. [Comment on relationship between caries prevalence and fissure sealants among 12-year-old German children at three educational strata. *Soz Praventivmed.* 2004.]

5. Fisher-Owens SA, Barker JC, Adams S, et al. Giving policy some teeth: routes to reducing disparities in oral health. *Health Aff (Millwood).* 2008;27(2):404–412.

6. Oral Health America. State of decay: are older Americans coming of age without oral healthcare? Available at: http://www.toothwisdom.org/action. Accessed December 5, 2016.

7. Hinton E, Paradise J. Access to dental care in Medicaid: spotlight on nonelderly adults. 2016. Available at: http://kff.org/medicaid/issue-brief/access-to-dental-care-in-medicaid-spotlight-on-nonelderly-adults. Accessed December 3, 2016.

8. Center for Medicare Advocacy. New report: expanded dental coverage needed to confront health crisis. Available at: http://www.medicareadvocacy.org/new-report-expanded-dental-coverage-needed-to-confront-health-crisis. Accessed December 5, 2016.

9. Grant R. In Kentucky's new Medicaid plan evidence takes a back seat. 2016. Available at: http://healthaffairs.org/blog/2016/08/25/in-kentuckys-new-medicaid-plan-evidence-takes-a-back-seat. Accessed December 5, 2016.

10. Purnell TS, Calhoun EA, Golden SH, et al. Achieving health equity: closing the gaps in health care disparities, interventions, and research. *Health Aff (Millwood).* 2016;35(8):1410–1415.

11. Northridge ME. Dental benefits: "Because Medicaid has, how do you call it? A limit." *Am J Public Health.* 2016;106(10):1726–1728.

12. Krueger RA, Casey MA. *Focus Groups: A Practical Guide for Applied Research.* 4th ed. Thousand Oaks, CA: Sage; 2009.

13. Boyatzis RE. Transforming Qualitative Information: Thematic Analysis and Code Development. Thousand Oaks, CA: Sage; 1998.

14. Healthfirst. Available at: http://healthfirst.org. Accessed December 4, 2016.

15. Neely M, Jones JA, Rich S, Gutierrez LS, Mehra P. Effects of cuts in Medicaid on dental-related visits and costs at a safety-net hospital. *Am J Public Health.* 2014;104(6):e13–e16.

16. Schrimshaw EW, Siegel K, Wolfson NH, Mitchell DA, Kunzel C. Insurance related barriers to accessing dental care among African American adults with oral health symptoms in New York City. *Am J Public Health.* 2011;101(8):1420–1428.

17. Griffin SO, Jones JA, Brunson D, Griffin PM, Bailey WD. Burden of oral disease among older adults and implications for public health priorities. *Am J Public Health.* 2012;102(3):411–418.

18. Metcalf SS, Birenz SS, Kunzel C, et al. The impact of Medicaid expansion on oral health equity for older adults: a systems perspective. *J Calif Dent Assoc.* 2015;43(7):369–377.

35

Building Innovative Models of Oral Health Care to Help Eliminate Disparities: The National Dental Association

Hazel J. Harper, DDS, MPH, Anne M. O'Keefe, PhD, JD,
Janet H. Southerland, DDS, PhD, MPH, and Nicole S. Cheek, DDS

HEALTH CARE DISPARITIES AND ORAL HEALTH

Despite advances in technology and research, glaring disparities exist among underserved and vulnerable populations. In 2000, the widely quoted US Surgeon General's report "Oral Health in America: A Report of the Surgeon General" stated, "Although major improvements have been seen nationally for most Americans, disparities exist in some population groups as classified by age, sex, income, and race/ethnicity."[1] Consider the following:

- Access to care is limited for 72 million children and adults who rely on Medicaid and the Children's Health Insurance Program (CHIP).[2]
- Only about one third of US dentists accept public insurance.[2]
- As of September 2015, 22 states did not provide any dental benefits to adults in their Medicaid programs beyond emergency procedures.[3]
- In 2017, there were more than 46 million children enrolled in Medicaid and CHIP.[4]
- In 2017, fewer than half (20 million) of children on Medicaid received dental care.[5]
- In 2012, more than 2 million dental-related emergency department visits were estimated to cost up to $1.6 billion.[6]
- As of November 6, 2018, there were 5,749 designated Dental Health Professional Shortage Areas (DHPSAs).[7]
- More than 63 million people in the United States reside in DHPSAs, and 65% of them have unmet dental needs.[7]
- To meet the needs of the underserved in the DHPSAs, 10,463 additional practitioners are needed.[7]
- Hispanic and African American dentists are proportionally less represented in the profession when compared with the US population; African Americans represent only 3.8% of practicing dentists.[8]

Research also shows that low health literacy is highly predictive of inefficient use of health services and poor health outcomes.[9] Surveys estimate that only 12% of the US adult population is proficient in health literacy, including awareness that poor oral health is linked to respiratory disease, cardiovascular disease, diabetes, and adverse pregnancy outcomes.[10] Tooth decay is the most common chronic childhood disease—four times as common as asthma among adolescents.[11] Vulnerable and underserved populations include but are not limited to the following:

- Racial and ethnic minorities, including immigrants and non-English speakers;
- Children, especially those who are very young;
- Pregnant women;
- People with special needs;
- Older adults;
- Individuals living in rural and urban underserved areas;
- Uninsured and publicly insured individuals;
- Homeless individuals; and
- Populations of lower socioeconomic status.[12]

The burden of poor oral health falls disproportionately on the poor and people of color.[13,14] This burden continues to lead to disparities among minority and underserved populations that adversely impact their well-being, health outcomes, and quality of life.

INNOVATIONS FOR CHANGE

In February 2007, Deamonte Driver, a 12-year-old boy in Prince George's County, Maryland, died of dental caries while his mother tried desperately to find a dentist to treat him. The family had recently lost its Medicaid coverage and was living in a shelter. Award-winning *Washington Post* reporter Mary Otto, in her article, "For Want of a Dentist," chronicled the terrible story of a boy who could have been saved by an $80 tooth extraction, but who died needlessly after $250,000 of brain surgeries that failed to save him.[15]

In the months that followed Deamonte Driver's death, then–Maryland Governor Martin O'Malley charged the state's legislators and policymakers to "fix the system" that had failed the child. Across the state, stakeholders in every sector collaborated to change Maryland's broken health system. Policies were reformed, legislation was enacted, funding was appropriated, and the state dental coalition was formed. Children's oral health became a top priority for the state, and mechanisms were put in place to accomplish the governor's mandate.

Members of the National Dental Association's (NDA's) chapter based in Washington, DC—The Robert T. Freeman Dental Society (RTFDS)—were deeply affected. In 2008, two RTFDS member dentists, Hazel Harper and Belinda Carver-Taylor, cofounded the Deamonte Driver Dental Project (DDDP) under the auspices of the NDA. They recruited their patients, colleagues, family, and friends and launched the DDDP. They worked with public officials at the local, state, and federal levels and secured almost $300,000 during the 2008 Maryland General Assembly to acquire a previously owned mobile dental unit (MDU) to screen, triage, treat what they could, and refer students throughout Prince George's County and the DC metropolitan area to dental homes within 15 minutes of their school. The project included the cooperation of principals, teachers, administrators, school nurses, and parents at the schools targeted for services from the MDU and a network of 50 dentists, called Dentists in Action, who all agreed to treat uninsured, underinsured, and Medicaid patients without regard to payment.

Born out of tragedy and developed out of necessity, the project was designed as a grassroots, school-based, mobile health community initiative to stamp out the epidemic of tooth decay by increasing access to care and providing early intervention. The DDDP was launched at Deamonte's school—The Foundation School, in Prince George's County, Maryland—where Governor O'Malley personally presented the DDDP with the Governor's Award for Innovations in Health. The award included additional funding to purchase, staff, and operate a new, state-of-the-art DDDP MDU for three years. Deamonte's mother, Alyce Driver, granted permission to name the project in memory of her son, and NDA members pledged to continue the crusade to address the life-threatening problem of lack of dental care for vulnerable children.

In the years that followed, Maryland went from nearly dead last in oral public health to number one in the nation, as reported in 2011 by the Pew Center on the States in "Children's Dental Health: Maryland. Making Coverage Matter."[16] The DDDP was cited in that report and the award-winning regional project also gained the distinction of being a national model for public–private partnerships. The DDDP continues to operate in Prince George's County, administered by the Maryland State Health Department. This project highlights the importance of coalition building to effectively address the needs of our most vulnerable populations.

THE CRUSADE CONTINUES: THE CREATION OF NATIONAL DENTAL ASSOCIATION–HEALTH NOW

The NDA's legacy of leadership and tradition of service paved the way for another program that has been promoted nationally. This program will continue to advance NDA's mission and achieve its goal of eliminating disparities through education, literacy, and community empowerment. Building on a track record of successful community collaborations, strong corporate relations, and enduring public–private partnerships, NDA–HEALTH NOW (Health Equity, Access, Literacy, Technology, and Hope—National Outreach on Wheels) was created to be the organization's signature project. Formed in

2012 with a planning grant from The Links Foundation, the NDA–HEALTH NOW project is a replication and expansion of the best practices of the model used for development of the DDDP.

The NDA–HEALTH NOW initiative provides resources and services to underserved communities and works to (1) increase health care access, (2) eliminate disparities, (3) increase health literacy, and (4) promote prevention. In expanding and improving the DDDP model, NDA–HEALTH NOW has expanded its scope to include medical, vision, and dental services for children, adults, and older adults. The project has strategic alliances with public school systems, health agencies, federally qualified health centers (FQHCs), recreation departments, hospitals, and senior citizen communities. It leverages the time, talent, and efforts of a massive network of volunteers from civic, social, and service organizations along with fraternities and sororities. The focus is on total health and prevention to increase awareness about the connection between oral health and overall health. Through community outreach programs, NDA–HEALTH NOW features interprofessional health teams (including oral health professionals, physicians, optometrists, nurses, physician assistants, and pharmacists), and fosters collaborations with community organizations, academic institutions, and faith-based entities. Ultimately, the project will feature mixed-use mobile health units equipped for medical, vision, and dental care provided by interprofessional teams.

Program Design and Development

The project is guided by recommendations made by the Institute of Medicine and the National Research Council of the National Academies. It is based on two widely accepted, evidence-based principles:

- Oral health is an integral component of overall health and must, therefore, be a core component of comprehensive health care; and
- Improving access to oral health care will prevent disease and improve overall health.

This project was designed to be community-led and community-owned. The goals of NDA–HEALTH NOW are to increase access to oral health services, improve health literacy, promote prevention in vulnerable populations, and eliminate disparities in oral and general health through public–private partnerships. The core components of this approach are collaboration, service, education, research, and policy recommendations. Project sites have been selected on the basis of the following:

- Identifiable high-risk and underserved populations;
- Existence of a local NDA chapter;
- Potential to collaborate with and expand existing community programs;

- Existence of oral health and other academic institutions; and
- A local NDA leader with the vision and political will to lead the effort.

The vision of this initiative is to engage community partners around oral health to form collaborative networks to create and implement strategies, build capacity, and have a collective impact on health and oral health policy.

Program development includes the identification of stakeholders within each targeted area, the formation of advisory committees, and the engagement of community partners. Partners include state and local government health agencies, FQHCs, hospitals, public school systems, community centers (recreation and senior citizens), civic and social organizations, corporations, foundations, and academic institutions. The project also partners with well-established national entities that have strong local chapters and grass-roots networks such as The Links, Kappa Alpha Psi Fraternity, Omega Psi Phi Fraternity, and the American Diabetes Association. The participation of academic institutions and student organizations is also important, especially collaborations with students in dentistry, medicine, nursing, pharmacy, optometry, public health, communications, business, law, and social work.

The role of the local advisory committees is critical for guiding program processes. In each NDA–HEALTH NOW partner city, the advisory committee determines the programming needs, priorities, goals, and strategies. They set the stage for collaborative, sustainable programs and provide input, direction, guidance, and support to the local NDA program directors.

Collaborators and Sponsors

Resources and in-kind support are provided by foundations, corporations, academic partners, and a volunteer network of NDA members and community organizations. These contributions have been invaluable in helping the NDA continue to advance its mission and expand its vision to encompass health and well-being, especially by focusing on reducing health disparities.

Corporate Sponsors

In the initiative's first five years of operation (2013–2018), corporate sponsors included Colgate, Henry Schein, DentaQuest, VOCO, ADI Mobile Health, A-Dec, Crest Oral-B, Air Techniques, Patterson Dental, GlaxoSmithKline, Philips Sonicare, CareCredit, and Sunstar. Foundation partners have included the Aetna Foundation, The Coca-Cola Foundation, the Energy Foundation, General Electric's African American Forum Affinity Foundation, the Harris Rosen Foundation, Henry Schein Cares Foundation, and the W.K. Kellogg Foundation.

Academic Sponsors

Academic partners are Columbia University (Schools of Dentistry and Nursing), Howard University (Colleges of Dentistry, Nursing, and Communications), Louisiana State University School of Dentistry, Morehouse School of Medicine, New York University (Colleges of Dentistry and Nursing), Texas A&M University College of Dentistry (formerly Baylor), University of California–San Francisco School of Dentistry, University of Central Florida School of Nursing, Valencia College Department of Dental Hygiene, and Xavier University Pharmacy School. Other partnering organizations include Hear-to-HEAL, Oral Health America, and the New Orleans Recreation Development Commission.

Collaboration With National Dental Association Members and Community Organizations

Colgate and the NDA represent one of the most successful, longstanding, public–private health partnerships in America and around the world. For nearly three decades, they have worked together to improve oral health in underserved and vulnerable communities. NDA members have volunteered with Colgate's award-winning Bright Smiles, Bright Futures mobile dental project for inner-city children since it began in 1989. Since then, Colgate Bright Smiles, Bright Futures has served more than 950 million children in 80 countries. The NDA–HEALTH NOW–Colgate collaboration is a major factor in the ongoing success and growth of the NDA–HEALTH NOW initiative.

The Links and the NDA became national partners in 2011. Since then, The Links has formed a National Oral Health Committee and has made oral health an integral part of its national health initiative. There are nearly 15,000 Links members with 288 chapters across the United States. In fact, many NDA women dentists are also Links members serving in leadership positions with both organizations on national, regional, and local levels. These cross-cutting positions help to enhance the expansion, replication, and sustainability of these efforts. Two NDA–HEALTH NOW programs that were created for The Links have been replicated in many venues. The first, Razzle, Dazzle Smiles for Life, the popular "taste and touch" interactive module for senior citizens and their caregivers, was created for and popularized by a Chicago Links chapter. The program has been conducted many times in its entirety or in part, and each time the event receives excellent evaluations from attendees. Another program created at the request of The Links Birmingham, Alabama, Chapter was the program for teens, What's a Selfie Without a Smile? This education module provides information on age-appropriate topics such as teeth whitening, tongue piercing, the dangers of sports drinks, wisdom teeth, and science, technology, engineering, and mathematics (STEM) careers. Webinars and strategic planning workshops have also been conducted.

The Greater New York Dental Meeting (GNYDM), with more than 50,000 attendees annually, provides extraordinary opportunities to support longstanding partnerships that improve health not only in New York but also nationally and internationally. In addition to providing the venue for lectures and hands-on oral health training for nursing students and volunteers, this partnership provides a tremendous opportunity for community service. For nearly 10 years, the Greater New York Smiles (GNYS) program has partnered with the Colgate Bright Smiles, Bright Futures program and the DentaQuest Foundation to host a community event for local children. This adventure features health profession role models and includes dental screenings and referrals, health and nutrition education, instructions for oral hygiene, oral health videos, a puppet show, and a variety of hands-on activities.

In 2018, permission was granted to expand the GNYS program to include the newest feature of NDA–HEALTH NOW—Step-Up-to-STEM—an age-appropriate interactive program focused on oral health. A contest was designed by the NDA to encourage dental students to create innovative programs. Two winning entries were selected, and the Harris Rosen Foundation awarded cash prizes to the winners. The contest winners were Student National Dental Association members Celeste Edwards (Louisiana State University) and Raymond Dawkins (University of Alabama). In July 2018, Step-Up-to-STEM made its debut in Orlando, Florida, at the NDA-HEALTH NOW community outreach program for 300 children at the Hughes Boys and Girls Club in the Parramore section of Orlando.

Implementation of the Plan

In 2012, The Links Foundation awarded a one-year planning grant to the NDA that supported project and infrastructure development and program creation and implementation. Two pilot cities were selected—Chicago, Illinois, and Dallas, Texas. These sites were selected because (1) local NDA members had credibility and longstanding relationships with community organizations and institutions, (2) Sheila Brown, MEd, DDS (Chicago) and Jocelyn Kidd, DDS (Dallas)—both NDA leaders and Links members—agreed to be the local HEALTH NOW project directors, and (3) both sites offered the potential for strategic alignment to improve and expand existing programs.

With the help of the planning grant, an action plan was proposed that made specific recommendations to do the following:

1. Identify stakeholders and recruit community partners;
2. Form local advisory committees;
3. Select the local project director;
4. Identify and prioritize community needs;
5. Establish specific, measurable, attainable, realistic, and time-based (SMART) goals;
6. Form partnerships and collaborations with existing programs to include oral health;
7. Develop and implement new programs to achieve defined goals; and
8. Develop plans for sustainability and replication beyond the first three years.

At the end of the grant cycle in 2013, the action plan had been completed, and the next three-year plan phased in the three additional HEALTH NOW partner cities of New York, New York; New Orleans, Louisiana; and San Francisco/Oakland, California. The goal was to provide support and resources for all five cities to have successful, sustainable, replicable programs by 2016. Funding from the W.K. Kellogg Foundation and The Coca-Cola Foundation supported the project in meeting and exceeding its goals.

In 2016, NDA–HEALTH NOW also conducted programs in the metropolitan Washington, DC, area and Atlanta, Georgia. In addition, the project supported NDA chapter programs in Nashville and Memphis, Tennessee, as well as in Upper Marlboro, Maryland. NDA–HEALTH NOW also supported Links programs in Austin, Texas; Birmingham, Alabama; Macon, Georgia; Gaithersburg and Prince George's County, Maryland; and Milwaukee, Wisconsin. By 2018, HEALTH NOW programs had also been hosted in Houston, Texas (Hurricane Harvey emergency relief effort) and Orlando. Globally, NDA–HEALTH NOW has supported programs in Kenya, Haiti, Jamaica, Guatemala, Greece, Pakistan, and Sudan.

Events and Outcomes

American Diabetes Association Programs

Participation in programs of the American Diabetes Association has increased awareness about the link between oral health and diabetes. On-site screenings and education at NDA–HEALTH NOW oral health kiosks have impacted thousands of participants participating in American Diabetes Association events. In New York City, in 2016, NDA–HEALTH NOW designed and activated the "dental zone" at the American Diabetes Association Convention, where 250 patients were screened, educated, surveyed, and referred. The "zone" was a collaborative effort of HEALTH NOW and Columbia University's College of Dental Medicine and School of Nursing. Participating students were astonished to see the number of people who were in desperate need of dental treatment. It was a powerful lesson that exemplified community-based learning and underscored the problem of lack of access for underserved populations. NDA–HEALTH NOW has also set up education stations at Diabetes Step-Out Walks in New York City; Dallas; Fairfax, Virginia; and Oxon Hill, Maryland.

More than 4,000 surveys exploring the public's knowledge about the link between oral health and diabetes have been collected at events in Dallas, New Orleans, New York, Chicago, and the DC-metro area. The Diabetes and Oral Health survey questionnaire creates opportunities for oral health professionals and students to engage and educate the public. Preliminary data from this survey are currently being compiled and will be used to develop oral health education messages and other specific interventions targeting persons with diabetes.

Greater New York Dental Meeting

In 2015, NDA-HEALTH NOW's New York community partners agreed to support the expansion efforts of the GNYS program, the community outreach initiative of the annual GNYDM, the nation's largest dental convention. The GNYS hosted 1,500 New York City third graders at the Javits Convention Center as a collaborative effort of the GNYDM and Colgate Bright Smiles, Bright Futures.

In addition to screenings and referrals performed in the Colgate van, NDA-HEALTH NOW recommended the phase-in of fluoride varnish applications as a preventive service and training opportunity for nursing students. However, permission to provide this preventive service must be authorized by the New York State Health Department. To support this effort, HEALTH NOW developed and conducted a nurses' training program at the GNYDM that spanned four days and included lectures, hands-on training for oral screening, volunteer orientation on the Colgate van, participation in the GNYS children's program, and guided tours of the GNYDM technical exhibit hall. The program was partially underwritten by the Aetna Foundation. New York Advisory Committee members provided resources, in-kind donations, speakers, trainers, and volunteers. The GNYDM provided the venue, including training areas, audiovisual setup, and technicians. Product donations were received from Sunstar, Henry Schein Cares, and Columbia Dentoform. Since 2015, when the program began, 139 nurses have completed the training.

Course evaluations revealed that of 100% of the responding nursing student attendees felt the training would make them a better health team member. When asked if this information and training should be required for all nurses and other nondental health professionals, 95% agreed that it should. When asked to rate, on a scale of one to five (with one being the lowest and five being the highest) how inclined they were to do oral examinations because of the training, the average response was 4.74. Of special significance was the fact that 100% of the pediatric nursing students agreed that this training would help them promote oral health with their pediatric patients.

Chicago Resource Directory

The Chicago Public School District was instrumental in the distribution of the first NDA–HEALTH NOW–Chicago Resource Directory in early 2015. The directory, designed to connect individuals with dental homes in their communities, was distributed to 664 Chicago schools that included 396,683 children and their parents or guardians. The publication is updated every six months and can be downloaded from the NDA Web site. It lists public and private dental facilities that accept Medicaid and uninsured adults and that offer sliding fee scales. The Directory also contains information about discount pharmacies, how to enroll in various health plans, and contact information for local, county, and state health departments. The production and first printing (5,000 copies) of the directory were made possible by the W.K. Kellogg Foundation, The Links Foundation, and Patterson Dental.

Dallas, Texas: Mayor's Back to School Fair

In Dallas, Texas, A&M University's (formerly Baylor's) College of Dentistry designs and directs the Dental Zone at the annual Mayor's Back to School Fair. The fair attracts 40,000 children, their parents, and a massive network of volunteers. Between 800 and 1,200 children's screenings and fluoride varnish applications are performed between 8AM and 2PM by dental student volunteers. Other volunteers include faculty members, administrators, predental students, dental assistant students, hygienists, and dental assistants. NDA–HEALTH NOW–Dallas provides services for the parents and guardians of the children served, including bilingual education, donated dental products, and a dental resource directory for uninsured and underinsured adults. Bilingual oral health–diabetes surveys are also collected.

Sustainability of National Dental Association–HEALTH NOW

The NDA has a history of strong, longstanding, productive partnerships with civic and social organizations, multicultural health organizations, corporations, and foundations. These partners bring complementary expertise, resources, and vision to the project. The project's sustainability plan includes the following:

- Collaboration with partners that are rooted and respected in the community,
- Alignment with existing community programs,
- Involvement of students at every level, and
- Formal agreements with partners.

NDA–HEALTH NOW collaborates with FQHCs, school systems, hospitals, health departments, recreation departments, academic institutions, and many others. Formal partnership agreements have been executed with the Henry Schein Cares Foundation, the General Electric's African American Forum, The Links, Kappa Alpha Psi Fraternity, and the National Optometric Association. These partnerships inspire creativity, provide a vast network of talented volunteers and experienced leaders, and contribute other value-added benefits and resources. Foundation partners such as the W.K. Kellogg Foundation, the Aetna Foundation, and The Coca-Cola Foundation have provided much needed financial resources and technical support. Corporate partners not only provide resources but also offer expertise in public relations and marketing as well as communications and information technology. They also facilitate networking with prospective new partners and they share the techniques and fundamentals of data-driven strategic thinking.

Educational/Screening Tools

Six educational modules have been developed for children, teens, adults, and seniors:

- Razzle, Dazzle Smiles for Life is a two-part program (didactic and interactive) for seniors and their caregivers as well as for nurses and nursing students.

- Mouth Body Connection is an adult instructional PowerPoint in English and Spanish.
- Passport to Total Health offers children a circuit of health education and oral health screening stations. For adults, it includes health education and health screenings by physicians, dentists, nurses, pharmacists, nutritionists, and others.
- What's a Selfie Without a Smile? is an education and STEM career module for teens.
- Inter-professional Community-Based Learning: Oral Health and Nursing is a program that provides didactic lectures as well as hands-on training to instruct nursing students how to perform basic oral screenings and deliver oral hygiene instructions.
- Step-Up-to-STEM consists of age-appropriate interactive STEM programs to engage and inspire children aged 4 to 17 years to become interested in STEM with an emphasis on oral health.

Instructional materials, promotional materials, templates, and other resources are available to community partners at the NDA Web site: http://www.ndaonline.org/healthnow/eventsupport.

Accomplishments and Achievements

In the first five years of operation (2013–2018), NDA–HEALTH NOW supported 115 programs in 15 cities and 7 countries. The programs, managed by dozens of community partners and a massive network of volunteers, have provided oral health services and education to more than 27,030 individuals, performed screenings and referrals for 19,792 people, applied fluoride varnish to 8,081 children, and collected data on general knowledge about the link between oral health and diabetes and the need for prenatal dental care from 4,343 respondents.

A cooperative agreement with the Henry Schein Cares Foundation has allowed the project to support student missionary trips and provide in-kind product donations to free clinics and global outreach programs in Kenya, Haiti, Jamaica, Guatemala, Greece, Pakistan, and Sudan. In addition, donated products from Henry Schein Cares and Colgate supported the NDA–HEALTH NOW Hurricane Harvey relief effort in Houston in 2017, providing products and support to 7,500 school children and their families. The achievements of these interventions include the following general accomplishments:

- Planning and implementing collaborative community service projects in HEALTH NOW cities;
- Identifying and recruiting stakeholders as community partners;
- Forming local advisory committees;
- Developing project Web sites with templates, resources, graphics, and examples;
- Compiling and disseminating resource directories;
- Recruiting community dental providers for "dental homes" to serve targeted populations; and
- Achieving the SMART objectives generated by advisory committees in each city.

Additional specific accomplishments include the following:

- "The Land of Healthy Smiles" an oral health education video, was produced by Iris Morton, DDS, a member of the NDA and The Links, in conjunction with the Howard University School of Communications' Department of Media, Journalism, and Film. The film earned third place in the 2013 MY HERO International Short Film Festival "Narrative Animation" category. The film was featured at the Film Festival on November 23, 2013, at the University of Southern California. The video has been used in HEALTH NOW cities and around the world.
- A "train-the-trainers" video was produced for NDA–HEALTH NOW–Chicago by NDA member David Miller, DDS, and national project partner, Oral Health America. The video was broadcast as a leadership training module for Chicago community partners.
- In 2016, NDA–HEALTH NOW received the American Society of Association Executives Power of A Award, the industry's highest honor, in recognition of the project's "valuable contributions ... outstanding accomplishments ... [and] efforts to enrich lives, create a competitive workforce, prepare society for the future, drive innovation and make a better world" (Chris Vest, CAE, written communication, June 8, 2016).
- In 2018, the Links and NDA–HEALTH NOW produced and presented the first joint webinar on oral health for the entire Links membership of nearly 15,000 women.
- In 2018, preliminary data collection began to expand the NDA–HEALTH NOW education component to include information about prenatal dental care. This expansion effort will include increased engagement of nurses, The Links member dentists, and other providers of maternal and child health.
- In 2018, the Dental Trade Alliance Foundation awarded a planning grant for the NDA–HEALTH NOW–Metro DC pilot project, Links to Oral Health for Expectant Mothers. This project will be "for women, by women"—a collaboration of NDA women dentists, the Washington, DC, Chapter of The Links, and other community organizations to improve birth outcomes and maternal and child health.

Lessons Learned and Plans for the Future

Important lessons learned include the following:

- Building trust is essential for successful community engagement and collaboration.
- Cultural and linguistic competencies are necessary.
- Oral health literacy is a matter of life or death for the community at large and, hence, should be required learning for nondental health professionals.
- Senior citizens and their caregivers desperately need education and services.

- Dental providers in underserved communities have special concerns and needs that must be addressed.
- Resource directories are vital for increasing access.

The project will continue to build on best practices that have shaped this initiative from the beginning, including collaborating with organizations that are rooted and respected in the community, aligning with existing community programs, strengthening and expanding public–private partnerships, partnering with academic institutions, and incorporating student participation. Plans for the future include the following:

- Designing community-based participatory research projects to better understand the social and behavioral determinants of health disparities and, based on the outcomes of this consumer research, implementing health policies that remediate the inequities; and
- Developing tools to evaluate and improve these public health interventions for sustained behavior change.

CONCLUSIONS

The systematic disenfranchisement of vulnerable communities has created a culture of marginalization. For generations, the voices of underserved populations have been muted. NDA–HEALTH NOW creates opportunities for those voices to be heard. The project's innovative community-driven programs will not only serve those communities but also bring about transformational change in health behaviors and health outcomes. The project will focus on service, education, collaboration, research, and policy recommendations.

By increasing awareness about the link between oral health and overall health, NDA–HEALTH NOW is planting seeds at the grassroots level for oral health advocates and oral health champions who are poised to make a collective impact. The knowledge and insights derived from the life experiences of those served will illuminate pathways to more responsive health care and a healthier nation. The NDA will continue its legacy of leadership and tradition of service to eliminate disparities and achieve oral health equity for all.

ACKNOWLEDGMENTS

We wish to acknowledge the vision and leadership of the following individuals for the role they each played in helping the NDA–HEALTH NOW dream become a reality: Kim Perry, DDS, MSCS, Dennis Mitchell, DDS, MPH, Pamela Alston, DDS, Stephen Brisco, DDS, Robert Edwab, DDS, Marsha Butler, DDS, Ernie Lacy, DDS, Dan Jones, DDS, Patrick Ferrillo, DDS, Alice Craft-Kearney, RN, Robert Johns, LaVette Henderson, Alvenia Albright, Derrick Humphries, Steve Kess, Beth Truett, Jim Kitch, and Millie Goldstein. The NDA won a 2016 Power of A Silver Award.

REFERENCES

1. US Department of Health and Human Services. Oral health in America: a report of the Surgeon General. Rockville, MD: National Institute of Dental and Craniofacial Research, National Institutes of Health; 2000:35.

2. Koppelman J. How to improve oral health outcomes for kids. Pew Dental Campaign. February 16, 2018. Available at: https://www.pewtrusts.org/en/research-and-analysis/articles/2018/02/16/how-to-improve-oral-health-outcomes-for-kids. Accessed August 24, 2018.

3. National Association of Dental Plans. Dental benefits basics—who has dental benefits today? 2014. Available at: http://www.nadp.org/Dental_Benefits_Basics/Dental_BB_1.aspx#_ftn1. Accessed August 24, 2018.

4. Statistical Enrollment Data System. Combined CHIP enrollment total report and form CMS-64.EC as of 5/30/2018. Available at: https://www.medicaid.gov/chip/downloads/fy-2017-childrens-enrollment-report.pdf. Accessed August 24, 2018.

5. Centers for Medicare and Medicaid Services. Annual EPSDT participation report, form CMS-416 (national) FY2017. August 2018. Available at: https://www.medicaid.gov/medicaid/benefits/downloads/epsdt/fy-2017-data.zip. Accessed August 24, 2018.

6. Wall T, Vujicic M. Emergency department use for dental conditions to increase. Health Policy Institute Research Brief. Chicago, IL: American Dental Association; 2015.

7. Health Resources and Services Administration. Designated health professional shortage area statistics as of Nov. 6, 2018. Rockville, MD: US Department of Health and Human Services, Bureau of Health Workforce; 2018.

8. American Dental Association Health Policy Institute. The dentist workforce—key facts, 2014–2015. Chicago, IL: American Dental Association; 2015.

9. Berkman ND, Sheridan SL, Donahue KE, Halpern DJ, Crotty K. Low health literacy and health outcomes: an updated systematic review. *Ann Intern Med.* 2011;155(2):97–107.

10. Kutner M, Greenberg E, Jin Y, Paulsen C. The health literacy of America's adults: results from the 2003 National Assessment of Adult Literacy (NCES 2006–483). US Department of Education, National Center for Education Statistics. 2006. Available at: https://nces.ed.gov/pubs2006/2006483.pdf. Accessed October 29, 2016.

11. Dye BA, Tan S, Smith V, et al. Trends in oral health status, United States, 1988–1994 and 1999–2004. *Vital Health Stat 11.* 2007;(248):1–92.

12. Institute of Medicine, National Research Council. *Improving Access to Oral Health Care for Vulnerable and Underserved Populations.* Washington, DC: National Academy of Sciences, National Academies Press; 2011:12.

13. Newacheck PW, Hughes DC, Hung Y, Wong S, Stoddard J. The unmet health needs of America's children. *Pediatrics.* 2000;105(4):989–997.

14. Bloom B, Jones LI, Freeman G. Summary health statistics for US children: National Health Interview Survey, 2012. National Center for Health Statistics. *Vital Health Stat 10.* 2013; (258):1–81.

15. Otto M. *TEETH. The Story of Beauty, Inequality, and the Struggle for Oral Health in America.* New York, NY: The New Press; 2016.

16. Children's Dental Health: Maryland. Making coverage matter. Pew Dental Campaign. 2011. Available at: http://www.pewtrusts.org/en/research-and-analysis/fact-sheets/2011/05/11/childrens-dental-health-maryland. Accessed October 29, 2016.

36

Lack of Public Awareness and Effective Lobbying by Special Interests Contribute to the Continuing "Silent Epidemic" in Oral Health in the United States

Wendell B. Potter, BS

Does the name Deamonte Driver ring a bell? It has been almost 12 years since his name made headlines,[1] more than a decade since people across the country were shaken when they heard what had happened to him or, more accurately, what had not happened. "Twelve-year-old Deamonte Driver died of a toothache Sunday."[1] Those were the first words of a story in the *Washington Post* on February 28, 2007, that made Deamonte Driver the poster child, quite literally, of an inequitable system of dental care in the United States.

Although the story was both heartbreaking and shocking, the reality was that Deamonte was just the latest victim of what former Surgeon General David Satcher had a few years earlier called a "silent epidemic." Satcher used that term in a seminal report that called attention to the "profound and consequential oral health disparities within the American population."[2]

After that unforgettable first sentence, reporter Mary Otto went on to write the following:

A routine, $80 tooth extraction might have saved him.

- If his mother had been insured.
- If his family had not lost its Medicaid.
- If Medicaid dentists weren't so hard to find.
- If his mother hadn't been focused on getting a dentist for his brother, who had six rotted teeth.[1]

By the time Deamonte's own aching tooth got any attention, the bacteria from the abscess had spread to his brain, doctors said. After two operations and more than six weeks of hospital care, the Prince George's County, Maryland, boy died.

THE "SILENT EPIDEMIC" OF DENTAL AND ORAL DISEASES

What undoubtedly surprised many readers was that tooth decay is not just a painful annoyance but a serious infectious disease that can, and often does, lead to death, even among children. And probably just as surprising to many was how difficult getting timely and appropriate care can be for people who lack dental benefits or who live in areas where few dentists practice and even fewer are willing to treat Medicaid patients.

In his 2000 report, Satcher wrote that "it (is) abundantly clear that there are profound and consequential disparities in the oral health of our citizens."[2] He added

> Indeed, what amounts to a "silent epidemic" of dental and oral diseases is affecting some population groups. This burden of disease restricts activities in school, work, and home, and often significantly diminishes the quality of life. Those who suffer the worst oral health are found among the poor of all ages, with poor children and poor older Americans particularly vulnerable. Members of racial and ethnic minority groups also experience a disproportionate level of oral health problems. Individuals who are medically compromised or who have disabilities are at greater risk for oral diseases, and, in turn, oral diseases further jeopardize their health. [2]

More than a decade and a half after Satcher's report, those disparities persist, even after the passage of the Affordable Care Act of 2010, which included dental care as an essential benefit for children.[3] Tooth decay is still the number-one chronic disease affecting children, and children of color are especially at risk. More than a third of elementary-school children have untreated tooth decay, and the rate is twice as high for Hispanic and non-Hispanic Black children and even worse for Native Americans. In addition, more than half of all kids on Medicaid did not see a dentist in 2011, in large part because only about one third of US dentists accept Medicaid.[4] In some states, the percentage is even lower. And, since 2000, the number of people living in dental shortage areas has nearly doubled, from 25 million to 49 million.[5]

So, clearly, despite Satcher's call to action, progress to reduce the disparities in oral health has been slow. That was made evident in a 2016 report by Surgeon General Vivek Murthy and the Department of Health and Human Services.[6] Murthy provided some encouraging statistics: more children are receiving dental sealants to help prevent cavities than in 2000, fewer teens have tooth decay, and more adults are retaining their natural teeth. But, he added the following:

> Poor oral health continues to disproportionately affect low-income individuals, the frail and vulnerable, and the traditionally underserved. One-quarter of preschool-aged children living in households below the federal poverty level have untreated tooth decay, compared with about one in 10 children living above the poverty level. As of 2012, more than 29% of non-Hispanic black adults aged 65 years and older had complete tooth loss compared with fewer than 19% of the overall U.S. population of the same age. [6]

Because so many US residents are unable to get the dental care they need in a timely and cost-effective way, increasing numbers of both children and adults wind up in hospital emergency departments when pain caused by diseased teeth and gums becomes unbearable. As Murthy noted, "Emergency room treatment for preventable dental conditions . . . is expensive and continues to increase."[6] That point has also been made by former Health and Human Services Secretary Louis Sullivan in a 2012 op-ed in the *New York Times*[7]:

> We know that too many Americans can't afford primary care and end up in the emergency room with asthma or heart failure. But in the debate over health care coverage, less attention has been paid to the fact that too many Americans also end up in the emergency room with severe tooth abscesses that keep them from eating or infections that can travel from decayed teeth to the brain and, if untreated, kill. [7]

Instead of decreasing since Surgeon General Satcher's 2000 report, the number of emergency department–related dental visits nearly doubled over the following decade and continues to increase. The American Dental Association (ADA) estimated that, in 2012 alone, emergency department dental visits cost the US health care system $1.6 billion, with an average cost of $749 per visit.[8]

There are other costs and consequences of America's continuing silent epidemic. People with diseased and missing teeth are at a disadvantage when applying for employment. Pregnant women with untreated decay can pass disease on to their unborn children. Toothaches also contribute to children missing school and to their parents missing work.

Arguably the biggest reason for the slow progress in reducing disparities in oral health is the lingering problem of access. As the framework for action that accompanied Surgeon General Murthy's report noted, "One of the greatest barriers to oral health care is a lack of dental services. This can be called the greatest unmet oral health need in the United States."[9]

REMEDIES TO FIGHT THE "SILENT EPIDEMIC"

As Murthy wrote, there are remedies. Among the recommendations are the following:

- Strengthen the oral health workforce,
- Expand capabilities of existing providers, and
- Promote models that incorporate other clinicians.

The good news here is that progress is being made, albeit slowly, in all three areas. The ADA launched a pilot project in 2006 to train what the ADA calls community dental health coordinators.[10] Their focus is education and prevention.

Midlevel providers, often called dental therapists (DTs), are another addition to the dental team that an increasing number of states and tribal communities are considering. Their scope of practice is considerably broader than that of community dental health coordinators. DTs have been practicing for many years in several other countries (since the early 1900s in New Zealand)[11] but only for a little more than a decade in the United States, starting in tribal communities in Alaska. Dental disease had become so prevalent among Alaska Natives, many of whom live far from a dentist's office, that tribal leaders decided to see if DTs could make a difference. The first four DTs to start treating patients in Alaska traveled to New Zealand in 2004 for their two-year training program, financed and coordinated by the Alaska Native Tribal Health Consortium. Subsequent students have been trained under the auspices of the University of Washington School of Medicine. Now more than 30 dental health aide therapists, or DHATs, as they are called in Alaska, are providing care to more than 45,000 people. As in other countries, they work as part of a broader dental team and are supervised by dentists. Their scope of practice ranges from education and prevention to uncomplicated extractions and fillings. When a patient requires care beyond their scope of practice, they refer the patient to a dentist.

Dental therapists began practicing in Minnesota in 2009 after state lawmakers passed legislation authorizing their training and licensure. In a 2014 report, the Minnesota Department of Health concluded the following:

- The dental therapy workforce is growing and appears to be fulfilling statutory intent by serving predominantly low-income, uninsured, and underserved patients.
- DTs appear to be practicing safely, and clinics report improved quality and high patient satisfaction with DT services.[12]

Maine, Vermont, and Arizona are the most recent states to allow DTs to practice, and several other states, including Washington State, are considering it. In a 2014 report to the legislature, the Washington State Board of Health concluded that the care DTs provide within their scope of practice "is at least as high in quality as care provided by a licensed dentist."[13] The report also suggested that not only would midlevel providers increase access to oral health care in the state, but they could also decrease the cost of providing it.

Although enabling legislation has not yet been enacted in Washington State, a DT began treating patients there in January 2016 after the Swinomish Native American community exercised tribal sovereignty and recruited one of the Alaska-trained DTs. In welcoming the DT to the community in January 2016, Swinomish chairman Brian Cladoosby noted that DTs have succeeded in large part because they are more likely to provide culturally competent care than other practitioners because they typically either grew up in or have lived in communities similar to those they serve (see Chapter 19).

CONCLUSIONS

Although Surgeon General Murthy did not mention specific practitioners in his 2016 report on oral health in America, DTs clearly are among the "other clinicians" who can strengthen the oral health workforce to improve access and reduce disparities.

Former Surgeon General Satcher not only has mentioned DTs in interviews and presentations in recent years but he has also been vocal in advocating that the expansion of the dental workforce should include them, as has former Department of Health and Human Services Secretary Sullivan.[14,15] "I think we need more dentists and I think we need more professionals who are not dentists but who can contribute to oral health services," Satcher said at a July 16–July 17, 2012 conference hosted by the Morehouse School of Medicine in Atlanta, Georgia (David Satcher, MD, PhD, oral communication, 2012). Both Satcher and Sullivan have encouraged the dental profession and policymakers to support adding DTs to the workforce. "Public officials should foster the creation of these midlevel providers," Sullivan wrote in his 2012 op-ed, "and dentists should embrace the opportunity to broaden the profession so they can expand services to those in need."[7]

REFERENCES

1. Otto M. For want of a dentist. *Washington Post.* February 28, 2007. Available at: http://www.washingtonpost.com/wp-dyn/content/article/2007/02/27/AR2007022702116.html. Accessed November 4, 2018.

2. US Department of Health and Human Services. Oral health in America: a report of the Surgeon General. Rockville, MD: National Institute of Dental and Craniofacial Research, National Institutes of Health; 2000.

3. Patient Protection and Affordable Care Act, 42 USC 18001 (2010). Available at: https://www.gpo.gov/fdsys/pkg/PLAW-111publ148/pdf/PLAW-111publ148.pdf. Accessed November 4, 2018.

4. Koppelman J. Millions of Medicaid dollars spent on dental emergencies. The Pew Charitable Trusts. June 19, 2015. Available at: https://www.pewtrusts.org/en/research-and-analysis/articles/2015/06/19/millions-of-medicaid-dollars-spent-on-dental-emergencies. Accessed November 4, 2018.

5. Childress S. Do you live in a "dental desert"? *PBS Frontline.* June 26, 2012. Available at: https://www.pbs.org/wgbh/frontline/article/do-you-live-in-a-dental-desert-check-our-map. Accessed November 4, 2018.

6. Murthy VH. Oral health in America, 2000 to present, progress made, but challenges remain. *Public Health Rep.* 2016;131(2):224.

7. Sullivan LW. Dental insurance, but no dentists. *New York Times.* April 8, 2012. Available at: https://www.nytimes.com/2012/04/09/opinion/dental-insurance-but-no-dentists.html. Accessed November 4, 2018.

8. Wall T, Vujicic M. Emergency department use for dental conditions continues to increase. Research Brief. Health Policy Institute, American Dental Association. 2015. Available at: http://www.ada.org/~/media/ADA/Science%20and%20Research/HPI/Files/HPIBrief_0415_2.ashx. Accessed November 4, 2018.

9. US Department of Health and Human Services Oral Health Coordinating Committee. US Department of Health and Human Services Oral Health Strategic Framework, 2014–2017. *Public Health Rep.* 2016;131(2):242–257.

10. Action for Dental Health, American Dental Association. About community dental health coordinators. Available at: https://www.ada.org/en/public-programs/action-for-dental-health/community-dental-health-coordinators. Accessed December 14, 2018.

11. Coates DE, Kardos TB, Moffat SM, Kardos RL. Dental therapists and dental hygienists educated for the New Zealand environment. *J Dent Educ.* 2009;73(8):1001–1008.

12. Early impacts of dental therapists in Minnesota. Report to the Minnesota Legislature, Minnesota Department of Health, Minnesota Board of Dentistry. February 2014. Available at: https://mn.gov/boards/assets/2014DentalTherapistReport_tcm21-45970.pdf. Accessed November 4, 2018.

13. Executive summary: Health impact review of HB 2321. Concerning mid-level dental professionals. Washington State Board of Health. November 6, 2014. Available at: http://sboh.wa.gov/Portals/7/Doc/HealthImpactReviews/HIR-2014-08-HB2321.pdf. Accessed November 4, 2018.

14. Former Surgeon General David Satcher says oral health epidemic persists; calls for pursuing options to expand access - including midlevel providers, dental therapists. *BlackNews.* July 19, 2012. Available at: http://www.blacknews.com/news/david_satcher_oral_health_epidemic_persists101.shtml#.W97Xs-RdkdU. Accessed November 4, 2018.

15. Dr. Louis W. Sullivan visits successful dental therapy program in Alaska. The Sullivan Alliance. September 12, 2012. Available at: http://www.thesullivanalliance.org/cue/news/pr/ak-dental-therapy-trip.html. Accessed November 4, 2018.

37

Revisiting Oral Health in America*

David Satcher, MD, PhD, and Joyce H. Nottingham, PhD, MS

Oral Health in America: A Report of the Surgeon General,[1] released in 2000 during my tenure as surgeon general of the United States, was the first ever Surgeon General's Report on oral health. Its purpose was to inform the American people about the importance of oral health and how crucial oral health is to overall health.

Although the Surgeon General's Oral Health Report acknowledged that progress had been made over the past 50 years, it also reported that significant oral health disparities exist between different racial/ethnic groups. For example, it had been predicted that by the year 2000, annually a little more than 30,000 Americans would be diagnosed with oral or oropharyngeal cancer (the seventh most common cancer among all American males and the fourth most common among Black males) and that approximately 8,000 people would die of these diseases.[2] Also poor children were found to suffer twice as many dental caries as their more affluent peers, and the disease was more likely to be untreated. The disparities were related to determinants of health, such as income, age, gender, race/ethnicity, access to care, and medical status.

According to the 2004 report *Factors Affecting the Health of Men of Color in the United States*[3] released by the Health Policy Institute of the Joint Center for Political and Economic Studies, Black men (51%) are more likely to have untreated dental problems than are White men (28%). In addition to serious periodontal disease, Black men, with 50% having untreated cavities, are 1.5 times more likely than are White men to have missing teeth. General health risk factors, such as tobacco use and poor dietary practices, also affect oral and craniofacial health.

The Surgeon General's Oral Health Report concluded that although common dental diseases are preventable, many people face barriers, sometimes insurmountable, that prevent their access to oral health care. The report outlined a collaborative National Oral Health Plan that is all inclusive and wide ranging in its approach to reducing oral health disparities. Furthermore, it emphasized the importance of focusing on people at the highest risk for specific oral diseases and improving access to existing care. One approach involved making dental insurance available to all Americans.

*This is a modified version of the article that appeared in the *American Journal of Public Health*. See: Satcher D, Nottingham JH. Revisiting *Oral Health in America: A Report of the Surgeon General*. Am J Public Health. 2017;107(suppl 1):S32–S33.

THE STATUS OF ORAL HEALTH IN AMERICA TODAY

So where are we today in terms of promoting oral health and preventing disease 18 years after the release of the first ever Surgeon General's Oral Health Report? The 2011–2012 National Health and Nutrition Examination Survey[4] found that, among children aged two to eight years, the prevalence of untreated tooth decay in primary teeth was higher for Hispanic and non-Hispanic Black children than for non- Hispanic White children. Other data showed that among Hispanic children aged 6 to 11 years, 27% had dental caries in permanent teeth, 1.5 times more than non-Hispanic White and Asian children had, at 18% each. Also, in those aged 6 to 11 years, non-Hispanic White children (at 44%) were more likely to have dental sealants than were non-Hispanic Black and Asian children (at 31% each). The study, thus, concluded, "Disparities in caries continue to persist for some race and ethnic groups in the United States."[4(p1)] It has been reported that almost half of Americans aged 30 years and older have periodontal disease, which is more prevalent among Blacks, the economically disadvantaged, the uneducated, and smokers.[5]

The American Cancer Society estimated that in 2016 close to 50,000 people would contract oral or orpoharyngeal cancer and that close to 10,000 people would likely die of these diseases—a significant increase over the 30,000 and 8,000, respectively, predicted for the year 2000. Their prevalence is greater among men than women, and the incidence is about the same for Blacks as Whites.[6] Death rates from all cancers combined are higher among Blacks than Whites.[7]

In terms of promoting oral health and preventing disease, the good news is that our understanding of common oral diseases continues to grow. We know that people living in communities with water fluoridation have 25% fewer cavities than do those living in communities without fluoridation. Children's access to dental care has improved because dental benefits are now required under the Affordable Care Act, which says that dental care for children is an "essential health benefit." Oral health has benefitted from our efforts to reduce obesity. For example, more emphasis is now placed on good nutrition and healthy lifestyles by programs, such as Fuel Up to Play 60, that encourage children to eat more fruits and vegetables, thus helping to prevent tooth decay and build strong bodies.

The bad news is that too many Americans continue to experience needless pain and suffering from diseases of the mouth because of oral health disparities. Some prevention services, such as fluoridated water, are not available to everyone; the potential danger of fluoridation is a growing debate.

CONCLUSIONS

The major challenge, expressed in the conclusion of *Oral Health in America: A Report of the Surgeon General*, "that not all Americans have achieved the same level of oral health and wellbeing "[1(p287)] is as relevant today as it was when the report was released in 2000.

We must accelerate efforts toward achieving this goal. Continuing to play a major role in the effort to eliminate oral health disparities and improve oral health for all, the Centers for Disease Control and Prevention, Division of Oral Health has made oral health an integral part of public health programs in the United States.

We must address the compelling need for a more diverse oral health workforce. Continued investment in research, such as that undertaken by the National Institute of Dental and Craniofacial Research Centers for Research to Reduce Disparities in Oral Health, is critical. Lastly, we must continue to expand initiatives to prevent tobacco use and promote better dietary choices.

Looking to the future, we are hopeful that at least the children's benefit, prioritized under the Affordable Care Act, will not be dismantled. Also, Medicare needs to cover routine and preventive dental care for our seniors. Despite the current social and political climate, we hope that progress will continue to be made toward eliminating oral health disparities and improving the oral health and overall health of all Americans.

REFERENCES

1. US Department of Health and Human Services. *Oral Health in America: A Report of the Surgeon General—Executive Summary.* Rockville, MD: National Institute of Dental and Craniofacial Research; 2000.

2. Greenlee RT, Murray T, Bolden S, Wingo PA. Cancer statistics, 2000. *CA Cancer J Clin.* 2000;50(1):7–33.

3. Leigh W. *Factors Affecting the Health of Men of Color in the United States.* Washington, DC: Joint Center for Political and Economic Studies; 2004.

4. Dye BA, Thornton-Evans G, Li X, Iafolla TJ. *Dental Caries and Sealant Prevalence in Children and Adolescents in the United States, 2011–2012.* Hyattsville, MD: National Center for Health Statistics; 2015. NCHS data brief 191.

5. Eke PI, Dye BA, Wei L, et al. Update on prevalence of periodontitis in adults in the United States: NHANES 2009 to 2012. *J Periodontol.* 2015;86(5):611–622.

6. American Cancer Society. What are the key statistics about oral cavity and oro-pharyngeal cancers? 2016. Available at: http://www.cancer.org/cancer/oralcavityandoropharyngealcancer/detailedguide/oral-cavity-and-oropharyngeal-cancer-key-statistics. Accessed November 26, 2016.

7. American Cancer Society. Cancer facts & figures for African Americans 2016–2018. 2016. Available at: https://www.cancer.org/content/dam/cancer-org/research/cancer-facts-and-statistics/cancer-facts-and-figures-for-african-americans/cancer-facts-and-figures-for-african-americans-2016-2018.pdf. Accessed January 17, 2017.

VI. VOICES OF DENTAL THERAPISTS: MODELS FOR SERVICE AND CAREER DEVELOPMENT

38

Dental Therapist Profiles: A Closer Look at Minnesota's Newest Team Member

Karl Self, DDS, MBA, and Amanda Nagy, MPH

In 2011, the first cohort of Minnesota dental therapists (DTs) graduated from their education programs and entered the dental workforce. In June 2018, there were 88 licensed DTs in the state. The purpose of this new provider is to help improve access to oral health care for underserved populations and to help these disadvantaged groups achieve better oral health. The legislation created both a licensed DT and a certified advanced dental therapist (ADT).[1] Licensed DTs are eligible to pursue certification as an ADT if they have obtained additional education and completed 2,000 hours of supervised clinical practice as a DT. The scopes of practice of these two provider types are very similar; the major difference lies in the levels of supervision. ADTs can perform their full scope of practice without a dentist present.

The implementation of dental therapy in Minnesota has occurred at a steady pace. There are more Minnesota employers looking to hire a DT then there are available DTs. Although the outcome evaluations of dental therapy's impact are ongoing, a 2014 report titled "Early Impacts of Dental Therapists in Minnesota"[2] found the emerging dental therapy profession to be a positive addition to the oral health care delivery system. Impacts related to underserved patients included an increase in visits by public-program patients, a reduction in wait times for an appointment, and a reduction in travel time. Clinic-related impacts included a significant savings in personnel costs, thus allowing clinics to expand capacity to serve more underserved and public-program patients, as well as an overall increase in productivity, which led some clinics to offer more complicated services than they were able to without the DT. Finally, the report noted that DTs were practicing safely and that there have been no quality-of-care–related patient complaints.

To fully understand how dental therapy is evolving in the state, it is important to look at the providers themselves. The following profiles introduce four DTs who are pioneering the growth and development of the field. They represent some of the diverse roles and impacts a DT can have on an oral health team, employment site, or community. Profile information was collected through written questionnaires and in-person interviews.

RURAL AND REMOTE

Bill Heitzman took a nontraditional path into the dental profession. He first worked as a middle-school science teacher in an urban public school, then as an engineering technician working on space-grade electronics. When asked why he wanted to become a pioneer DT, he put it simply: "I wanted to serve people by applying science to help people live healthier lives." Heitzman was admitted into the second dental therapy cohort at the University of Minnesota School of Dentistry and graduated with his degree in 2012. He received his ADT certification in 2016.

After graduation, Heitzman was surprised by some of the challenges he faced as he transitioned to practice:

> At the time it seemed like no one knew what dental therapists could do, or how to integrate them into practice. We had all worked hard to develop our clinical knowledge and skills and earn our credentials; we just needed some forward-thinking dentists to give us an opportunity.

So, early in his DT career, Heitzman left the Twin Cities Metropolitan area to work in one of the most remote counties within the state. His employer, Grand Marais Family Dentistry, is located 253 miles northeast of Minneapolis, Minnesota, and 42 miles southwest of the Canadian border in the rural town of Grand Marais, Minnesota (population 1,253). He states that he feels very fortunate to work with a progressive and receptive dentist who values his clinical judgment and skills. "The clinic is a team-centered care environment where everyone on the team has a role to play in keeping our patients healthy."

The patient care he provides consists of 70% restorative care, 25% urgent/emergency care where assessment and treatment is provided during the same visit, and 5% treatments including fluoride varnishes, sealants, extractions, recementing crowns, and repairing dentures. Heitzman's patient base consists of 70% Medicaid and uninsured patients; this is a significant increase from the clinic's 57% Medicaid/uninsured patient mix before his arrival.

Grand Marais is a vibrant arts community that offers miles of trails and streams to explore and has been deemed the "coolest small town in America" two years in a row. Unfortunately, like many rural areas, it has struggled to provide dental care to the whole community, and, as such, its county is a designated dental health professional shortage area.

Fortunately, the community is also dedicated to meeting the oral health needs of its youth. Grand Marais Family Dentistry collaborates with the nonprofit Oral Health Task Force to provide oral health screenings in schools and two "free days" at the clinic for those aged 0 to 26 years to receive care. In the 2015–2016 school year, Heitzman provided 337 screenings at four area schools. Heitzman has a positive impact on his clinic and community by increasing the volume of underserved patients that can receive high-quality primary care services. Owner and dentist Alyssa Hedstrom echoes that sentiment:

> Having an advanced dental therapist on your team is like having an associate. You have a colleague and professional that you can collaborate and share the workload with. It allows a small rural practice to serve more patients and see everyone. It's great.

INTERPROFESSIONAL PRACTICE

Kelly Meyer works as a dually licensed dental hygienist and ADT at Hennepin County Medical Center (HCMC). HCMC is a renowned level-one adult and pediatric trauma center located in Minneapolis (population 407,207). It is also classified as a safety-net hospital and teaching institute. The dental clinic at HCMC consists of more than 20 oral health providers, including two ADTs. Meyer received her dental therapy degree in 2011 and became certified as an ADT in 2013. Meyer understands the needs of the patient base and the hospital setting, as she worked as both a dental assistant and dental hygienist for HCMC before enrolling in the first cohort of Metropolitan State University's Advanced Dental Therapy Program:

> I chose to become an ADT because I have a passion for public health, and the ADT scope of practice was the perfect complement to my existing career in dental hygiene.

Meyer currently provides dental care for the pregnant patients enrolled in HCMC's Maternal Oral Health Program, Bright Start. There is a dental operatory located within the Obstetrics Clinic where roughly 45% of the care provided is for restorative service; the rest is evenly divided between diagnostic procedures, periodontal care, and extractions. In 2015, 90% of the patients seen were women of color and 80% were on public health insurance. Meyer typically sees approximately eight patients a day for their periodontal and restorative needs. "Dental therapy allows me to expand the services I provide to an underserved population, and I welcomed the increased responsibility."

Meyer collaborates daily with other midlevel providers (nurse practitioners and nurse midwives), nursing staff, physicians, and a variety of language interpreters in the hospital. She describes HCMC as a "prime example of how dental therapists can collaborate with other medical professionals, and integrate dental and medical care to meet all patient needs." Meyer also collaborates with rotating dental therapy students, dental assisting students, dental hygienists completing Restorative Expanded Functions requirements, and dental residents. Meyer stated that "this increases collegiality and creates better reception of the ADT into the dental work force. The dental residents learn how to integrate the ADT into everyday practice and how to create a treatment plan delegating care to the ADT."

As an oral health provider who has been in the field for almost 20 years, Meyer is excited about where the field is today. She looks forward to a higher degree of utilization of DTs in Minnesota and other states in the future.

HOMETOWN COMMUNITY

As one of the youngest ADTs, Lydia Diekmann knew at an early age that her passion was to work with teeth. Before enrolling in the dental therapy program at the University of Minnesota School of Dentistry, Diekmann was on the predental track with the goal of becoming an orthodontist. After learning about the new dental therapy field from her hometown dentist at a routine care appointment, Diekmann's focus quickly changed. "It was at that moment I decided to pursue dental therapy. I never really wanted to be 'the boss.' As a dental therapist I can still have just the right amount of responsibility without managing the business side of a dental office."

After graduating with her dental therapy degree in 2013, Diekmann started working at her hometown dental office Shetek Dental Care in the southern, rural town of Slayton, Minnesota (population 2,152). "I knew I wanted to work in the rural town I grew up in because of the great community support there. Everyone knows your name, your parents' names, and who your grandparents are. Now I am able to support the community by providing an increased access to dental services." Shetek Dental Care has eight treatment rooms; the team consists of one dentist, an ADT (Diekmann), two hygienists, and three dental assistants. Patients know Diekmann as the restorative provider, as 72% of her work is restorative care. Having a DT as a part of the dental team has allowed the clinic to see a larger volume of patients, and wait times for restorative appointments have been drastically reduced. Before Diekmann joined the team, an appointment for a filling would have been scheduled three months out. Now patients are able to be seen for restorative work in as quickly as one week.

With Diekmann's ability to complete fillings for the clinic's patients, owner and dentist Gary Plotz has reduced the percentage of restorative services he provides from 22% to 6% and is able to focus on the more complicated procedures only a dentist is trained to complete. This benefits the rural community by keeping the care within the clinic and not needing to refer patients farther away for continued care. Diekmann and the team at Shetek Dental Care are also making a positive impact on her rural community through education and prevention. One such effort involves supporting fluoride application in collaboration with the local Special Supplemental Nutrition Program for Women, Infants, and Children. Another effort focuses on mentoring dental hygiene and dental assisting students who are completing their externship programs.

Diekmann has continued to develop within her profession by becoming certified as an ADT in 2016. The ability to provide care without the dentist on site benefits patients and allows Diekmann more available appointment times, especially for children.

Twenty-eight percent of her work involves assessments and preventive care for children through age 12. She says

> Being a dental therapist is everything I have wanted. I continuously find new ways to grow as a provider, as each patient and each new day brings its own challenges and accomplishments.

EDUCATION AND PRACTICE

Danae Seyffer first became interested in the dental field her junior year of college following a routine visit to her dentist. After exploring both the dental and hygiene professions, Seyffer applied and was accepted into the dental hygiene program at the University of Minnesota School of Dentistry. Soon after being admitted into the hygiene program, Seyffer learned about the new dental therapy profession:

> Dental therapy was designed to help underserved populations and that really hit home for me. My father grew up in rural Missouri and my mother in Thailand. Neither of them had dental insurance and the only times they visited the dentist was when they experienced pain. I saw the impact that it had on them and knew that dental therapy was my calling and my way to help others.

She declined her hygiene acceptance and was enrolled into the first dental therapy cohort at the University of Minnesota School of Dentistry.

Seyffer felt honored to be "among some of the strongest pioneers for the profession. DT is a step in the right direction in order to make sure that those in need have access to quality care." Her professors noticed Seyffer's intelligence, strong clinical skills, and passion while in the program. After receiving her dental therapy degree in 2011, Seyffer was asked to return to the School of Dentistry to instruct students in the school's pediatric clinic. She started as an adjunct clinical professor within the pediatric clinic, and her teaching responsibilities have expanded. Seyffer currently serves as a clinical assistant professor for the school's dental therapy division. Her responsibilities include teaching courses such as pediatric dentistry to dental hygiene and therapy students, but an important part of her position is being a DT faculty presence and modeling the oral health team concept for the school's patients, students, and staff.

Seyffer, a certified ADT, divides her time between the School of Dentistry and the Community University Health Care Center (CUHCC). CUHCC is a federally qualified health care center that provides medical, dental, and mental health care services to low-income children and adults in Minneapolis. Recent data highlight the success of the dental program to reach underserved populations:

- 96% have household incomes below 200% of the federal poverty level,
- 70% are on public health insurance,
- 21% are uninsured, and
- 71% are people of color.

The majority of Seyffer's patients are aged younger than 18 years, and 85% are from minority and/or immigrant cultures. Clinically, the care she provides is relatively evenly split among diagnostic (27%), preventive (37%), and restorative (34%) services. Seyffer is also an important part of the clinic's interprofessional efforts. She identifies the dental status of patients scheduled to see a pediatric nurse practitioner. Once identified, she works with the nurse practitioner to either perform or schedule the appropriate follow-up care that the patient requires. In addition, she works with the medical team to counsel youth and their parents on good oral hygiene habits and nutrition for a healthy mouth. "Childhood is one of the most influential periods of a person's life. I believe if we work hard to educate children and their parents/guardians about the importance of good oral hygiene and instill those behaviors at a young age that we can make a lifelong impact." Seyffer is excited to continue to use her dual position to increase dental therapy's involvement in interprofessional care and to stimulate students' passions to care for pediatric populations.

CONCLUSIONS

These profiles spotlight the efforts of four DTs practicing in Minnesota. These four are truly a microcosm of all DTs in Minnesota. All DTs in Minnesota have worked hard to overcome the challenges of integrating a new provider into the existing oral health care team. DTs in Minnesota not only serve a vital role in increasing access to oral health care for the state's most vulnerable populations but they are also paving the pathway for future DTs and the profession in general. These pioneers have been excellent ambassadors for this new profession. They have also taken an active role in educating their colleagues on the value DTs bring to the health care system and in highlighting their role as a team player. Those who enter the field come with a passion to practice dentistry and serve their communities, knowing that their chosen occupation is controversial within the dental community both locally and nationally.

Although dental therapy has not yet been embraced by the dental profession as a whole, a group of early adopting dentists in Minnesota is giving DTs the opportunity to demonstrate their value to reducing health disparities and to increasing access to care. These four profiles highlight diverse ways in which DTs are adding value to the health care delivery system as well as the passion and commitment of those who choose to enter a health profession whose mission is to improve the health of underserved and disadvantaged populations.

ACKNOWLEDGMENTS

The authors would like to thank the profiled dental therapists and their practices for allowing us to share their stories.

REFERENCES

1. Revisor of Statutes, State of Minnesota. MN Dental Therapy and Advanced Dental Therapy Statute. Pub L No. 150A.105 and 106 (2014). Available at: https://www.revisor.mn.gov/statutes/?id=150A. Accessed September 30, 2016.

2. Minnesota Department of Health. Early impacts of dental therapists in Minnesota. St. Paul, MN: Minnesota Department of Health; 2014.

Contributors

Krishna Aravamudhan, BDS, MS, American Dental Association
Oscar Arevalo, DDS, ScD, MBA, MS, Nicklaus Children's Hospital
Terrence Batliner, DDS, MBA, Colorado School of Public Health
Camden Bay, PhD
David Beckmann, MD, MPH, Massachusetts General Hospital
Tera Bianchi, MSW
Jo-Ann Blake, MPH, RDH
Colleen Brickle, RDH, EdD, RF, Normandale Community College
Melissa Burroughs, BA, Families USA
Jean Marie Calvo, DDS, MPH, University of California San Francisco
Jeffrey Chaffin, DDS, MPH, MHA, MBA, Delta Dental of Iowa
Elisa M. Chávez, DDS, University of the Pacific
Nicole S. Cheek, DDS, National Dental Association
Donald L. Chi, DDS, PhD, University of Washington
Chairman M. Brian Cladoosby (Spee Pots), Swinomish Indian Tribal Community
Marya Cohen, MD, MPH, Massachusetts General Hospital
Mary L. Conicella, DMD, FAGD
Nicole C. Cranston, DDS
John Da Silva, DMD, MPH, ScM, Harvard School of Dental Medicine
Maria C. Dolce, PhD, RN, State University of New York at Stony Brook
R. Bruce Donoff, DMD, MD, Harvard School of Dental Medicine
Julianne Doucette, DNP, CPNP-PC, Rush University College of Nursing
Neile Edens, PhD
Janalyn C. Edmonds, PhD, RN, CNE, Howard University
Ivette Estrada, MA, MPhil, Columbia University College of Dental Medicine
Caswell A. Evans, DDS, MPH, University of Illinois at Chicago
Cheryl Fish-Parcham, MSW, Families USA
Ingrid Forsberg, DNP, FNP-BC, Rush University College of Nursing
Paul Gates, DDS, MBA, BronxCare Health System
Raymond Gist, DDS
Jennifer Goldberg, JD, LLM, Justice in Aging
Ariel P. Greenblatt, DMD, MPH, New York University College of Dentistry

Hazel J. Harper, DDS, MPH, National Dental Association
Sharon Nicholson Harrell, DDS, MPH, FAGD, FICD, FirstHealth of the Carolinas
Lisa Gaarde Hartsock, MPH
Denise Muesch Helm, RDH, EdD, Northern Arizona University
Karin Herzog, DDS, MSD
Sherry Hirota
Robert A. Horn, PhD
Judith A. Jones, DDS, DScD, MPH, University of Detroit Mercy School of Dentistry
Molly Jung, MPH, Johns Hopkins University School of Public Health
Matthew Jura, MSPH, University of California San Francisco
Kata Kertesz, JD, Center for Medicare Association
Jane Koppelman, MPA, Pew Charitable Trusts Dental Campaign
Aubri Kottek, MPH, University of California San Francisco
Daniel J. Kruger, PhD, University of Michigan
Carol Kunzel, PhD, Columbia University College of Dental Medicine
Wey-Wey Kwok, JD, Center for Medicare Advocacy
Simona C. Kwon, DrPH
Curtis Le
Huong Le, DDS
Charo Ledón, Acción Buenos Vecinos
Dane Lenaker, DMD, MPH, Southeast Regional Health Consortium
Julia Liou, MPH
Mikel Llanes, MD, University of Michigan Medical School
Sarah Lowman, MPH
Nicholas S. Makrides, DMD, MA, MPH
Amy Manion, PhD, CPNP-PC, Rush University College of Nursing
Richard Manski, DDS, PhD, MBA, University of Maryland School of Dentistry
Stephen A. Martin, MD, EdM, Harvard Medical School
Camesia O. Matthews, DDS
Kristen McGlaston, MS
Sara S. Metcalf, PhD, State University of New York
Elizabeth Mertz, PhD, MA, University of California San Francisco
Michael Monopoli, DMD, MPH, MS, DentaQuest Foundation
La June Montgomery Tabron, W.K Kellogg Foundation
Amanda Nagy, MPH
Mary E. Northridge, PhD, MPH, NYU Langone Dental Medicine, New York University
  College of Dentistry
Joyce H. Nottingham, PhD, MS
Jan Odiaga, DNP, CPNP-PC, Rush University College of Nursing
Anne M. O'Keefe, PhD, JD

Jessica L. Parker, EdD, RDH, Northeastern University
Steven P. Perlman, DDS, MScD, DHL (Hon), Boston University Henry M. Goldman
  School of Dental Medicine
Wendell B. Potter, BS, To Be Fair, Inc.
David Preble, DDS, JD, CAE, American Dental Association
Thu Quach, PhD, MPH, Asian Health Services
Kathy Ramsey, BA, RHIA
Carol Raphael, MPA, MEd, Manatt Health Strategies
Robert Restuccia, MPA
Marguerite Ro, DrPH, Public Health—Seattle & King County
Bianca Rogers, BS, Oral Health in America
David Satcher, MD, PhD, Morehouse School of Medicine
Eric W. Schrimshaw, PhD, Columbia University Mailman School of Public Health
JoAnna Scott, PhD
William Seaman, PhD
Karl Self, DDS, MBA, University of Minnesota, Minneapolis
Claudia A. Serna, DDS, PhD, MPH, New York University–Lutheran Dental Medicine
Jay D. Shulman, DMD, MA, MSPH, Texas A&M University, Dallas
Lisa Simon, DMD, Harvard School of Dental Medicine
Rebecca Singer-Cohen, MPP, The Pew Charitable Trusts
Tiffany Sitlin
Patrick D. Smith, DMD, MPH, University of Illinois at Chicago College of Dentistry
Janet H. Southerland, DDS, PhD, MPH, University of Texas Medical Branch
Louis W. Sullivan, MD, The Sullivan Alliance to Transform the Health Professions
Flavia Teles, DDS, DMSc
Matthew Tobey, MD, MPH, Massachusetts General Hospital
Scott L. Tomar, DMD, DrPH, University of Florida
Sarah Tomlinson, DDS
Christopher Toretsky, MPH, University of California San Francisco
Henrie M. Treadwell, PhD, Morehouse School of Medicine
Chau Trinh-Shevrin, DrPH
Beth Truett, BS, MDiv, Oral Health in America
Marko Vujicic, PhD, American Dental Association
H. Barry Waldman, DDS, PhD, MPH, Stony Brook University
Adreanne Waller, Washtenaw County Public Health
Darien Weatherspoon, DDS, MPH, National Institute of Dental and Craniofacial
  Research
Jennifer Webster-Cyriaque, DDS, PhD, University of North Carolina at Chapel Hill
Cynthia Wides, MA, University of California San Francisco
Patrick Willard, MA, Families USA

Beatrice Williams, BA
Rachael Williams, AB, Massachusetts General Hospital
Kasey Wilson, MSW
Cassandra Yarbrough, MPP, American Dental Association
Albert K. Yee, MD, MPH, Community Catalyst
Stella S. Yi, PhD, MPH

Index

A

ACA. *See* Affordable Care Act
academic community's role in access
  Medicaid stigma, 181–182
  nursing curriculum adding oral health, 189–192
  profile of dental therapy educator, 333–334
  social responsibility instilled, 32
  special needs patient skills, 60–61
  sponsorship of community health care, 306
  student rotations in correctional facilities, 211–214
  See also dental schools
Access to Baby and Child Dentistry (ABCD) program, 15, 20–21
ADA. *See* American Dental Association
Adams, Jerome, xii
adult dental care
  Black men, 81–85
  decline in, 27, 65, 238
  disparity statistics, 301
  emergency room use, 71–75. *See also* emergency department visits
  incarcerated, 54–55
  Medicaid exclusion
    Black men and dental health, 83
    enrollment numbers, 301
    older adult perspective, 294–298
    percentage of states excluding, 287, 301
    policy recommendations for access, 34, 35, 77, 96, 120
    states' option to exclude, 7, 27, 66, 83, 120, 136, 219, 232–233
    states reducing or eliminating, 28
  patients with disabilities, 60–63
  See also older adults
Aetna and National Dental Association, 183, 184–186, 309
Affordable Care Act (ACA; 2010)
  ADA support of "free-standing" insurance, 31
  children's dental care, 208, 231, 318, 324
  chronic health conditions, 195–196
  Indian Health Care Improvement Act reauthorization, 156, 157, 158
  innovations in health care, 237
  Medicaid expansion for dental care, 83, 231
    dental hygienist visit increase, 240
  numbers of uninsured, 195
  preventive dental care lacking, 208
African Americans. *See* Black populations
Alaska

ADA opposition to access to care, 157
  Community Health Aide Program, 137, 154, 157, 159
  Dental Health Aide Therapist Program
    dentist–therapist team, 146–148
    establishment of, 145, 320
    exported to Washington state, 138
    Kellogg Foundation Community Catalyst, xii
    process, 146
    safe, effective dental care, 3–5, 137, 146, 147
  dental therapists
    Community Health Aide Program, 137, 154, 157
    educational requirements, 140
    effectiveness of, 35, 137, 138, 151, 155–156, 166
    Medicaid reimbursement, 159
    numbers practicing, 209
    practicing, xiii, 10, 136, 166, 179
    salaries, 139
    training, 155
  lack of oral care, 3, 145
    racial/ethnic disparities, 4, 70, 145, 153
Alaska Native populations
  dentists on DTs and CDHWs, 268–277
  disability rates, 58
  diversity of workforce, 255
    minority dentist perspective, 268–277
  HIV infection and early dental care, 106
  prevalence of dental disease, 4, 70, 145, 153, 209
    children's untreated tooth decay, 318
  student financial aid, 256
Alaska Native Tribal Health Consortium (ANTHC), xiii, 145, 146, 155, 320
alcohol use and oral cancer, 92
altruism of professional community, 31–32
American Dental Association (ADA)
  Code of Ethics and Professional Conduct, 31
  community dental health coordinators, 35, 208, 266, 319
  cost savings from dental coverage, 237–238
  fluoridation endorsement, 282
  Medicaid reimbursement lobbying, 208
  Medicare dental benefit designs, 223–224
  membership by minorities, 269
    opposition to community dental health workers, 270, 271, 274, 275
    opposition to dental therapists, 270, 271, 273, 275
  opposition to access to care, 31, 156–157
  opposition to dental therapists, 10, 156, 157, 209, 275
  untreated caries rates lower, 138